# NO W
# TO TREAT
# A FRIEND

# NO WAY
# TO TREAT
# A FRIEND

## Lifting the Lid on Complementary and Alternative Veterinary Medicine

*Niall Taylor BVM&S, GPCert (SAM) MRCVS*
*Alex Gough MA, VetMB, CertSAM, CertVC, PGCert MRCVS*
*Foreword by Emma Milne BVSc MRCVS*

5m Publishing

First published 2017

Published by
5M Publishing Ltd,
Benchmark House,
8 Smithy Wood Drive,
Sheffield, S35 1QN, UK
Tel: +44 (0) 1234 81 81 80
www.5mpublishing.com


A Catalogue record for this book is available from the British Library

ISBN 9781910455913


Book layout by Servis Filmsetting Ltd, Stockport, Cheshire
Printed by Replika Press Pvt Ltd, India
Photos as credited in the text

To Alison, Tom and Charley – for inspiration, encouragement and patience.
N.T.


To my family, for putting up with another long project!
A.G.

# *Contents*

# Foreword

## By Emma Milne BVSc MRCVS

WHEN I was asked if I would write the foreword for this book I jumped up and down and shouted, 'Oooh, yes please, yes please!' I immediately thought of a case I'd had in practice where a client of mine had gone for a second opinion after I had said his dog's teeth were in a poor state. He was a young dog in for routine vaccination and health exam so I recommended the owner should think about cleaning and properly examining the teeth in the next few months before they got worse.

I didn't know the owner had gone for a second opinion and if I had known it would have been fine. All clients have the right to ask for another vet's opinion. The health of our pets is a serious business and this client was terrified at the thought of an anaesthetic and wanted to avoid it if possible. Now when a client comes to you seeking a second opinion it is professional to contact the first vet and ask for the history. I never heard from the holistic, complementary practice my client had chosen for the second opinion. In fact the first I knew was when, about six months later, the owner came back to me because the dog was unable to open its mouth, eat or even drink.

The vet they had been to see a few weeks before had said there was nothing wrong with the dog's teeth and all he needed to do was switch the dog to a raw meat and bones diet and the teeth would clean right up. Unfortunately, because dogs are about 40,000 years away from being wolves and because bones can break wolves' teeth too, this plan had not helped. I couldn't examine the dog's mouth because of the pain he was in so we admitted him and anaesthetised him. His entire mouth – cheeks, tongue, palate and gums – were completely lacerated, ulcerated and infected. It must have been agony. His teeth were in an even worse state than before and with all the new damage from the bones his anaesthetic ended up being about twice as long as it would have been in the first place.

The thing is that it would be easy to hear this story and think the moral of it is that all complementary medicine and raw, bony diets are bad. But the problem is that this is just an anecdote. It's one thing that happened to me. Sure, it made a lasting impression on me, my client and the poor dog that was involved but it is NOT evidence. In the grand scheme of the debate on this hot topic it means virtually nothing. I realised in my eagerness to share it with you that I was exactly the same as all the internet zealots quoting individual experiences where homeopathy or a raw food diet have appeared to help. It means NOTHING.

I am a scientist, I adore science and I love trying to understand this beautiful, amazing natural world we live in. It's hard. Science is undoubtedly hard to understand and my meagre brain can only grasp a fraction of it. But the great thing about science is that you can prove stuff. You can show the same thing time and again. When someone asks me to put my faith in something because they cannot prove it alarm bells start clanging in my head like a campanologists' leaving party.

In 1796 two things were 'discovered' that have both made huge differences one way or another to human and animal medicine. Both discoveries have spawned million pound industries. They both involved taking a little bit of something very harmful, tinkering with it and using it to try to cure people of disease. One of the discoveries was made by Samuel Hahnemann and it was homeopathy. The other discovery was by Edward Jenner and it was the smallpox vaccine.

It's not a big stretch to see how the concept of how a vaccine works might lead to weird and wonderful experimentation by others in an era of very little scientific knowledge. But we are lucky, we have the wonderful power of hindsight and hundreds of years of advancement. We now know that unequivocally, I repeat, *unequivocally*, vaccinations have saved millions and millions of lives and have eradicated entire killer diseases. Homeopathy has not.

I have to be honest, that last statement is just my opinion. With the science I understand I do not believe homeopathy can work but I don't pretend to know all the facts. Since my encounter with the dog I told you about I have now spent many years with clinical nutrition as my main job. I do feel qualified to quite categorically say that feeding raw meat and bones to dogs because they are descended from wolves is like me saying I will feed raw chicken and the like to my kids because before Man discovered fire that's what we ate. It's dangerous nonsense.

The best scientists are the ones who know they still have much to learn, the ones constantly questioning what we think we know instead of blindly following accepted ideas. By reading this book you are fact finding and looking at evidence. It's what we should all strive to do. I'm no genius, I'm just a lover of facts, so I will send you on your journey of discovery with the wisdom of the brilliant Tim Minchin. Take a moment to revel in these words from the wonderful song, *If You Open Your Mind Too Much Your Brain Will Fall Out*:

… if anyone can show me one example in the entire history of the world of a single homeopathic practitioner who has been able to prove under reasonable experimental conditions that solutions made up of infinitely tiny particles of good stuff dissolved repeatedly into relatively huge quantities of water have a consistently higher medicinal value than a similarly administered placebo … I will give you my piano, one of my legs. And my wife!

# *Preface – Who We Are, How We Got Here and Why*

Taking a leisurely stroll down the average high street in the average town today it is impossible not to notice the plethora of New Age, or spiritual, or holistic fare on offer.

Restaurants – natural, organic and wi-fi- and gluten-free – and emporiums offering Tibetan Pulsing, Intuitive Healing, Soul Therapy Meditation and States of Consciousness Guidance all rub shoulders with shops with names such as Natural Earthling, Enlightenment or Simply Yin Yang. In one town in the English county of Somerset, handmade tofu and high colonic irrigation are both offered from the same establishment – whether provided by the same or different persons isn't made clear on the sign. And then there is the constant presence of alternative medicine – homeopathy, acupuncture, reiki, chiropractic, herbal and crystal healing (Elestial or otherwise).

The list is endless. We have it seems an insatiable appetite for all things mystic, ethereal and other-worldly. And why not? The promises on offer are beguiling, especially when we are told there really is more to life than this – the mundane, the ordinary. For some the world seems to get more complicated and incomprehensible every day and these kindly sales-people are there to offer simple solutions – comfortable certainties to give us back control over our lives. Maybe we would be a bit happier at work after a good soul cleansing; perhaps a thorough detox would put a bit more of a spring in our step and help us get through the day. After all, we tell ourselves as we enter our PIN number, what's the harm, these things are so popular, there must be something in them. Often there is little or no objective evidence of any benefit from these things beyond the good feelings that may result, but nevertheless we are willing to suspend disbelief and not demand or even look for evidence because we want the good feelings to be true – to ask for proof would be churlish. It might even break the spell.

And of course, it follows naturally that if we feel able to benefit from these things then we will also want our animal companions to benefit in the same way.

But nothing is as simple as it seems and, to coin a phrase, if something looks too good to be true, it probably is. There are problems with most, if not all of these supposed cures and fixes. At best many don't deliver on promises made, at worst some cause harm – either direct physical injury or indirectly, by attempting to treat or prevent serious physical ailments in lieu of proper medicine. And it might be said that would be quite bad enough in a population of rational, adult humans. But the problems are compounded when it comes to making health decisions for those companions who show us unconditional trust and depend on us to act on their behalf and do what is best for them: the animals in our care, in our homes and stables and on our farms. It is they who make being an 'owner' such a special and demanding privilege and it is for them, for their faith and loyalty, that we are writing this book.

There are indications recently of a growing frustration in veterinary and scientific circles over irresponsible claims from practitioners of Complementary and Alternative Veterinary Medicine (CAVM). There are claims it can cure cancer, some veterinary surgeons maintain dowsing (radionics) is an effective diagnostic tool, while others report CAVM can be successfully employed in the treatment and prevention of other serious diseases including hormonal disorders, epilepsy, and bacterial and viral infections.

In parallel with these claims there is a continuing trend of exaggeration and distortion of the evidence base for CAVM and a denial of serious scientific studies that have time and again, after the removal of methodologically inadequate trials and the exclusion of bias, found most of it to be no more effective than a blank placebo. The potential ethical and welfare concerns could not be more clear. The treatment of real diseases with ineffective therapies means our patients are put at risk.

Yet those who profit from CAVM seem oblivious to such concerns, and this attitude is starting to generate a backlash from heretofore tolerant science-based practitioners up to now content to let sleeping dogs lie whether as a result of a simple lack of interest in the subject, concern for the ideals of clinical freedom, or a general feeling of collegiality and a reluctance to speak out against one's peers – a sense of honour and fairness of which the profession is rightly proud. There is now a realisation though that these courtesies are becoming increasingly one-sided and, rather than being reciprocated in the form of a mutual respect and modest recognition of the limitations of non-science-based practices, are instead being met by attacks and attempts to mislead the profession and the public about what can be achieved by CAVM and scaremongering about the risks of conventional medicine.

This rising tide of concern (of which this book is a part) has come about, not simply because of the lack of evidence for CAVM, nor even the plentiful evidence it is ineffective, though both these things are damning enough in and of themselves as we will see, but also because this lack of evidence is coupled with a lack of any realistic mechanism for its various claimed actions (despite what we are told might be 'just around the corner'). This is not because of any ignorance amongst its critics – a simplistic lack of understanding of the principles behind CAVM – or a failure to comprehend abstruse and ultimately self-defeating post-modernist and social-constructionist views about the nature of science and reality, but as a result of careful consideration by a number of commentators who, while not practising CAVM in all its aspects (considering to do so would be highly unethical) have nevertheless devoted a great deal of time to its objective study and have found it wanting.

When perusing the popular literature on the subject it seems it is largely practitioner advocates of CAVM who currently have things their own way, with large numbers of websites, books and articles in glossy magazine extolling its virtues in unquestioning and often rather gushing terms. By publishing this work the authors hope, in a small way, to redress the balance.

This book is intended to be a readable exposé of the fallacies underpinning much of CAVM. It will be helpful to anyone with an interest in the subject – its history, philosophy, use and evidence base, and will allow readers to draw their own conclusions about whether, and which, CAVM is right for their pets and livestock. Many of the arguments come from debates the authors have taken part in in various forums, in the veterinary press and face to face with alternative veterinary practitioners over many years.

As well as (we hope!) reasoned arguments and the presentation of evidence, we fight fire with fire so to speak, turning one of CAVM's most powerful propaganda tools, the anecdote, against it by recounting tales and case histories gleaned from colleagues around the world that give a powerful illustration of the harm that can be caused by CAVM and also of the simple, incontrovertible fact that will come as no surprise to any veterinary surgeon in practice anywhere in the world today – animals sometimes get better on their own.

We begin, in the first part, with a discussion of the nature of both veterinary and human forms of complementary and alternative medicine as well as of science and understanding, including some of the ways bias and logical fallacies can unconsciously skew the way we perceive the world around us, particularly in matters of apparent cause and effect. How these limitations can manifest is discussed briefly in a chapter on historical veterinary treatments, some of which were barbaric, and most of which were ineffective yet they had a following among the animal-owning community of their day every bit as loyal and evangelical as that of contemporary supporters of homeopathy, raw feeding and the rest. We will also discover why ineffective treatments can appear to be effective in animals, a patient group on the face of it immune from the effects of wishful thinking.

The second part is given over to discussions of some of the main individual practices and beliefs themselves that encompass the 'alternative' mind-set; therapies such as homeopathy and acupuncture, and the questionable views held by the anti-vaccination and raw feeding lobbies.

Finally, we have appended a list of references for each chapter and a brief glossary explaining some of the less self-evident terms used.

Writing this book, aimed at a general readership as well as veterinary surgeons, involves putting our heads above the parapet. Given previous experiences in debating CAVM, and knowing how its critics are treated, we fully expect personal attacks on social media and one-star reviews on Amazon from advocates of non-science-based medicine who may or may not even have read the book. But we also hope some of the ideas we put forward might strike a chord with some and promote an understanding of the truth behind Complementary and Alternative Veterinary Medicine.

§

## About the Authors

I qualified from Edinburgh Veterinary School in the summer of 1982 at a time when it was the ambition of virtually every veterinary student in the country to go into general practice. And that is exactly what I did – it's why I went into the profession in the first place and it's what I have been privileged to be able to do ever since.

In my early years in practice I worked largely with farm animals, doing mainly what is known as 'fire-engine' stuff, attending sick animals, trimming feet, calving cows, lambing ewes and testing livestock for the ever present scourges of tuberculosis and brucellosis. Latterly I have found my career reflecting global changes in the farming sector and I now concentrate exclusively on companion animal species, from dogs, cats and rabbits to sugar-gliders and ferrets, snakes and lizards. I've even been asked to treat a stick insect and once had to remove a large piece of gravel from the mouth of a goldfish – one of my most satisfying cases.

As well as the anticipated roles of surgeon, medic, dentist, proctologist, radiologist, ultrasonographer, paediatrician, geriatrician, podiatrist and so on, what I wasn't expecting when I entered practice was that I would also be required to be a bereavement counsellor, tax collector, personnel manager, amateur accountant, building designer and maintenance man, anaesthetic machine repair man, diplomat, barrack-room lawyer and webmaster. I even make the tea on occasions.

And I love every minute!

CAVM made its first real impression on me many years ago, when I was working in rural southern England. Up to that point I had never taken much interest in the subject and if senior professional colleagues said there was something in it, I was prepared to take their word for it. Life was too busy to do otherwise.

Then one day I was asked by the boss to accompany a homeopathic veterinary surgeon who had been called in by one of our farm clients to have a look at his herd of dairy cows, which was suffering unacceptably high rates of mastitis – a painful condition affecting the udder and which can cause considerable financial loss for the farmer. I was to be liaison for our practice.

When the referral vet arrived at the farm I made the introductions and accompanied him as he carried out his assessment of the premises and livestock.

I watched as he prodded the cows that were brought to his attention by the farmer. Much seemed to be gained from pressing spines and there was no recourse to the usual, more risky (and muckier), methods of examination involving thermometers, stethoscopes and the obtaining of milk samples.

Finally the referral veterinary surgeon reached into a medicine bag and produced two small, brown glass vials containing clear liquid – one for the mastitis, he said, and the other for some ringworm we had discovered in a batch of calves. 'Strong stuff', I thought, as the farmer was told to empty the contents into the water supply for each groups of animals being treated. They were labelled carefully and the farmer was instructed, in serious tones, to ensure they were not mixed up.

Then came the moment that has stuck with me to this day. The homeopath turned to me, 'Still,' he grinned, 'it wouldn't matter if they were mixed up, after all, they're both water!' To say I was amazed would be an understatement. Did he *really* mean these remedies were simply water, and how could a few drops mixed with several thousand gallons of drinking water possibly have any effect on an entire population of animals?

After that, I began to take much more of an interest in CAVM. I wanted to find out what was so special about this 'water'. I read articles in the popular press and in scientific journals, I corresponded with practitioners and discovered more about the scientific process. Eventually I came across the *Task Force For Veterinary Science*, an early attempt by concerned veterinary surgeons to collate the evidence surrounding the claims of CAVM practitioners in an accessible location online. But the more I read there and elsewhere, the less convincing the evidence for CAVM seemed to be.

In 2003 I happened to see a letter in the veterinary press from a group of veterinary surgeons expressing concerns regarding two cases where dogs, treated homeopathically, were seen to suffer greatly. The responses from the homeopathic community seemed to me to be dismissive, they appeared to show little concern and were actually quite condescending. It was made clear the respondents felt there was no case to answer, and the problem lay solely in critics' lack of understanding of the subject.

When I entered the debate by writing a letter myself I was urged to consult three scientific papers that I was told would give me the 'firm, properly conducted, blinded research' I had asked for. Now, I thought, I was getting somewhere. The papers were Kleijnen (1991), Boissel (1996) and Linde (1997). It took me some time to track them down (my internet skills were sorely lacking in those days), but when I did it was a terrible disappointment!

The three references were meta-analyses and literature reviews that scrutinised previous studies investigating homeopathy. In every case the authors found there was a risk of bias in the trials, they were of low quality and those that had the most rigorous protocols were the least likely to find in favour of homeopathy. In other words, the better the quality of the trial, the less likely the results will be favourable to homeopathy. The author of one of the trials even went as far as complaining in a later publication, 'our 1997 meta-analysis has unfortunately been misused by homoeopaths as evidence that their therapy is proven' (Linde and Jonas, 2005). If this was a homeopath's idea of 'firm, properly conducted, blinded research' I thought, then there was something dreadfully wrong with their understanding of science. How on earth, I asked myself, could anyone believe the results of these studies showed homeopathy was effective when clearly, to an impartial observer, they did precisely the opposite?

Shortly afterwards I joined the US-based ALTVETSKEPT-L discussion group and also became a member of the satirical British Veterinary Voodoo

Society, set up to counter the claims of veterinary homeopaths in the UK by highlighting the fact that veterinary voodoo has precisely as extensive and convincing an evidence base behind it as veterinary homeopathy – which is to say none at all! Sometimes laughter is the best medicine.

More recently (and more seriously) I took and passed a year-long course in Complementary and Alternative Medicine with the Open University (module k221, if anyone is interested), with an extremely pleasant and patient acupuncturist as my tutor. But although I learned much from it and was able to meet and talk with practitioners of CAM in the field of human medicine I continued to be struck by the virtual absence of the sort of evidence-based debate I was used to when discussing medical topics in other areas, the habitual distortion and misinterpretation of such evidence as there was and, furthermore the number of sheer factual errors in the coursework.

The more I discovered, the less sense the whole subject made. In short, the claims of miracle cures and consistent benefits from CAVM simply did not match the evidence – to this day I have never found a single trial or paper that supports homeopathy in the way claimed by proponents.

The main evidence on offer seemed to be stories – 'I gave a dog a homeopathic remedy and it got better', that sort of thing. And even as an undergraduate at vet school I had known that was insufficient evidence with which to support a claim – animals sometimes get better anyway, even without treatment. So what, I asked myself, is the difference between homeopathy and no treatment at all, if there is no actual objective evidence to tell us?

The sincerity of those who practised homeopathy and other forms of CAVM was never in doubt; clearly they believed the things they practised. But how could these highly trained professionals (including a veterinary colleague I worked with for many years and held in high esteem) be wrong, I wondered? Was there something I was missing?

So, as is often the case with those who are puzzled about such matters, I began to take a wider interest in how we know things, the nature of truth and reality, the way we humans perceive the world around us, and how that process can go wrong. And it turns out it is perfectly possible for people to be wrong in the face of overwhelming evidence – it is all part of being human. We are in many ways 'hard-wired' to make such errors, and the first step in properly understanding the real world around us is to be honest with ourselves about this.

Finally, after some ten years in the planning, I was approached by Sarah at 5M publishing and, at last, started to put virtual pen to virtual paper. I was honoured when Alex, who I had corresponded with on a number of forums on the subject of CAVM over the years and whose balanced and rational style I respect greatly, agreed to be co-author. In many ways for me this is the culmination of all those years of studying and collecting evidence, articles and opinions on the subject of CAVM in general and homeopathy in particular. As recreational activities go, while not quite on a par with extreme sports, it is nevertheless fulfilling, fascinating and at times frustrating. And it certainly gives a revealing insight into the way the human mind works.

Currently (when not writing this book!) I run the *Rational Veterinary Medicine* website and blog (www.rationalvetmed.net), dedicated mainly to collating the various reports and papers which homeopaths and other practitioners of CAM claim supports their cause. I also continue to contribute letters and articles in the veterinary press elsewhere. Like Alex, I am a founder member of the Campaign for Rational Veterinary Medicine (CfRVM) which has, as its central aim, the critical assessment of veterinary homeopathy by the UK veterinary profession's governing body, the Royal College of Veterinary Surgeons (RCVS), with a view to imposing limits on its use and on the reckless and unsubstantiated claims of veterinary homeopaths.

I currently live and work in the beautiful south-west of England with my wife, Alison, our two children, two dogs and three cats.

Niall Taylor, 2017

§

My veterinary training was ordinary and unremarkable, and touched little on the more esoteric subjects that are the realms of Complementary and Alternative Medicine (CAM). I knew of superstitions and pseudosciences such as tarot and astrology, but had little awareness that there were similar ideas being used in medicine and veterinary medicine. I graduated in 1996, when the internet was in its infancy, before Facebook and Twitter and Wikipedia, and information on non-mainstream practices was generally only found in the more mystical corners of bookshops and libraries. I had heard of homeopathy, acupuncture and herbal medicine, but knew little of the evidence for or against, and truth be told didn't much care – it was hard enough learning about all the stuff that worked, without worrying about things that probably didn't.

My first inkling that complementary and alternative veterinary medicine was a real thing, and a potential problem, was when I was participating in extra-mural studies or 'seeing practice' with a veterinary specialist in cattle health. He was explaining to me the concept of somatic cell counts in the monitoring of mastitis. Cell counts are measures of the level of white blood cells found in milk, which are a proxy measure for the level of mastitis in a herd, and have an influence on the quality of the milk produced. Farmers are therefore penalised financially for high cell counts, and an important part of dairy farming is to keep them as low as possible.

The vet I was observing was an expert in this field, and had lots of useful advice for farmers, and for vet students, on how to improve cell counts. However, like many things in biology, there is a large degree of variation in cell counts, the source of which is not always obvious. In similar ways, there is randomness in the occurrence of seizures in epilepsy, or the waxing and waning of immune-mediated diseases such as allergic skin disease, and when a frequency or severity of a condition is at a high point from natural varia-tion, there is a tendency for this parameter to return near to the average point over time. This concept, known as regression to the mean, is discussed in more detail in Chapter Four. To illustrate the natural fluctuation in somatic cell count, my mentor discussed an anecdote in which, contrary to his advice, a farmer had used homeopathy to treat mastitis in an attempt to improve his poor cell counts. Lo and behold, the cell counts dropped, and my mentor was impressed, despite his scepticism of the usefulness of a few millilitres of a potion in the herd's water. After the rather smug farmer had departed though, a farm hand approached my mentor and whispered to him, 'Don't tell the boss, but I accidentally dropped that stuff on the ground. They never got a drop of it.'

Although the anecdote was intended to educate me about mastitis and cell counts, it got me thinking about homeopathy. After I graduated, with the internet starting to take off, I became exposed to clients with an inter-est in alternative medicines, but a cursory glance at the available evidence left me unenthusiastic about recommending them. The proponents of alternative medicines were so vociferous in promoting them that I felt it sensible to educate myself about the pros and cons. I joined an email list, ALTVETSKEPT-L, run by Dr David Ramey, author of *Complementary and Alternative Veterinary Medicine Considered*, and the late Dr Robert Imrie, in around 1998 and have been a member ever since. It was on this list that I met my co-author and fellow sceptic, Niall, and though we have corre-sponded and spoken on the phone for many years, we only met for the first time on agreeing to write this book together.

The ALTVETSKEPT-L list introduced me to a large body of evi-dence, primarily in the human field, but in the veterinary field where the evidence existed, showing that CAVM was usually ineffective or useless. It also introduced me to concepts such as the aforementioned regression to the mean, the placebo effect, logical fallacies and cognitive biases.

Of course, debating with people who share your position already can reinforce erroneous beliefs, so I have attempted to engage with people holding opposing views, and supporting CAVM. Most people who use social media will be familiar with the anger and passion with which people espouse their views in that arena, whether it be on CAVM, politics, conspiracy theories or whether Rooney still deserves to hold his place in the England team. Back in the late '90s, my first exposure to this level of irrational emotion occurred at the time that pet vaccinations had hit the national press, in a sensationalised safety scare (see Chapter Nine).

Interested in what the campaigners were saying, I joined a pet anti-vaccination email list, intending only to lurk. The owner of a new puppy, unsure of the right course of action, asked the group for advice on vaccinations, and was hit by a barrage of emails telling her to avoid vaccination like the plague, unless she wanted her puppy to die a horrible death. I sent the new owner a private message, giving her my opinion on how safe vaccinations were, and she was grateful, as I think she was also taken aback by the ferocity of the group's responses. Soon though, I felt unable to refrain from arguing against the misinformation that was being circulated on the list. I spent an interesting day off being bombarded with angry and abusive emails, most of which I replied to, always keeping my tone polite. Politeness was not enough to save me though, and I was banned from the list for my dissent.

Curious as to what they would say when I had gone, I re-joined under a different name, and found I was being discussed in various derogatory ways – I didn't know what I was talking about, I wasn't a vet, I was a vet, but I was a disabled Danish vet, which was why I was at home and able to respond to their emails so much. I replied along the lines of 'Hello, it's me again, I'm not a disabled Danish vet, but even if I was, I don't see how that would invalidate my arguments.' Of course I was promptly booted again.

I have also engaged alternative practitioners in debates on *vetsurgeon.org*, a large vet-only forum, with debates on raw food diets (see Chapter Seven) being typical of the standard of debate with CAVM practitioners – full of anecdote, speculation, and so much raw emotion and *ad hominem* attacks that the debate had to be relegated to a 'controversial section' of *vetsurgeon*, away from the main forum, since the tone of the debate was such that the moderator was worried it would scare people away. In contrast to raw food proponents, homeopaths currently seem to be attempting to avoid debate in public forums, though letters to the *Veterinary Times*, many by Niall and myself, are often replied to by supporters of homeopathy.

In 2003 I joined the newly resurrected British Veterinary Voodoo Society (BVVS) (www.vetpath.co.uk/voodoo). This had originally been conceived in 1990, by veterinary surgeon George Tribe, as a counter to the British Association of Veterinary Homeopaths' application to become an official specialist division of the British Veterinary Association (BVA) (an application that was declined). The second incarnation of the BVVS was intended to highlight the fact that the Royal College of Veterinary Surgeons (RCVS) maintained a list of veterinary homeopaths, despite their qualifications not being officially recognised by the RCVS. The BVVS (of which Niall was treasurer, though sadly it collected no money), asserted that if this was acceptable for homeopaths, it should also be acceptable for voodooists, for which a similar evidence base of efficacy existed. The society's aims were listed as:

- To have the list of homeopaths removed from the RCVS Register.
- To have the advertising of homeopathic 'educational' courses banned from official BVA publications.
- To call on our universities to cease inviting homeopathic veterinary surgeons to lecture to undergraduates.

It was successful in the first aim, and after the retirement of key members, it became quiescent.

More recently Niall and I have been founder members of the Campaign for Rational Veterinary Medicine (CfRVM) (www.vetsurgeon.org/microsites/private/rational-medicine) which was set up 'to argue the case that 21st century veterinary treatment should in all cases be based on rational, established scientific principles.' Our petition to the RCVS, which is ongoing, asks for a public position statement from the RCVS on homeopathy, and asks that the RCVS requires veterinary surgeons who prescribe homeopathic treatment to abide by the Advertising Standards Authority rules, and to get owners of animals to be treated with homeopathy to sign a consent form giving the College's view on the inefficacy of homeopathy. A concurrent petition to the RCVS, not produced by the CfRVM, is calling for a complete ban on vets prescribing homeopathy, and at the time of writing has collected more than 1,000 signatures.

It was after I had already developed a scepticism about CAVM that my aunt, a vegan and a passionate animal rights advocate with a profound interest in CAVM, refused antibiotic treatment when she had septicaemia, treating herself with homeopathy instead. She died from the disease.

Where am I now? As I read more about the usefulness of CAVM (or lack of it), my interest shifted from whether CAM worked, to why people believed in it so vehemently, in the face of all logic and evidence. I explore this subject in Chapter Four, but it teaches a lot about human nature and psychology. Not only has it led me to question the beliefs and the motivation for beliefs of CAVM practitioners, but also my own. When I select a diagnostic test or treatment, or I interpret the results of the test or the response to treatment, I constantly question myself. Is the owner observing a real improvement? Am I, or am I just hoping that the animal is getting better? Is my test definitive, or is there room for doubt? What is the evidence base behind the efficacy of the treatment? Am I practising at a higher level of evidence base than a homeopath? These are healthy questions to ask. To be self-critical is to do our best by our patients and their owners.

And if I do one thing differently than many vets, having studied CAVM for twenty years now, it is this. When a delighted client tells me how pleased they are that their beloved pet is better, I often say, yes, it looks like the medication worked. Either that, or they got better on their own.

Alex Gough, Somerset 2017

§

## Note to the Reader

The spelling 'homoeopathy' was used in British English until recent times. Now the US spelling 'homeopathy' has been widely adopted for reasons of conformity in the digital age. In this book we have used the newer spelling throughout but you will see occasional examples of the older, British, spelling in direct quotes and in the titles of books and papers.

# Acknowledgements

The authors would like to extend grateful thanks to the following people and institutions for their generous and invaluable help at various points on our journey:

Simon Baker, Richard James, Morag Kerr, Andrea Lynch, Jason McDermott and David Ramey. Fellow members of the Campaign for Rational Veterinary Medicine: Martin Atkinson, Danny Chambers, Arlo Guthrie, Phil Hyde, Mike Jessop, Brennen McKenzie, Alison Price and Martin Whitehead. Clare Boulton and all the patient and helpful people at the RCVS knowledge library and information service. Sarah Hulbert from 5M publishing for her faith and perseverance. The Crown at Wells for beer, coffee and conviviality.

Finally, all the veterinary surgeons and nurses across the world who have lent their support and kindly contributed their own stories over the years.

# *Introduction*

HENRIETTA was a typical Bichon Frise. Not typical as in being a primped and preened powder-puff type of Bichon, but typical as in personality. She was spirited and happy-go-lucky, nothing daunted her, least of all her diminutive frame; to her, size most assuredly did not matter a jot, she had the heart of Lassie and the courage of Rin-Tin-Tin. She didn't so much walk, as bounce everywhere with her long, fluffy ears streaming out behind her as she shot from place to place with bright eyes and an eager expression, looking for the next adventure. And she loved people – she just couldn't wait to see the vet, she was one of those rare dogs who actually tried to pull her owner into the consulting room behind her. Which was handy really as her owner, Sandy Ross, wasn't particularly light on his feet these days, having suffered for a number of years with a nasty debilitating disease that ate away at his nervous system.

Today though things were a bit different as she came into the consulting room. Although she was still bright enough, some of the spring had gone from her step and Sandy said she was a little 'whiny' at times. She seemed to have some water-works problems too, and was passing a bit more urine than normal, including occasionally indoors – most out of character. Also she was getting a little picky about eating, which again was unusual, as her generous waistline attested. And she had been sick that morning.

Her vet, Ewan, a bluff Aberdonian, more used to dealing with burly farmers than the rather frail-looking Sandy and the effervescent Henrietta, was nevertheless extremely thorough and performed a detailed examination. Henrietta appeared to be suffering some of the signs of a false pregnancy and there were a few other unusual features that, he suggested, some blood and urine tests would help clarify. Sandy wasn't sure though – after all, the signs had only come on recently, this could just be a bit of a tummy upset. So they agreed to try some simple medication in the first instance and see if that and a little 'tincture of time' would do the trick.

And at first things seemed to look up. After three days Sandy phoned to say he thought Henrietta was brighter and seemed to have got over her gastric problems, although she was still drinking quite a bit. Sandy then informed Ewan he had taken Henrietta to an *applied kinesiologist* who, after getting Sandy to hold a sugar cube in one hand while placing his other hand on Henrietta's head, had informed Sandy she might have diabetes. Biting his tongue somewhat, Ewan refrained from pointing out this was why he had originally advised tests and instead suggested Henrietta came in to have a blood sample taken and to collect some urine.

A week after Ewan had first seen her Henrietta was even more subdued as she arrived to have her blood sample, although she perked up at the sight of her favourite vet. Sandy reported she was drinking constantly now, although her tummy upset had cleared up. In fact, she now seemed desperate for food, yet her weight was falling.

It was a matter of a moment to take a blood sample from the ever cooperative Henrietta, and a urine sample was forthcoming courtesy of a short walk around the chilly car park. Twenty minutes later Ewan had the results. Henrietta had *diabetes mellitus*, a condition (occasionally triggered by false pregnancy) affecting the pancreas resulting in the body being unable to produce the hormone insulin. Insulin controls the level of sugar and other substances in the blood and, without it, blood levels would increase catastrophically. Sugar is the body's main energy source and with it all locked away in the bloodstream, rather than where it was needed inside cells, the patient would effectively starve to death in the midst of plenty.

It wasn't all bad news though. Ewan told the stunned Sandy that with the right treatment there was a good chance Henrietta's condition could be controlled. All that was required was injections of insulin once or twice daily, something that Sandy wouldn't find difficult, having grown up around animals and well used to injecting the sheep on his father's croft when he was younger.

Insulin injections are best given in the morning so, early the following day, Sandy returned with his faithful companion and was shown how to give the injections, how to store the drug correctly and given advice on diet and exercise, both also useful in managing this condition. As the conversation continued, Ewan thought he noticed Sandy's attention was wandering. Putting this down to an understandable concern about Henrietta's well-being, Ewan continued, a nurse helping him with the advice and the injection. Finally, after Ewan had finished, there was a pause, Sandy looked uncomfortable. And then Ewan's face fell as Sandy dropped the bombshell – he wasn't going to use the insulin, he said.

Instead he told Ewan he was going to treat Henrietta using a combination of herbs – lemon balm and rosemary oil – and homeopathy. After all, he said, he'd been using them on himself and they had helped, so why wouldn't they do the same for his little dog.

No amount of pleading would change his mind. Why use unproven remedies, protested Ewan, when they had exactly the right treatment here that was known to work and work well and could easily give Henrietta years of happy life, rather than the weeks or months she would have without it. But Ewan's words were in vain, the best he was able to do was to get Sandy to agree to take the insulin home, and to bring Henrietta back in a week to measure her blood glucose levels again.

The week went by and Henrietta didn't turn up. Ewan phoned a couple of times but got no reply. Life was busy and the weather harsh, and time passed all too quickly. Ewan hoped no news was good news.

He was wrong.

Finally, five weeks later, in the middle of a freezing cold night, Ewan's phone rang. It was Sandy – Henrietta wasn't looking good. A relative was able to bring Sandy and Henrietta to the surgery where Sandy told Ewan he had been using homeopathy and herbs to treat Henrietta and hadn't given any of the insulin that he had taken home. Ewan's worst fears were realised. Henrietta was a shadow of her old self. Gone was the rushing around and the pulling to get into the consulting room. Instead she just lay, thin and huddled, on Sandy's lap. It was all she could do to wag her tail when she saw her old friend Ewan. The spark in her eyes was going out and she seemed to be in pain. She was so ill, this time Ewan had difficulty finding a vein to take the blood sample, but eventually he was able to confirm his suspicion this was an advanced form of diabetes called *ketoacidosis* – Henrietta's body was burning its own tissues to stay alive; and it was killing her.

The prognosis was hopeless, but Sandy was desperate to try something. So Henrietta was admitted to the hospital overnight, for intensive treatment including an intravenous drip, painkillers, antibiotics and something to stop her being sick.

The next morning there was no improvement. If anything, Henrietta was worse. Ewan's notes describe her as 'sunken-eyed, dull and unresponsive'. After a phone call to Sandy, Ewan was given permission to end her suffering by ending her life. Despite everything, she still managed a wag of her tail as he gave the injection.

§

The story above is true, although some details have been changed for reasons of confidentiality. When I spoke to Ewan about the case afterwards, he remarked that Sandy had seemed vulnerable. His own debilitating illness had meant he was easily taken in by the words of alternative healers, people who said they were his friends and who told him they knew best and that he didn't need drugs, either for his own condition, or Henrietta's.

And why shouldn't he believe them? After all, every day Sandy, like the rest of us, reads stories in newspapers, magazines, books and on the internet about the wonders of Complementary and Alternative Medicine (CAM). There seems no limit to its power. And not just from crank websites either, doctors and veterinary surgeons also claim great things for it – that CAM can treat, and cure, many serious diseases. Science-based medicine has failed, we are told, drugs are poison, so why use them when we can give you gentle, natural remedies that work in harmony with the body's own healing force, no side effects guaranteed.

So, of course, those who are in distress, those who are vulnerable, those who are trusting like Sandy, will take these people at their word. And that's when things go wrong.

This book is for all the Henriettas of the world.

§

# PART ONE

*Science and belief in medicine, the nature of understanding, how it can go wrong and what happens when it does.*

# CHAPTER ONE

# What Is Complementary and Alternative Veterinary Medicine?

COMPLEMENTARY and Alternative Veterinary Medicine (CAVM), the animal-oriented part of the wider field of Complementary and Alternative Medicine (CAM), is a diverse and varied subject. Enter the phrase into the internet search engine of your choice and you will get more than 650,000 hits; miss out the word veterinary and you get nearly 6 million.

Look closer at your search engine hits and in a very short space of time you will discover dozens of separate varieties including (in vague order of popularity): homeopathy, Bach flower remedies, tissue salts, homeopathic colour remedies, acupuncture, acupressure, aquapuncture, moxibustion, herbal medicine, nutraceuticals, chiropractic, magnet therapy, animal reflexology, orthomolecular and mega-vitamin therapy, ayurvedic medicine, reiki (wild and ordinary), laser therapy, aromatherapy, zero balancing, chakra balancing, qi-gong, crystal healing, pranic healing, energy healing, intuitive healing, spiritual healing, and the intriguingly named TAT.

In addition there are some areas that, while not strictly CAVM, nevertheless fall under the same alternative umbrella, being only loosely, if at all, based in science. These include the more far-fetched claims made for certain diets (often those involving feeding raw food to animals such as the Bones and Raw Food (BARF) or the Raw Meaty Bones (RMB) diets), the vaccine/anti-vaccination 'debate' and several diagnostic techniques such as kinesiology, dowsing, animal communicators, pet psychics and mediums, and Kirlian photography.

But what exactly is CAM, how is it defined, indeed can it be defined at all? Before getting into the meat of the subject in later chapters, in this first chapter we will take a brief look at important matters of definition and identity and try to tease out a few common threads from this motley collection of practices and beliefs. We'll try to discover if there is a common denominator by considering the views of those 'insiders' who practise it and those 'outsiders' who are perplexed by it. We'll have a look at the definitions arrived at by various legal, medical and professional bodies and we'll see if CAM can be defined by what it is alleged to do, or how it is claimed to do it. And, most importantly we will discover the difference between CAM and CAVM.

In later chapters we will discover how CAM *actually* manages to achieve the things it does, or at least appears to.

§

## Mechanisms – Vital energy

Although each individual practice has its own jargon to describe it, many are *vitalistic* in nature – claimed by practitioners to act by influencing so-called vital-energy. This energy is generally held to be ancient and integral with life itself and examples include the *Qi* of the acupuncturists the *vital-force* of the homeopaths and the *innate intelligence* of the chiropractor. Even some raw-feeding advocates believe in the *life energy* of raw, but not commercially prepared food, as you will discover in Chapter Seven.

These arcane energies are sometimes given a modern gloss, enabling proponents to have the best of both worlds by laying claim to both the provenance of ancient spirituality as well as the latest science. Currently the most popular contender drafted in to impart credibility is quantum physics with its counter-intuitive concepts and quirky (to the non-expert ear) terms such as strangeness and charm, entanglement and inter-connectedness, all echoing much of the obscure language used in CAM. This is nothing new, and in past ages other genuine phenomena that at the time seemed to defy understanding, such as magnetism or electricity, have been co-opted to lend a scientific respectability to non-scientific therapies.

Strangely though, it is usually the case that someone who believes in one type of CAM will believe in many other forms as well, despite the fact the ostensible mechanisms may be different or even contradictory in nature. Homeopathy, for instance, claims that most, if not all conventional drugs will interfere with the effects of a homeopathic remedy yet it is rare to hear that acupuncture, which also claims to influence *vital energy*, suffers (or even causes) the same adverse effect. Acupuncturists, who manipulate the mystic *Qi* by the precise placement of needles along defined pathways, are usually quite content also to employ homeopathy, which claims to manipulate a more diffuse, less constrained *vital-force* simply by means of tablets or drops. Herbalists know full well that the potency of their tinctures increases as they become more concentrated after prolonged infusion or distillation yet at the same time (with a few worthy exceptions) are often to be seen employing homeopathic remedies that instead are required to be diluted in order to achieve the same boost in potency. Crystal therapists seem happy that the life force can be manipulated by the proximity of their chosen gems as well as the remedies of the homeopath or the hand-wavings of the Reiki practitioner – no contradiction is perceived.

A purported mechanism of action – *vital energy* – which is as obscure as CAM itself is an inadequate and circular explanation for anyone hoping for an objective definition of the subject. Defining a set of practices by saying they manipulate a force that has stubbornly remained undetectable by science and is perceived only by practitioners themselves tells us little of what individual practices claim to do or how they claim to be able to do it.

## Effects

Another way of trying to make sense of CAM is to look at each therapy in terms of what it actually does (rather than what it claims to do) in the real world.

At one extreme there is the overtly fraudulent. For instance the stock-in-trade of the Psychic Surgeon is deliberate deception as simple conjuring tricks are employed to introduce various pieces of animal organs by sleight of hand into a bogus surgical field to be passed off as tumours or other masses, removed via an incision that heals instantly, leaving no trace. There is no possibility Psychic Surgeons can believe they actually do what they claim since they have purposely to conceal the piece of tissue before 'healing' commences. Their performance is done in the full knowledge, by the practitioner, that they are deceiving their patients.

Then there are modalities that have no material effect but whose practitioners genuinely believe in the power of what they do. These techniques appear to involve doing nothing at all to the patient, for instance homeopathy (which relies on sugar tablets or plain water for its effect), crystal healing, reiki and distant healing. In such cases, although the practitioners may be sincere, there is no way, given what we know about how the universe works, that their remedies or techniques can be effective. Any effect associated with their use is due to the factors discussed in Chapter Two of this work but is disingenuously portrayed by practitioners and users alike as being as a result of, rather than in spite of, the alternative treatment.

Finally, there are practices where something material is unquestionably done to the patient but it is uncertain whether the intervention is helpful or even relevant to the health of the patient. Herbal remedies we know contain plant material brimming with active ingredients often in quite unpredictable, occasionally harmful quantities. Acupuncture needles, when inserted into patients during a brain scan, are clearly seen to have an effect on the brain. Chiropractic involves vigorous manipulations and twisting, often accompanied (in human patients certainly) by an impressive array of clicks and pops; clearly something is happening in all of these cases. The debate with this group of techniques centres around their perceived benefits and, to a lesser extent, the supposed mechanisms that underlie them.

The evidence for any useful effect from almost all of these practices (particularly outside specialist publications) is, to be polite, equivocal in the extreme, as we will see in subsequent chapters. The exception being herbal medicine, where effects are widely recognised but where debate centres around the suitability or otherwise of using remedies that are crude and unrefined relative to conventional pharmaceuticals and which therefore may have unpredictable effects.

## Official and legal definitions

The American Veterinary Medical Association (AVMA), describes CAVM as 'a heterogeneous group of preventive, diagnostic, and therapeutic philosophies and practices. The theoretical bases and techniques of CAVM may diverge from veterinary medicine routinely taught in North American veterinary medical schools or may differ from current scientific knowledge, or both.'[1]

The British Small Animal Veterinary Association (BSAVA), in its position statement says: 'Complementary and alternative therapies are a diverse group of practices and products not considered part of conventional (mainstream) medicine.'[2]

The USA's National Centre for Complementary and Alternative Medicine (NCCAM) describes CAM as 'a group of diverse medical and health care systems, practices, and products that are not presently considered to be part of conventional medicine.'[3]

In 2000 the UK's House of Lords conducted a comprehensive inquiry into Complementary and Alternative Medicine, which looked closely at the reasons for its popularity as well as matters of training, regulation, research and funding. In the remit for the inquiry CAM is defined by what it isn't, rather than what it is:

*'Complementary and Alternative Medicine (CAM) is a title used to refer to a diverse group of health-related therapies and disciplines which are not considered to be a part of mainstream medical care.'*

Unable to discover an adequate, all-encompassing definition for CAM, the Select Committee instead elected to consider a list of therapies, grouped into three categories.

The first group comprised the 'Big Five'; those that the report referred to as 'professionally organised alternative therapies'; namely homeopathy, acupuncture, herbal medicine, chiropractic and osteopathy – these are also broadly the most popular therapies.

The second group encompassed complementary practices, used alongside conventional medicine without making any diagnostic claims. These included Bach flower remedies, Maharishi Ayurvedic Medicine, aromatherapy, body work therapies, reflexology and shiatsu.

Group three comprised a larger number of alternative practices that the committee considered had a particularly weak evidence base, including Anthroposophical, Ayurvedic and Chinese Herbal Medicine, crystal therapy, dowsing, iridology and radionics. The alternative disciplines in groups one and three were defined as those that '... purport to provide diagnostic information as well as offering therapy.'

The committee's findings also highlighted the tolerance of the state to CAM as enshrined in legislation: 'The Common Law right to practise medicine means that in the United Kingdom anyone can treat a sick person ... provided that the individual treated has given informed consent . . . The Common Law right to practise springs from the fundamental principle that everyone can choose the form of health care that they require.'[4]

## Definition by exclusion – CAM as the outsider

'Alternative medicine is a large residual category of health care practices generally defined by their exclusion and "alienation from the dominant

7

medical profession."' Ted Kaptchuk, *A Taxonomy of Unconventional Healing Practices.*[5]

It suits the agenda of many its supporters to define CAM as having been purposely sidelined by 'The Establishment' in a series of legislative turf wars over the years. The story goes that a scheming and self-interested medical elite has colluded and conspired with cronies in government and big business to ensure CAM practitioners are kept to the margins while The Establishment keeps its hands on the levers of power and its nose in the trough.

This argument is frequently heard in debates with proponents of CAVM and raw feeding in the veterinary press and on discussion forums when anyone who is critical of such things is condemned as being 'in the pay' of either the large pharmaceutical companies or the manufacturers of commercial pet foods. Such accusations are made wholly without evidence, of course, but they do serve as a useful device by which proponents can deflect the argument away from more awkward questions of efficacy and safety.

But just how accurate is this claim that the practices we regard as CAM were purposely abandoned as the medical establishment (physicians, surgeons and apothecaries) managed to use political and financial clout to get its foot in the door of state orthodoxy at the expense of equally deserving disciplines? How true is it that CAM is oppressed, the outsider looking in?

## The 1858 Medical Act

The nineteenth century was a time of great progress, in industry, science and medicine. Lister's writings on the importance of disinfection, Pasteur's work on germ-theory, the invention of vaccination, the development of anaesthetics, were all signs of a growing rational basis for medicine and a gradual turning away from the unproven methods of previous ages; not just the damaging practices of *heroic* medicine such as firing, purging and bleeding, which we will look at in more detail in later chapters, but other 'irregular' practices – homeopathy, animal magnetism, mesmerism and phrenology.

There is no doubt that scientific and medical bodies resisted the use of such practices, but this resistance was, to quote the *London Journal of Medicine* of 1851, 'not one of policy but of principle'. Objections were founded on science and common-sense rather than self-interest.[6]

In the UK the chief piece of legislation blamed for the alleged marginalisation of CAM is the 1858 Medical Act. Mike Saks of the University of Lincoln, UK is quite clear about its significance, and where the blame lies: 'Alternative medicine did not officially exist in Britain before orthodox medicine came into being with the 1858 Medical Registration Act'.[7]

In reality, what passed for the medical establishment prior to the 1858 act in the UK was an unsustainable mess, with an ossified medical elite, and general practitioners of all hues disenfranchised and largely disregarded – the mood of the country was such that something had to change.

With growing scientific confidence and public pressure on the medical establishment for improved accountability and safety came the demand for better organisation and greater inclusivity in the practice of medicine. Likening the situation in medicine prior to the act to end the corrupt rotten boroughs – the 'Gattons' and 'Old Sarums' – of the political system at the time, historian Michael Roberts argues that science-based practices of the time were slowly emerging from the prevailing chaos of the '"medieval", guild-based corporations of the profession, with their increasingly dysfunctional occupational demarcations into physicians, surgeons and apothecaries'. This was so much the case that some modern commentators now see legislation such as the 1858 Act as simply endorsing a prevailing trend of increasing professionalisation and specialisation in medicine that was inevitable anyway, even without parliamentary and legislative help.

But if the medical establishment thought it was going to get things all its own way in the drafting of the act it had another thing coming. Unorthodox practitioners had the backing of highly significant figures in parliament. At the time homeopathy was the darling of the nobility during a period in British history when aristocratic and Royal patronage was a major influence in politics. The chief advocate of homeopathy in Britain at that time was Dr F Quin, the physician of Prince Leopold of Saxe-Coburg, who dined regularly with royalty and may himself have been an illegitimate son of one of the wealthiest families in the country. Other blue-blooded lobbyists for 'irregular' medical practitioners included the Lords Ebury and Elcho and the Dukes of Edinburgh and Beaufort. Even the President of the General Board of Health and sponsor of the act itself, William Cowper, was a staunch supporter of unorthodox medicine who 'took a lifelong practical interest in homoeopathy, osteopathy and herbal medicine combined with a settled sense of the limits of practical utility of "orthodox medicine."'[8]

These big guns were more than enough to defeat any aspirations that unorthodox practices could be excluded by the newly emergent medical authorities and the final result was a compromise – far from the witch-hunt portrayed by present day CAM supporters. The act was eventually passed only on condition that medical authorities were specifically prohibited from barring any practitioner because he happened to hold views that differed from the mainstream. The freedom of the individual practitioner was thus sanctified in law, and consumer choice and the free market prevailed. This continued in subsequent revisions, such as in 1886 when fresh attempts by the medical establishment to regulate or exclude unqualified 'quacks' were defeated.

### The US 1938 Federal Food, Drug, and Cosmetic Act

In the United States the situation was, if anything, even more straightforward. Homeopathic remedies were actually granted equal status in law with conventional pharmaceuticals following the passing of the 1938 Federal Food, Drug, and Cosmetic Act (FDCA). The introduction to chapter two of the act even defined the term *drug* as meaning 'articles recognised in the official United States Pharmacopœia, official Homœopathic Pharmacopœa of the United States, or official National Formulary.'[9]

In part this seems to have been as a result of influence by the sponsor of the act, homeopath and amateur historian, Senator Royal Samuel Copeland, but at the time the homeopathic establishment was also working with the orthodox medical authorities in order to exclude from practice one William Frederick Koch, a medically qualified peddler of what were widely regarded by the establishment – homeopathic and conventional – as quack cures for cancer. Appeasement of the homeopathic lobby in this way would have been a shrewd move in the fight against what were seen as the real quacks – Koch and his followers.

The drafting of the 1938 legislation was as much a turf war between different types of unorthodox medicine – homeopathy, chiropractic, osteopathy and Christian Science healers – as it was between mainstream and unorthodox practices and it certainly represents collusion of homeopathic and mainstream authorities in the suppression of another unorthodox practitioner.

The simplistic view favoured by many CAM proponents today, that legislation was concocted by The Establishment to exclude unorthodox practices, is far from reality. In the UK we have seen the purpose of the 1858 act was as much to break down the prevailing orthodoxy as it was to either legitimise or exclude specific medical practices, and in the US homeopathy was actually recognised in law as a form of drug on a par with orthodox science-based pharmaceuticals. Furthermore, CAM generally and homeopathy in particular has always had the backing of significant influential figures, which continues to this day – hardly the picture of institutional oppression painted by some commentators.

CAM is not, in fact, excluded as a matter of principle by any 'establishment', be it legislative, political or medical. On the whole the law has gone to some lengths to accommodate individual freedom of choice and maintain a free market in matters of health care.

To claim that CAM is excluded simply for being alien or different, or can be distinguished from science-based medicine solely by virtue of orthodox medicine's 'legitimation by the state'[10] is putting the cart before the horse. The reason CAM continues to be excluded is because it fails to reach the scientific standards required by the rest of the medical profession – in most cases it simply doesn't work.

## Definition by requirement – CAM as a social construct

CAM can be considered as representing a lifestyle choice, an attitude or state of mind. In the 2000 House of Lords report mentioned above, one contributor, Dr Thurstan Brewin, suggested the popularity of CAM was dictated by fashion. Indeed, it is common to hear someone say they 'chose' to use alternative medicine or they 'believe' in energy pathways or the *life essence*; homeopathic texts, even today, talk of individuals 'converting' to homeopathy. The use of CAM is a statement about an individual user – it says something about their approach to life, their need for choice, and it aligns them with others of a similar persuasion.

There is an element of relishing the *otherness* about much of CAM and a delight in simply being different for its own sake, to the extent of resisting integration with science-based practices, 'for some groups of CAM practitioners, the growth of "integrative medicine" represents an undermining of counter-cultural values ...'[11]

For some, CAM's anti-establishment overtones permit a modest rebellion against the conformity of modern life while still allowing its benefits to be retained – protest with a safety net. As CAM researcher and commentator Dr John Astin puts it: '... in contemporary American society there is an emergent subculture that can be broadly defined in terms of involvement in various forms of esoteric, spiritual pursuits ... CAM may be a reaction to and a way to counter what people experience as an overly rationalized life experience ...'[12]

In this respect CAM has more in common with a belief system than with science-based medicine. After all, when did anyone ever claim they were 'becoming an antibioticist', only started 'believing in insulin' after a friend tried it, or was 'converting to hormones'. Such things are real-world entities, with no requirement for belief or faith from anyone.

For sceptics however, to look on CAM as a simplistic take it or leave it choice, a mere indulgence, is to miss much of what it means to many users. There is an unquestionable need in human and, arguably, veterinary medicine for forms of health care that go beyond the conventional, science-based mainstream. This may be for reasons of personal conviction, or simply the need for reassurance and human contact such as might be conveyed by massage, aromatherapy or reiki, irrespective of any actual objective, biomedical effect. It may be a (human) patient desires the feeling of self-determination in health care choices that using CAM can bring and which is sometimes lacking in increasingly stretched, occasionally quite impersonal, mainstream medical systems.

Science-based medicine and some of the diseases it treats can be overwhelming for individual sufferers, so it is not surprising people with serious illness will reach for aromatherapy with its pleasing perfumes and calm relaxing ambience, or homeopathy with its lengthy consultation and history taking. It's not always easy to talk to a busy doctor, surgeon or even a family member about serious illness. In some circumstances a patient may not even want to, they may have had enough of facts and figures, of drugs and debilitating treatments, of survival statistics and risk-benefit assessments; they may even have had enough of sympathy. They may just want someone who has the time to listen to them, even if it is a homeopath asking if they have an irrational fear of clams or how close they prefer to sit to the fireplace, or a crystal therapist asking with which gem they feel the greatest affinity.

## Choice, trust and responsibility

Only the hardest of hearts surely, could argue with those seeking consolation in complementary therapy under such circumstances. The problems start though, when therapists begin to believe they can not only provide solace during the course of a serious disease but that they can actually treat such diseases alone and unaided. And, as veterinary surgeons, this problem is all the more acute when such practitioners believe they can treat diseases in animals.

Unlike their owners, animals are unlikely to benefit from lengthy, sympathetic chats or exhortations to 'think positively'. Neither are dogs and cats, with a sense of smell many orders of magnitude stronger than our own, likely to appreciate being drenched with pungent oils or having to hang around too long in a room reeking of incense and burning herbs.

One of the most humbling things about being a veterinary surgeon is the recognition of the enormous trust animals place in us, their human caregivers. They rely on us to act in their best interests and we owe it to them not to permit our own personal beliefs or philosophical rationalisations to get in the way of getting things right.

In short, animals don't have the luxury of making lifestyle choices and that, finally, is the difference between CAM and CAVM – and that's where this book comes in.

# CHAPTER TWO

# Why CAVM Appears to Work in Animals

IF only one thing is achieved from the writing of this book its authors would most of all hope it will, once and for all, dispel the facile myth that CAM must be effective since it appears to be successful in cases involving animals.

This assertion, happily promoted by proponents of CAM who have little practical knowledge of the natural course of disease and injury in animals (and a few who ought to know better), rests on the argument that while an apparent response following the administration of non-science-based treatments in adult humans could conceivably be the result of the will to believe – the placebo effect – this cannot be the case in veterinary species since animals do not have the ability to anticipate the outcome of any treatment and therefore cannot influence such an outcome by means of wishful thinking.

For instance, according to homeopath Dr Harris Coulter 'the use of homoeopathy in veterinary medicine is of particular interest because the psychosomatic factor in treatment is largely excluded'.[1] Peter Adams, another homeopath, states confidently, in the case of animal treatment, 'the patient is not even aware of receiving any medication so the placebo effect can be discounted'[2] and Gerhard Koehler asserts that responses in animals associated with the use of homeopathy '... show how ridiculous it is to call homoeopathic treatment "suggestive" ... it is the objective result which counts in this field.'[3]

As this chapter will show, these (non-veterinary) authors are completely wrong; there are numerous ways an ineffective treatment can appear to have caused an improvement in our animals when in fact there has been no such benefit. Contrary to the assertions of those who profit by using CAM, there is no such thing as a purely 'objective' result, even where animals are

14

concerned.[4] This, as might be imagined, has serious ethical and welfare implications in veterinary medicine, particularly when bogus treatments are used in lieu of effective medicines in serious conditions, for instance when attempting to relieve pain or control infection in animals.

In an enlightening article, Canadian-born professor of psychology the late Barry Beyerstein, described 'At least ten kinds of errors and biases [which] can convince intelligent, honest people that cures have been achieved when they have not.'[5] While Professor Beyerstein's points were made concerning human medicine, many of them apply equally well to animal patients and there are also quite a few additional ones which are specific to veterinary practice, as will be seen below as we explore the reality behind the tired old canard that usually runs along the lines of, 'well, our dog's rash got better after homeopathy, so it can't be mind over matter, can it?'

## The disease may have run its natural course or resolved spontaneously

The body is perfectly capable of dealing with the vast majority of illnesses without external assistance. Evolution has gifted us a powerful immune system and a number of most effective mechanisms capable of ameliorating or resolving a wide variety of diseases. Many organs are capable of regeneration following injury. The skin will grow into large deficits to heal with minimal scarring, the liver will regenerate to full function following massive damage, certain fractures will knit, giving a functional result, without any form of surgical intervention, the heart can maintain its output and function despite defects such as valvular insufficiency. Animals' lack of the psychological problems associated with trauma in humans and their apparent stoicism in the face of pain means in some instances even major injuries and disease will resolve themselves naturally in time if medical or surgical intervention is withheld or unavailable.

In her enchanting book *Country Tales – Old Vets*, author Valerie Porter recounts a story told by Evelyn Day, a veterinary surgeon who practised in Stanford in the Vale, in the south of England, for more than thirty years from 1946. Evelyn recalls the case of an Alsatian dog who was brought to her with a broken leg. In this instance the owner was unable to afford the fees for a referral to a specialist orthopaedic surgeon to carry out a surgical repair so instead Evelyn ordered that the dog's activity was temporarily curtailed to limit movement across the fracture site and made sure that pain relief and good nursing was provided. Within six weeks, recalls Evelyn, the fracture had healed as a result of these measures alone.[6]

In my own practice a similar case occurred where a young cat was brought to us after having been missing for four weeks or so. The owners noticed it was a little lame in a hind leg so it was X-rayed. We found that the thigh bone had been fractured, probably not long after he had gone missing, and the ends of the bones had overlapped one another, and were now starting to heal in place. No money was available to arrange the referral to an orthopaedic specialist that would have been required to separate the fracture fragments and then reset them in the correct position. So, since the cat was virtually pain-free by that stage and only minimally lame it was decided to leave things well alone. After another week or so being confined to barracks the lameness resolved completely and he went on to lead a completely normal, happy life.

While these illustrations aren't to suggest this method of 'benign neglect' is to be condoned as a routine method of treating long-bone fractures they do make the point that sometimes even what can appear to be quite hopeless cases can heal surprisingly well without vigorous intervention. Even today a minority of fractures, particularly pelvic fractures in cats, once the initial assessment has been done will be treated entirely successfully by the simple means of providing pain relief and six weeks' close confinement.

Other examples of conditions that can present as severe yet may resolve with minimal or no active intervention include gastroenteritis, cystitis and lower urinary tract disease in cats, lameness caused by sprains or bruising, some abscesses in cats, upper respiratory tract infections (cat 'flu' and kennel cough) and mild spinal disease. In uncomplicated cases spontaneous recovery can appear almost miraculous.

One of the most striking examples of exactly the sort of condition that, though severe in appearance, will often resolve spontaneously and could wrongly appear to offer convincing proof of the effectiveness of CAVM is known as vestibular syndrome.

These cases have a most dramatic and upsetting presentation. The patient is often an elderly dog who will have seemed completely normal one moment then suddenly, within the space of a few minutes, started to drool, occasionally vomit, hold her head to one side, to stagger around, often walking compulsively in circles and tending to fall over, unable to direct her movements and clearly very distressed, with an anxious, pleading expression on her face as she tries to make sense of her predicament. All the while, on closer inspection it will be seen her eyes are rolling around in her head, shifting uncontrollably from side to side, a phenomenon known as *nystagmus*.

16

This condition is caused by sudden damage to the vestibular apparatus, that part of the sensory system that is responsible for maintaining balance. Various theories over the years have been proposed to account for why this damage happens but current thinking has returned to the idea that the most likely cause is a small 'stroke' or bleed in a specific part of the nervous system, although infection and trauma are also sometimes implicated in cases of vestibular syndrome.

In most cases, particularly those of peripheral vestibular syndrome, associated with damage to the inner ear and cranial nerve VIII, the prognosis is extremely good. With symptomatic treatment, rest and good nursing considerable improvement is usually seen within twenty-four to forty-eight hours and a virtually complete recovery is frequently made within the same period again. Despite this though, many websites and texts will quite needlessly recommend CAVM treatments for this condition.

If, say a homeopathic remedy is given or a chiropractic adjustment delivered during the course of vestibular syndrome, or any of the other conditions listed above, and is followed (coincidentally) by almost complete resolution within a short period of time, it will be nigh on impossible to convince an observer this 'treatment' was not in some way responsible for the final outcome. Thus the erroneous idea that homeopathy, chiropractic or whatever, has 'cured' the disease is reinforced (and relayed with great enthusiasm to anyone who will listen) when in fact such treatment has been irrelevant to the outcome, which would have been the same regardless.

Not every case will resolve unaided, however, and all the conditions above still require veterinary treatment of one sort or another. The correct treatment of diseases known to be self-limiting is geared towards offering palliative support, especially pain relief, but also other things including fluid therapy or medication to counter nausea, with a view to improving patient care. Clearly, if CAVM is used to the exclusion of conventional drugs, although the final outcome may be similar, healing may be delayed and the animal subjected to needless discomfort in the interim, particularly if denied proper analgesia.

## Many diseases have a waxing and waning course

Other diseases, while not of the sort that will completely resolve with minimal intervention, nevertheless have occasional periods of remission. At such times often quite marked symptoms can abate, occasionally for weeks, or even months, giving the false impression of a genuine improvement, if not cure.

Allergic skin conditions are common in the dog. One of the worst is known as atopy where a dog has a genetic predisposition to become allergic to normally innocuous substances present in the environment such as pollen, house dust mites and fungal spores to which it is exposed by either breathing them in or by direct contact with the skin. Atopy causes an irresistible compulsion on the part of the sufferer to itch and scratch so vigorously that, if not treated, the skin will eventually become sore, raw and bloody.

It starts insidiously, often obvious only at a certain time of year – it may be worse for instance when the pollen of a particular plant is more plentiful as it comes into flower. For this reason it is described as having a seasonal course.

As it grows older, an affected dog may in turn grow more sensitive to an ever increasing range of allergens. Consequently the allergy season will start earlier and end later until the affliction appears almost permanent. Nevertheless it is still prone to periods of waxing and waning for a number of reasons. Environmental conditions can change and variations in temperature and air quality will improve or worsen the clinical signs; for instance, periods of greater or lesser humidity will affect the numbers of house dust mites and fungal spores with which the sufferer comes into contact.

At the same time, other influences (known as *flare-factors*), while not affecting the degree of allergy per se, will increase the general tendency to scratch. For example, exposure to direct irritants – plants such as stinging nettles or ivy, or certain washing powders and carpet cleaners – will all add to the mix, conspiring to bring about changes in severity over time.

Consequently any treatment, including any form of CAVM, given at a time when the symptoms of atopy are at their height will stand a reasonable chance of being followed by an improvement (a phenomenon discussed in Chapter Four, known as regression to the mean). Whether or not the treatment had anything to do with the consequent improvement, or indeed had any effect at all, the impression to an owner desperate for an answer will be that CAVM has helped bring relief.

Addison's disease is a hormone imbalance, usually affecting dogs, which results from an under-active adrenal gland, hence its proper name; *hypo-adrenocorticism*. More colloquially, it is often referred to by frustrated veterinary surgeons as the great pretender, since it has the knack of throwing up a wide variety of symptoms that resemble other conditions. It can present almost identically to straight-forward gastroenteritis, with inappetence and bloody diarrhoea; it can resemble cardiac disease by causing lethargy, weakness, exercise intolerance and a slow, irregular heartbeat; and will occasionally look like kidney failure when it causes vomiting, dehydration and weight loss – even some of the results of blood tests will be similar.

The deceptive nature of Addison's disease is made all the more so by the tendency of clinical signs (if mild) temporarily to improve spontaneously or with minimal treatment. Since one of the jobs of the adrenal glands is to help cope with stress (by producing the hormone cortisol) when, as in Addison's disease, this ability is impaired the dog is no longer able to properly cope with stress. This means symptoms will wax and wane depending on what is happening in the sufferer's life at any one moment. For example, if a long car journey is undertaken, or a trip to a grooming parlour or the veterinary surgery, these will all cause stress to a greater or lesser degree. Thus, a dog affected with undiagnosed Addison's may start to become ill – to appear dull, go off his food or develop diarrhoea. If the attack isn't too severe however, once the trip is over and routine is restored, stress levels fall, the signs may well abate and as a consequence the dog will appear to return to normal, even though the underlying hormone imbalance is still present.

So, in the early stages of this condition the impression could very easily be gained that say, a dose of rescue remedy or a session of reiki given after what looked like signs of gastroenteritis, heart or kidney disease or even simply depression has produced a cure when really all that has happened is a trigger factor has been removed and the effects of the Addison's disease have abated, albeit temporarily, but completely independently of any treatment with CAVM.

And this may continue for months, with CAVM falsely appearing to give positive results, while all the time the underlying problem is getting worse, until a full-blown Addisonian crisis hits and urgent, life-saving (and this time genuinely effective) treatment is required.

Even certain types of cancer can have a waxing and waning course that can deceive us into believing there has been a clinical improvement when there has been no such thing. The mast cell tumour, for instance is a common cancer affecting dogs, often growing in or just below the skin. It may take the form of a small lump that can lie dormant for many months. If knocked or scratched however, these tumours will produce large amounts of highly active substances such as histamine, resulting in a large, local swelling many times the size of the original tumour.

These swellings arise extremely quickly and can be quite spectacular in appearance, sometimes they are accompanied by vomiting as the histamine travels in the bloodstream and affects the stomach. It would be easy in these circumstances for an owner to convince themselves this was the 'beginning of the end' and believe their pet was close to death as a result of cancer. Left to their own devices in the early stages of a mast cell tumour's development however, these signs will invariably subside. Again, if any form of CAVM is given before this improvement happens it would be hard afterwards to convince an onlooker they haven't just witnessed a cure for cancer. Of course, the original cancer persists after the reaction has subsided and although the mass may be small, it will eventually give rise to serious problems if left, requiring a more conventional, evidence-based approach.

And the list goes on – the number of conditions in animals that seem to come and go of their own accord is a long one, as any practising veterinary surgeon will tell you. Juvenile lameness in the dog can 'disappear' between 12 and 18 months of age, only to come back in a much more serious form years later; feline lower urinary tract disease causes great distress to the affected cat, who will be seen straining to pass tiny amounts of blood-stained urine, yet can be back to normal in a few days – until the next time when the same signs could be as a result of a life-threatening blockage. Forms of bronchitis will come and go depending on air quality, colitis cases have good days and bad days depending on stress levels or what diet is given (or what food patients have managed to acquire for themselves!) A whole range of immune-mediated conditions such as polyarthritis and certain neurological and muscular disorders can all occasionally seem to have been put on this earth with the sole purpose of deceiving clinicians and owners alike into thinking treatments are effective when they are not as symptoms come and go, varying in intensity from one day to the next.

Yet, despite the occasional remission most, if not all of these conditions are progressive, getting gradually worse over time. Some, like the mast cell tumour or Addison's disease, will respond well to treatment if caught early but if they are left untreated other than by ineffective alternative remedies, with coincidence being passed off as success, the consequences can be severe and real treatment, when it comes, may be too late to be of any benefit. Yet in the interim CAVM can claim credit where none is due.

## Use of a provisional or working diagnosis

Much as we might wish otherwise, inevitably, in veterinary medicine standards of diagnostic investigation are not always as rigorous as those in the human medical field. Cost constraints, finite resources and concerns about not wishing to inflict potentially uncomfortable tests or invasive treatments on an elderly or frail animal are (entirely understandably) limiting factors in many cases. This means in general practice veterinary surgeons may have to rely on a presumptive, working diagnosis only or have to shortlist a number of possibilities based on limited evidence, and treat speculatively.

Consider the case of a dog with a lump between its toes. This is a common presenting sign that can have one of several explanations. If, for whatever reason, it is not possible to perform the laboratory tests that would give a definitive diagnosis the veterinary surgeon may instead choose to discuss a range of potential diagnoses with the owner. The possibilities would include a cyst, a wound, an abscess (possibly caused by a foreign body such as a grass seed), or occasionally even cancer. If a full investigation is still not an option the veterinary surgeon will more than likely go with whichever diagnosis seems the most probable on purely clinical grounds; if the lump is discharging pus it is not unreasonable to proceed as if the cause was a bacterial infection. If the mass is discharging freely the best advice may be to treat it by bathing the area to encourage the lesion to drain further. If the condition was simply a local infection this, along with suitable pain-relief, may be all that is required to effect a cure – the lump will subside once the infection has drained. If, at the same time however, an owner had chosen to administer an alternative remedy he or she could very easily become convinced that this remedy was the cause of the 'cure' when in reality it was nothing of the sort. In some cases, if the limitations of working with a provisional diagnosis have been misunderstood ('the vet said it might be an abscess but I could tell what she really thought ...'), the owner may even get the idea that CAVM has cured his or her dog of cancer.

## Misdiagnosis by veterinary surgeon, owner or owner's friend

Interpretation of the clinical examination, imaging (such as X-rays or an MRI scan) or laboratory analysis is not always cut and dried. There are very few conditions for which there is one completely conclusive diagnostic sign, most diagnoses rely on a multitude of tests as well as one's clinical impression. So even trained professionals will occasionally make a misdiagnosis. A good practitioner will work with this possibility always in mind, continually reviewing a case in the light of new information or an unexpected turn of events and reappraising the diagnosis accordingly, rather than ascribing atypical developments to non-rational treatments.

A recent case of mine involved the removal of several suspect skin masses in a dog. Initial laboratory analysis suggested cancer. This didn't concur with my clinical impression and, following a conversation with the pathologist at the laboratory that had carried out the analysis, the findings were reinterpreted in the light of more detailed information as being the result of harmless inflammation. The owner, however, having heard the provisional results, had self-referred to a veterinary homeopath, who set about treating the 'cancer' and incidentally a self-limiting post-operative swelling called a seroma, homeopathically.

Needless to say, treatment of the seroma was completely 'successful' and the 'cancer' never returned (i.e. the result was exactly the same as if no homeopathy had been involved). Whether, having been informed of the revised laboratory report, the veterinary homeopath still claimed a cure for cancer I don't imagine will ever be known with any certainty.

The natural tendency of concerned owners to self-diagnose or to trust the diagnosis of acquaintances who may have had a pet with similar symptoms greatly adds to the potential number of misdiagnoses and consequently to the number of apparent 'miracle cures'. For instance, a dog with a cough due to a viral infection may present very similarly to a dog in the initial stages of heart disease, which also often causes coughing. If, at this stage, the owner of a dog with a viral infection is told by the owner of a dog with heart disease that their dog had the same condition and deteriorated rapidly following the initial diagnosis, requiring detailed investigations and costly lifelong treatment; and later the dog with the viral infection is treated homeopathically then – when it self-cures in a week or two – behold, a miracle, homeopathy has cured a failing heart.

## Concurrent use of conventional medicine

So-called 'complementary medicine' can be the most galling of all to the genuine practitioner when homeopathy or other forms of CAVM, used concurrently with conventional medicine, is credited entirely with the cure. This is particularly likely to happen in the case of conditions that are slow to respond to treatment. After some time on conventional treatment, an owner, concerned about the apparent lack of response, may turn to a practitioner of non-science-based medicine who initiates treatment that is followed, as a consequence of entirely natural variations in the speed of response to treatment, by an improvement. After this it would be well-nigh impossible to persuade someone the CAVM had been irrelevant to the outcome and that if they had simply allowed further time for the conventional drug to work, the final result would have been the same.

The habit of CAVM practitioners of promoting their various specialities by means of uncorroborated anecdote means we can never be certain which are full and factual accounts and which conceal inconvenient facts. As we will see elsewhere in this volume, the role played by conventional medication can be happily airbrushed out of the picture if it serves the purpose of promoting CAVM.

## Non-specific effect of CAVM treatment ('collateral benefit')

The term 'homeopathy' is a value-laden one that carries considerable kudos among certain groups of consumers. As a result of canny marketing over many decades this simple word is now loaded with ill-deserved feel-good connotations – safe; natural and simple; harmony, not harm; cooperation, not confrontation and so on. There is also a strong element of self-empowerment – making a positive personal choice, bringing health care decisions back into the hands of the individual and away from what are perceived as faceless health services and grasping pharmaceutical multinationals.

So with all these pre-packaged and positive perceptions already in place, it's not surprising that some manufacturers will endeavour to jump on the bandwagon by including the word 'homeopathy' at every opportunity on the packaging of their latest range of over-the-counter nostrums, even when the product may actually have very little connection with Samuel Hahnemann's 200 year old invention (see Chapter Ten).

Skin creams and eye ointments or gels such as Calendula or Arnica, while possessing not a trace of the eponymous base ingredient, as would be expected in a correctly formulated homeopathic remedy, nevertheless contain many other ingredients that will have some degree of therapeutic effect. Eye drops may contain antiseptics and moisturisers that will provide relief in cases of minor irritation regardless of any supposed homeopathic effects. Homeopathic skin creams contain water, oils, astringents, moisturisers and antiseptics, many or all of which will have a beneficial effect on superficial wounds, areas of dermatitis and minor bruising, particularly if applied according to directions such as 'Apply a thin layer of cream to affected area and massage gently as soon as possible after minor injury.' In other words, as your grandmother might have said; just rub it better; no homeopathy required.

'Arnica' mouthwashes are little more than solutions of salt with key words such as 'Homeopathic', 'Hepar sulph' 'natural' and so forth written on the label to disguise the fact that, for the same antiseptic effect, one would be as well to reach for ordinary table salt from the kitchen cupboard rather than an overpriced but largely identical equivalent from the medicine chest.

And it's not just homeopathic gels and unguents that benefit vicariously from the presence of entirely conventional, non-homeopathic ingredients; other forms of CAVM benefit from effects unrelated to their supposed 'alternative' modes of action. The manipulations and measured tones of the chiropractor will have much the same tension-relieving effect, regardless of the existence or otherwise of so-called vertebral subluxations, and the needling of animals will produce a rise in natural, pain-relieving endorphins irrespective of the presence or absence of invisible energy pathways or disturbances in the flow of *Qi* as proposed by acupuncturists.

The non-specific effect of some products are not always to the benefit of patients of course, there have also been cases of 'collateral damage' occurring following the use of CAM and CAVM treatments. In 2015 the company Petco was forced to withdraw a dog-calming medicine from sale after customers raised concerns about the risk of adverse effects on the health of their pets. With a 13 per cent alcohol content, any calming effect observed was more likely to have been a result of alcoholic intoxication than homeopathy.[7]

In the area of human health, the supposedly safe homeopathic preparation Zicam Cold Remedy contained so much Zinc that amounts exceeded the toxic threshold and when used as instructed, in a vain effort to reduce the duration of the common cold, some 130 users were instead permanently robbed of their sense of smell.[8]

## A desire to believe on the part of owner and practitioner

Beyerstein describes this as the 'psychological distortion of reality' and it applies as much when an owner's animal is under treatment as it does when the owner is. It can be seen as a kind of enhanced form of the caregiver placebo effect, discussed in more detail in Chapter Five.

Even when there are few if any objective improvements in an animal treated by CAVM, owners and veterinary surgeons who have a strong psychological investment in alternative medicine will, unconsciously and with the best of intentions, often manage to convince themselves their animal has been helped regardless. To have received no relief after committing time and money to, and having a deep, personal belief in, alternative treatment is difficult to admit to oneself and others, so there is strong pressure to find some redeeming value in such treatment and so avoid losing face.

There may also be an unspoken complicity between owner and practitioner with neither party willing to disappoint the other with negative findings or comments. Of course, an animal cannot make an informed choice and plays no part in this cosy consulting room conspiracy; it will either get better in spite of, or suffer as a result of, their caregivers' ideologies.

## Some conditions are as a result of owner concerns and preconceptions

Dogs, as a species, have co-evolved with us over tens of thousands of years, they have been our companions and protectors since the late Mesolithic period, and in many ways they know us better than we know ourselves. They are ultra-sensitive to our moods and humours.

In 2008 authors Nina Cracknell and Daniel Mills of the University of Lincoln published a paper that looked at the effects of homeopathic remedies in alleviating the fear of firework noise in seventy-five dogs over a four-week period during the height of the firework season.[9] In their conclusion the authors found all the indices of stress looked at in the trial improved dramatically after treatment. The intensity and severity of fearful behaviours such as running around or freezing on the spot, drooling, panting, trembling and even self-harming improved in around two-thirds of cases – a level that suggested true statistical significance.

The really interesting aspect of this trial though, is not the effect associated with the homeopathic remedy, but the fact that homeopathy and an identical-looking placebo both gave the same results. Regardless of whether they had been using the homeopathic remedy or an inert equivalent, the behaviour of the dogs in both groups improved to such an extent that fifty-three of the participating owners said they were satisfied with the treatment and fifty-five would be likely to want to use it again.

In their comments on the results the authors speculated, 'an expectation of improvement could cause owners to report some degree of improvement regardless of the treatment used' and pointed out, 'Many authors have commented on the importance of owner behaviour influencing fear responses in the dog.'

Anyone who knows dogs knows how exquisitely sensitively they are attuned to the body language of both other dogs and humans. Their level of perception greatly exceeds that of their human companions and in some cases can seem almost miraculous; akin to mind-reading. So it is highly likely the dogs' fearful behaviour during this trial was caused, at least in part, by the anxieties of their owners. When fireworks are anticipated, a dog will perceive only that their owners – the 'pack-leaders' – are anxious and worried. They would have no understanding of the fact this was natural human concern for the well-being of their canine companion, not the fireworks as such. All they would comprehend would be the pack had cause to fear something, and that would trigger behaviour of the sort under study, which in turn would cause the owners even more anxiety and so the cycle would continue. If, on the other hand, an owner believed his or her dog had been given a medication that would reduce or eliminate its fear of fireworks, this means the owner's own anxiety will be reduced, which in turn will be sensed by the dog who will thus be less anxious themselves.

No matter how carefully nonchalant we try to be it is simply not possible to fool a dog into thinking there is nothing wrong when there is. They beat us hands down every time, just ask anyone who has ever tried to get a dog into the car to take them to the vets – somehow, no matter how clever or casual we think we are being, they always know it's not a trip to the park!

And it is a small step from knowing this to realising that when a worried owner gives a worried dog a remedy intended to calm it, that remedy will have an effect on both dog and owner, greatly to their mutual benefit but irrespective of any physical properties of the remedy.

§

## The miracle cases

As we have seen in the preceding section, most CAVM depends on its apparent effect, not on the ability to manipulate the body and its healing powers by means unknown to science, but simply by claiming success for improvements and resolutions in animals that would have happened anyway. However surprising and unlikely these improvements may seem, they are nevertheless witnessed every day by veterinary surgeons in practice around the world.

In the section that follows (and at various points elsewhere in the book) there is a selection of real examples of such cases. Although some of the details of the cases have been changed for reasons of confidentiality, every one of them is true, involving real animals, owners and veterinary practitioners. Some were recorded by the authors, many more were provided by other veterinary surgeons with similar concerns. To those contributors we extend our grateful thanks.

In some of them, often following apparently serious injury or disease, having not been expected even to survive for more than a brief period following diagnosis, some individuals have defied expectation and lived happily for many a year. These tales have been included for the purpose of illustrating that these 'Miracle Cases' are real, actually quite common and, of course, not miracles at all but the result of well understood, everyday processes. The average general practitioner, if he or she is honest with themselves and others, will admit this quite happily. It is one of the ways we all learn, with a view to modifying and improving our approach to future cases, often by accepting the prompt that further study is needed in certain areas. Acknowledging these things demands a degree of humility but in the long-term we and our patients are better for it.

In the case of practitioners of CAVM however, possibilities such as those listed in the first section of this chapter seem rarely, if ever, to be considered. Instead of recognising say spontaneous improvement or the need to revise an initial diagnosis – perhaps one that was based on limited information – such practitioners will claim the 'Miracle Cases' for themselves, as proof-positive for the effectiveness of their chosen modality. They will then go on to post such stories on websites, talk about them at conferences and write books about them, while quietly forgetting all those other cases where the 'Miracle' didn't happen and an animal may have suffered as a result of not receiving effective treatment.

Ironically, this reflects an excessive and altogether misplaced faith in the power of Mankind over disease. Contrary to the CAVM practitioner's pretensions to 'holism' and 'natural healing' their attitude actually suggests a denial of the 'natural' ability of the body to heal itself unaided, whether by science-based or non-science-based medicines. In homeopathy, this conceit goes all the way back to its inventor, Samuel Hahnemann himself, who wrote, in his *Organon of Healing*, 'Natural diseases ... cannot be overcome and extinguished by the *vital force* without the help of a therapeutic agent.'[10]

Simple anecdotes are, as we will learn in Chapter Five, a powerful and beguiling tool in the hands of an alternative practitioner determined to promote themselves by relating stories that support the idea that his or her preferred form of CAVM is effective. But such anecdotes can also be deceptive and, although we should not doubt the literal truth of such stories, we should also be aware of certain factors that make them less than trustworthy as evidence in favour of CAVM. The stories are selective – unconsciously authors may omit certain crucial points for reasons of clarity or to better make their case. Also, the stories themselves are selected to support a specific point of view while others that don't suit the agenda may be left out.

The accounts that follow are intended to turn the tables somewhat by illustrating the point that for every anecdote about a 'Miracle' following homeopathy, acupuncture, radionics or anything else, there are dozens of near-identical cases that happen spontaneously, without the need for any form of CAVM – these are the 'ones that got away', which you won't read about in any CAVM website or textbook. The point is, to use a statistical cliché, correlation does not imply causation. In other words, just because two events happen together, it doesn't mean one has caused the other, no matter how strong our urge to believe otherwise might be – coincidences happen, whether we like it or not.

§

Manhattan was a big cat, one of the biggest, and what's more he had the scars to prove it. It wasn't that he was the aggressive type – he was actually a very gentle giant – it just seemed that every other cat in the neighbourhood felt it was their duty to 'have a go' whenever his impressive physique wandered too close to their territory. As a result he had been seen at the clinic on a regular basis for a variety of bites and scratches in the past – injured feet, infected ankle joints, that sort of thing. Luckily they had all responded to fairly basic treatment with antibiotics, painkillers and antiseptic washes.

This time though, things were different. He first presented a few days after his owners had heard the unmistakable sounds of a cat fight from their back garden following which Manhattan had appeared indoors looking ruffled and with a bleeding wound by the base of his tail. After a day or so of uncharacteristic depression and lack of appetite, they brought him to the veterinary surgery for a check-up. On first examination the small, innocuous looking wound was noted; a common enough sequel to a cat fight. What was less usual though was the excessive amount of bruising around it, way out of proportion to the size of the wound itself. The whole area was extremely painful to the touch. Suspecting the fight had caused the rupture of a large blood vessel and infection, the attending veterinary surgeon prescribed antibiotics and painkillers and instructed his owners to keep a close eye on the situation.

Sure enough, a few days later they became so concerned they got back in touch and the veterinary surgeon's suspicions about the injury were confirmed. This time instead of a small puncture wound, a large, gaping hole had appeared at the side of the base of the tail and, peering past the one tiny strip of skin remaining, a deep cavern could be seen where the infection had tracked forward, undermining and damaging muscle and tendon as it went, leaving an enormous defect and extending to within a few millimetres of the spinal cord. The whole area was infected, oozing pus and, being at the base of the tail, was constantly moving – every time Manhattan twitched his tail, any attempt at healing was immediately undone. The surrounding skin was so badly damaged, and the cavern so vast, as to make stitching the wound closed impossible. All that could be done was to leave it open to encourage drainage, while the owners continued to keep the area as clean as possible. But it was explained, as tactfully as possible, that a wound as large and as deep as this would be extremely unlikely to heal on its own, particularly given its location. There was a distinct possibility Manhattan's tail might, unfortunately, have to be amputated in order to allow the wound to come together. A follow-up appointment was made in a week's time and the case vet began to prepare mentally for a high amputation.

The day of the appointment came and the change was staggering – a mere eight days after presenting with a hole so big healing had seemed impossible, against all the odds the wound was now reduced to a small, shallow area of healthy pink tissue, virtually closed and well on its way to complete resolution. There were smiles and astonishment all round as he was checked over, before returning home with no further treatment required. Within a short space of time Manhattan was back to normal and able to get back to duty, keeping the neighbourhood in order once again, with barely a scar to show for his ordeal.

§

Practice staff had known her for years as Mrs Elspeth Spencer. The general opinion was although she was occasionally demanding and a little 'other-worldly', her heart was in the right place. Some months ago however she had attended a week-long retreat at a '*Spiritual Awakening and DNA Consciousness*' centre at a remote location in southern England (or Pagan Heartland as Mrs Spencer preferred to call it). Since then her 'other-worldliness' had reached new heights; she had taken to wearing flowing, sky-blue robes and now insisted on being referred to by her new Goddess name, *Lakshmi*.

Today though, reality had intruded in no uncertain fashion – her dog,

Anubis, had a sore bottom. As she swept into the consulting room with a tinkling of ankle bells and a whiff of incense, Susie, her veterinary surgeon, sighed inwardly and prepared for battle; from the set of her jaw she could tell *Lakshmi* was in confrontational mood.

Some twenty minutes later, with the help of a muzzle and a skilled veterinary nurse, Susie had made her diagnosis. Anubis had an infected anal gland that, instead of draining the usual way, along the natural duct, had ruptured to the skin surface in a painful, smelly mess right next to his anal sphincter, a very uncomfortable predicament. Susie and the nurse had clipped and cleaned the area to allow better drainage but more treatment would be needed and Susie suggested to *Lakshmi* that, as well as some pain relief, Anubis would benefit from a course of the antibiotic Antirobe, ideal for infections of this sort.

At this, the former Mrs Spencer furrowed her brows and adopted a far away, steely gaze. Her hand reached through her robes and she extracted a chain, to which was affixed a teardrop-shaped crystal of purple amethyst. *Lakshmi's* eyes screwed shut in concentration as she twirled the crystal over Anubis's nether regions. Finally her eyes snapped open and she declared 'I'm getting a NO for Antirobe'.

Patiently, Susie began to explain about anaerobic infections and the need for a suitably targeted antibiotic but before she could utter more than a couple of words *Lakshmi* fixed Susie with an uncompromising glare and, holding the crystal between them, as if warding off a malign influence, boomed, 'I am a fully qualified Radionics Healer!'

This was clearly going to be her last word on the subject. For Susie it had been a long day and the thought of a war of words with Mrs Spencer held little appeal. She decided to try another tack.

'Well,' she said thoughtfully, 'We could try some Clindamycin instead. It's a bit of a long-shot, but it might just do the trick'. Once again the crystal twirled and sparkled in the fluorescent lights of the examination room. This time *Lakshmi's* face relaxed into an aspect of smug beneficence. 'Oh my dear, this is much better, I'm getting a YES for that one.' Her look and the pitying tilt of her head spoke volumes. Susie returned an enigmatic smile.

*Lakshmi* and Anubis set off for home a few minutes later, both happy and relieved, a pack of Clindamycin safely stowed in the former Mrs Spencer's hand-crafted vegan leather handbag.

Susie tells me Anubis's infection responded extremely well to treatment. Whether *Lakshmi* ever discovered that Antirobe and Clindamycin were simply different names for the same drug she never asked, and as far as is known, *Lakshmi's* faith in the power of radionics persists, undiminished, to this day.

§

A veterinary surgeon from the south coast of England writes:

*One of our clients owns an ancient tortoise named Arnie. At 89 years of age he is without doubt the oldest animal on our books!*

*I saw him last June as he hadn't eaten or passed a motion since waking out of hibernation in April. That meant he hadn't eaten anything or had a bowel movement since starting hibernation eight months previously. His owner had tried everything which usually helped get him going – warm baths, allowing him out in the warm sun every day (it was an incredibly hot summer that year) and providing a heat lamp the rest of the time but nothing made any difference. He wouldn't even be tempted with his favourite food – peach slices. She had owned Arnie most of his (and her) life and she was getting worried, he'd never been this bad for so long before, she said. When I examined him he seemed a good weight but his eyes were dull and glassy. I was very worried about the old boy and was just considering what equipment would be needed to give him fluids and a laxative via stomach tube when he started to get a bit agitated on the consulting table, his hind legs stretched out and went into a kind of spasm.*

*At first I thought he was having some sort of terminal crisis because of starvation but then he started to pass great quantities of gelatinous sticky clear liquid and then a big mass of white, chalky uric acid (which reptiles produce instead of urine) followed, after a moment, by a single, solid, colossal stool. The stink was dreadful and the whole thing was disgusting but I swear you could see the relief on his face as he got rid of the last bits of that accumulated waste. All I had to do was pick him up and clean him off – perfect timing!*

*It occurred to me though, what if I hadn't got ready to pass a stomach tube and I'd performed a bit of Reiki on him instead – waving my hands around and adjusting his Chakras and so forth – and then he had obliged as he did, right in front of me, at that very moment. How impressive would that have been, and who would have believed, after eight months and with such 'perfect timing' that it wasn't the Reiki which had cured him?*

§

A young Labrador was referred to a veterinary teaching hospital having had seizures on and off for the past year. They had been increasing in frequency, particularly during the last few months, until he was having one seizure every few weeks. He had blood tests that looked at his general health and his liver in particular and everything seemed normal so in all likelihood the problem was in the brain itself. After examination at the neurology and neurosurgery department, the consultants prescribed potassium bromide, a well-established and effective drug for the treatment of idiopathic epilepsy but mentioned in some cases such as these other types of drug were occasionally required in addition if the initial treatment wasn't wholly effective.

Once they got back home however, the owners decided not to give the medication and instead to wait and see what happened. Miraculously, after all that investigation and a diagnosis by some highly qualified veterinary surgeons the dog simply stopped having fits without any treatment at all.

§

Liz, a veterinary surgeon from Essex, England sent this tale to me:

*A 10 year old cat was presented to us with a sore eye. The owner reported seeing a blob of matter on the eyeball the previous night and had been bathing it ever since, trying to get it off. When the eye was examined under magnification we could see it had been damaged. There was a penetrating wound in the cornea (the clear part at the front of the eye) and a corresponding red spot on the iris (the coloured part inside the eye) immediately underneath it. The blob of matter on the surface was tissue or clotted material from deeper in the eye protruding through the wound and acting as a plug – this was what the owners had been trying to remove (eek!) It was obvious a thin, sharp object had punctured the eye and gone into the eye far enough to injure the iris inside before coming back out again – the cat running or jumping on to a thorn was the most likely explanation.*

*We advised referral to a specialist ophthalmic surgeon at this stage. The corneal injury was deep and likely to have needed suturing. Without this there was a great risk the eye would fully perforate and require removal. Also, the infection and contamination which had been introduced into the eyeball would need to be addressed.*

*For various reasons however, this wasn't an option so, against our better judgement, we had to manage the case using antibiotics by injection and in the form of eye drops, as well as eye lubricants and painkillers.*

*Two days later, and much to my surprise, the wound was still stable and plugged and the eye was starting to mount a healing response. Two weeks after that he was doing very well indeed. The 'blob' was greatly reduced and his eye*

32

*was fully functional and healing well with a proper, organised line of scar tissue across the cornea as a permanent reminder of his lucky escape.*

*And no complementary or alternative medicine was involved at any stage in this miracle case!*

§

A middle-aged cairn terrier named Angus had developed glaucoma in his right eye. The severity and speed of onset was so great that treatment (not always terribly effective in cases of glaucoma at the best of times) made little difference. Angus became blind in the affected eye and because this was a painful condition the reluctant decision was made to remove it. The operation was performed shortly afterwards.

It is easy to imagine the devastation the owners felt when, two years later during a routine check-up with the ophthalmic specialist who had treated the glaucoma in the first eye, the same condition was diagnosed in the other, remaining one. Glaucoma causes an increase in pressure in the affected eye, leading to pain and blindness as a result of damage to the extremely fragile retina at the back of the eye. To combat this pressure build-up, Angus underwent some very hi-tech laser surgery to try to slow down the production of fluid within the eye.

Despite this pioneering procedure and follow-up with medication however, a month later at his post-operative examination the ophthalmologist gave Angus's owners some bad news – he had lost the sight in that eye too. He was now totally blind.

Nick, the veterinary general practitioner who contacted me regarding this case and who had arranged the initial referral described to me the conversation he had with the owners after this diagnosis. It was a very sad and difficult time and they were seriously considering euthanasia as it was hard for them to comprehend how Angus could lead anything like a happy life while not being able to see.

Eventually they decided between them to give it a bit more time to see if Angus could adapt. After all, Nick explained, dogs have other senses such as hearing and smell that they rely on far more than we humans. Time went on and Angus had two more follow-up examinations with the ophthalmologist, both of which confirmed his blindness.

Then, over four months after the diagnosis of glaucoma in his remaining eye, when Angus's owners came back to see Nick for a check-up they could hardly contain their excitement. They announced that Angus was now able to see again!

Nick, while not wishing to dash their hopes, was pessimistic. He knew that even completely blind dogs can navigate with uncanny accuracy and was worried this apparent improvement may have been more wishful thinking than anything else. When he examined the eye though, he felt there might have been some improvement, as the owners had said. Still not wanting to give false hope, he explained the retina was so delicate that blindness in these cases is inevitably irreversible, particularly after such a long period of time, and the chances of this being a genuine improvement were vanishingly small. The ophthalmologist hadn't so much as hinted there was any chance he would recover his sight. Another appointment with the specialist was arranged for a week or so later.

And, incredibly, following the examination, it was very good news – Angus's sight had indeed returned. The written report from the specialist was uncharacteristically upbeat, not at all the cautious, measured tones usually seen in such documents. Clearly they were as overjoyed as Angus's owners (and Nick) at this miraculous turn of events.

## Down on the farm

Homeopathy At Wellie Level (HAWL – www.hawl.co.uk) is an organisation of homeopathic veterinary surgeons and farmers set up to teach homeopathy to farmers, particularly those with organic units. As is usual for such organisations, their website and newsletters abound with enthusiastic anecdotes from veterinary surgeons and farmers about alleged successes following homeopathy, with little or nothing in the way of good quality evidence to support the wider implications of the claims made.

A number of testimonials involve the problems of livestock giving birth (dystocia), with farmers proclaiming the usefulness of homeopathy at this difficult and often very fraught time. Some births can be challenging, requiring considerable skill and physical strength, things can go wrong very quickly and there is an understandable sense of urgency, verging on outright panic at times.

One HAWL anecdote describes how a farm owner, on seeing his herdsman struggling to calve a cow with a narrow birth canal, took over and began to give a homeopathic remedy to the cow at ten-minute intervals. The delivery of a live calf some forty-five minutes later was hailed as certain proof of the effectiveness of homeopathy.

But to any veterinary surgeon with experience of large animal work this sequence of events is not in the least astonishing, regardless of the use of homeopathy. Any farm vet you speak to will be able to describe countless cases where a cow, having difficulty giving birth and with an inadequately dilated birth canal, managed to deliver successfully simply by means of allowing more time, taking things slowly and being patient. The steady pressure on the birth canal initially from a calf's forelegs and later its nose and head, coupled with careful manipulation by the veterinary surgeon or stockman will, more often than not, gradually cause the birth canal to dilate, perfectly naturally, sufficiently for the calf to be delivered with firm but gentle traction. This is by no means a miracle, far less proof that homeopathic remedies, diluted as they are to non-existence, can help farm livestock during the birthing process.

The same also applies to other animals, including sheep. In my first job in a practice in Cornwall two farmers turned up at the surgery, unannounced, within a few minutes of one another, each with a ewe in the back of his van that they had been trying to lamb for some time without success. Unfortunately for them, this was a busy farm practice and all the vets were out on rounds, none of us was going to be able to return to base for some hours. What happened next was relayed to us later, by the receptionist.

After a bit of muttering about how irresponsible it was of a veterinary practice not to ensure a vet was permanently stationed at the surgery twiddling their thumbs waiting for just such an eventuality, the farmers got to talking. When they discovered their identical predicaments one offered to have a look at the other's ewe and 'have a go' himself. The receptionist fetched warm water, disinfectant and lubricant and after a few minutes, to everyone's surprise, the ewe was delivered of live twins. Flushed with success, the second farmer offered to return the favour and duly 'had a go' with the first farmer's ewe. Sure enough, after a minute or two a large singleton was delivered. As they drove down the lane away from the clinic both farmers were reportedly beaming with delight at having not only successfully increased their livestock populations but, far more importantly, having got one over on the vet by cleverly avoiding a bill for services rendered. All it had taken to lamb their ewes was time and a bit of a ride around the countryside in the back of a van.

On another occasion I was called out to attend a calving by a farmer who had a lifetime of experience of calving cows and was very good at it. I remember the call distinctly as I was attending the local blood donor clinic with my family at the time so it took a while to extricate myself and dash back to the surgery to collect the Caesarean kit, which I was certain I would need as it was practice legend that any cow this particular farmer couldn't calve just couldn't be calved. So it was about half an hour before I arrived at the farm and got out of the car to put on the waterproof clothing that is essential when calving a cow.

As I was hopping around, wrestling with a last, recalcitrant boot, I saw the farmer striding towards me across the yard, wiping his arms down with handfuls of straw as he approached. I was expecting a short briefing on the problem to hand and to be pointed in the direction of the calving pen, but instead was delighted to hear him announce he had decided to try again while he was waiting and had finally managed to calve the cow in the time it had taken me to arrive; both mother and daughter were doing well, all it had taken for an uneventful calving had been a little more time. So, with smiles all around I was able to hop back into my car and return home in double-quick time to wait for the next call. I never did manage to give blood that day.

It can't be stressed enough that none of these cases is at all unusual to anyone with experience of farm animal practice – they wouldn't so much as raise an eyebrow at a gathering of large animal practitioners. In many cases of dystocia in any species, all that is required for a successful birth is time and patience – sitting down and having a cup of tea will be as much help as homeopathy or indeed, any other form of CAVM.

## A cure for cancer?

One of the most egregious claims made for CAVM and homeopathy in particular is that it can cure cancer. In the UK at least this claim is made apparently with the full blessing of the governing body for veterinary surgeons, the Royal College of Veterinary Medicine (RCVS).[11]

It is emphatically not possible for cancer to be cured by means of alternative remedies no matter what might be read on the internet about those miracle cures 'your doctor (or veterinary surgeon) doesn't want you to know about'. There are plenty of recorded cases where unfortunate (human) cancer victims have died as a result of being fatally misled by unscrupulous purveyors of everything from homeopathy to antineoplastons; laetrile to coffee enemas. Yet despite these salutary tales, practitioners continue to exploit relatives, patients and owners so desperate for a cure they will do and pay virtually anything if they are told there is even a chance of success.

A diagnosis of cancer can be overwhelming, so much so that to some people the situation can seem hopeless from the outset. But often cancer can be controlled, even cured, very effectively and often very simply. Every time a veterinary surgeon surgically removes a mast-cell tumour, melanoma, mammary carcinoma or a spindle-cell tumour at an early enough stage, with wide enough margins they are 'curing cancer'. This is a daily occurrence.

There are, however, cases where cancer has been diagnosed but where surgery that is likely to be curative is not possible either because of a difficult location or because of the extent of the tumour by the time of diagnosis. Yet even then, very occasionally events will defy expectations as tumours either seem to regress completely or do not progress as aggressively or rapidly as would normally be anticipated.

At least one case has made it into the veterinary mainstream scientific literature in a report describing the case of an elderly Labrador retriever who was diagnosed with a large, cystic brain tumour that was causing her to have seizures and to circle compulsively. By the time surgery was due to be performed to reduce the size of the mass a month later, the dog had made a miraculous recovery despite only having had symptomatic treatment to control seizures and reduce inflammation. The surgeon had expected her to be unable to walk but instead she was not only able to walk quite happily but was bright and lucid. Surgery was cancelled and an MRI scan confirmed the lesion had shrunk dramatically. She went on to live happily for more than a year afterwards before being euthanased for an unrelated condition.[12]

Other stories of apparently spontaneous resolution of cancers are by no means uncommon. I received a report recently from a veterinary referral hospital of one dog who was diagnosed on CT scan by one of the foremost imaging experts in the UK – no less than an RCVS-recognised specialist – as having pancreatic cancer that had spread to her lungs. No dog would be expected to live more than a few weeks following this diagnosis yet a year later, when another practice performed radiographic and ultrasound examinations, no trace of the growth was found, and two years after the initial diagnosis she was still symptomless and described as 'going strong'.

Osteosarcoma, a type of bone cancer, is a distressing form of the disease that can cause great pain, weaken bone and lead to fractures. They are highly aggressive tumours that spread rapidly, with a predilection for the lungs. Tragically, cases often involve dogs that are relatively young. It is generally accepted there is no cure, although survival times vary. Even when the amputation of an affected limb is performed it is done chiefly as a pain-relieving measure, not with any expectation of cure, and only increases life expectancy from two months without surgery to little more than six months with it. Intravenous chemotherapy after amputation might give a patient on average just under a year of life following diagnosis.

As a relatively new graduate I diagnosed a dog with osteosarcoma in a hind leg, and this was confirmed by a specialist orthopaedic surgeon. Statistics such as those above were not then as readily available as they are now and I went ahead with amputation of the affected limb thinking it seemed an obvious thing to do in the circumstances. He survived for years, living a normal lifespan before finally dying in his sleep at the age of 15. Believe it or not, his name was Lucky!

In another case, a dog was diagnosed with osteosarcoma of the jaw, which both owner and veterinary surgeon elected to treat conservatively with non-steroidal anti-inflammatory drugs and occasional antibiotics. Despite this limited treatment she lived for an amazing two years following diagnosis and, according to the owner was 'very well in herself' throughout.

Sometimes it is only possible to surgically remove part of a malignant tumour if the area it has grown in is too inaccessible or when radical surgery would give rise to more problems than the original cancer itself. The expectation with this approach is that results would provide only a temporary, palliative, improvement in the level of comfort before the tumour returned.

In one such case a cat developed a swelling of its third (inner) eyelid. Suspecting a malignancy, the veterinary surgeon involved removed as much of the eyelid as possible but it was obvious that obtaining 'clean margins' (i.e. getting back to healthy tissue) was going to be impossible without removing the whole eyeball, something for understandable reasons the owners didn't want done, since even that wouldn't have guaranteed every cancerous cell would have been removed. Laboratory analysis confirmed the worst suspicions of vet and owner, the mass was a malignant carcinoma, almost certain to grow back even more aggressively than before. Yet despite this gloomy prognosis the cancer stayed away. A full examination twelve months after surgery revealed no sign whatsoever of the tumour and the cat went on to live to a ripe old age.

§

Miss Brenda Marshfield, the proud owner of Tigger, an appropriately named, somewhat hyperactive Weimaraner, had noticed a lump on the skin over his elbow. It was one of these cases where the problem only became apparent gradually. For one thing Tigger wasn't the type of chap to be pinned down and closely examined – life was far too much fun for that – but also the lump was exactly where many dogs of a certain age have a harmless area of thick, somewhat hairless skin anyway. So it was a while before it dawned on Brenda something was wrong and that what she had taken to be a patch of dry skin had taken on a life of its own and started to grow into an obvious lump. Fortunately, she wasn't one to hang around where lumps were concerned, and Tigger was presented to her usual veterinary surgeon within a few days.

On first examination it was clear something was wrong, the skin of the upper front leg and over most of the elbow was thickened, raised and quite reactive. Initial suspicions weren't hopeful – the appearance and speed of growth of the lump suggested it could be cancerous. Normally a small biopsy would have been taken for a screening test at this point but Tigger, true to his exuberant (though loving) nature was having none of it! So Brenda and her vet decided the best thing would be to remove as much of the lump as possible under anaesthetic, send that for analysis and then, based on the lab results, come up with a plan about what to do next.

On the day Tigger bounced in for his operation things went well, the anaesthetic was smooth and uncomplicated. A large portion of the lump was removed, but some just had to be left behind. The difficulty of operating near the elbow, where there is very little free skin to close an incision and a real risk of wound breakdown as the region – being over a joint – is highly mobile, made surgical conditions less than ideal.

Eventually though, after a little difficulty the wound was closed and the lump was sent for laboratory analysis. By the time the stitches were due to be removed the report had come back. As suspected, this was indeed cancer; a particularly nasty malignancy called a grade-two mast-cell tumour, which could cause problems all over the body such as vomiting and itching, as well as being in the habit of popping up elsewhere, requiring multiple surgeries and – most worryingly – tending to grow back after removal unless the surgical margins were wide enough.

Unfortunately in this case they weren't, and the laboratory confirmed some cancer cells had been left behind; another nasty trick of the mast-cell tumour is to grow out beyond what appears to be the edge of the lump, thus escaping the surgeon's knife. The mass had only been partly removed. This is a common tumour, and from past experience, her veterinary surgeon had to advise Brenda that without further treatment Tigger was likely to have only a few months to live, before the cancer returned to make life so unbearable that euthanasia would be the kindest option.

After the news was broken, and the tears had dried, another long and difficult discussion ensued. Finally, after all options had been considered, it was decided not to refer Tigger for extensive surgery and reconstruction, followed by a regime of chemotherapy. Even after all that there would be no certainty of a cure and Brenda felt she couldn't put Tigger through any more surgery.

Neither Brenda nor her vet knew precisely what to expect, but what did happen was beyond either of their wildest hopes. Tigger remained comfortable and happy, there was no sign of any regrowth of the cancer. He got his few months, and more – he lived, bouncy and totally contented, for over three more years! This was a completely unheard of result and one that baffled even the cancer specialists. Brenda and her family didn't worry about that though – they just knew they had Tigger for three years more than they ever had the right to expect.

§

A veterinary surgeon from Liverpool contacted me about a case she had seen of a tumour that is commonly found in the mouth, throat and nose, the squamous cell carcinoma. A lovely flat-coat retriever named Rowan had first presented with coughing and retching that hadn't responded to the usual remedies. After a while her breath started to smell so it was decided to examine her throat under anaesthetic, something that is almost impossible to do thoroughly in the conscious patient. Sadly, after induction of the anaesthetic, as soon as Rowan's mouth was opened to insert an endo-tracheal tube down her windpipe, it was obvious there was a large growth on one of her tonsils that was partly obstructing her throat. After a phone call to her owners to get permission to proceed, the growth was carefully grasped with curved forceps and the bulk of it removed. There was no prospect of it being removed completely from such a difficult site.

Shortly afterwards the results were back from the laboratory and they confirmed the mass was a squamous cell carcinoma. It was no surprise to the veterinary surgeon the report finished with the phrase 'dirty margins' – she already knew a significant proportion of the tumour had been left behind.

There was an initial discussion with the owner about the possibility of referral to a specialist oncologist for radiotherapy or chemotherapy but Rowan's owners felt it wasn't fair to put her through such an ordeal. It is well recognised though that non-steroidal anti-inflammatory drugs (NSAIDs), routinely used for pain relief, can also have an inhibitory effect on the growth of some tumours, so they decided it would be worth a try. Besides, Rowan would need to be on them anyway to reduce the discomfort following surgery and, if the tumour grew back, to control the pain. It was simply a case of extending treatment.

On this regime Rowan was fortunate enough to live long enough to experience some of the problems of old age – a touch of deafness, a slight blurring of vision and the occasional skin tag. She was never again, despite all their worries, troubled with that inadequately removed tumour in her throat, it stayed away for good. Eventually she was put to sleep at home for an unrelated urinary problem more than five years after initial diagnosis.

In one of the most astonishing cases involving suspected cancer, a standard poodle was presented to me as the owners had suddenly become aware of a lump in her neck. When I examined it sure enough there was a large, sausage-shaped firm mass, roughly 2×8cm in size under the skin of the neck. It didn't seem to be painful or inflamed and there was no discolouration or anything else to suggest bruising or trauma. The mass was plain to see and feel and the owners were baffled as to how they could have missed it previously. After discussing the possibility of this being cancer in view of its speed of appearance and its situation (neck surgery can be highly challenging, not to say risky) we scheduled investigative surgery with a view to possibly removing it or at least obtaining a sample that would allow a definitive diagnosis.

When the owners presented her for the operation only two days later they were, once again, astonished – the lump had disappeared as quickly as it had first arrived. With some incredulity I checked for myself to find they were quite correct, there was not a trace of the mass, no matter how carefully I probed the area; it had completely gone! Think what would have been said if homeopathy, or acupuncture or some other form of CAVM had been applied during that initial consultation, who could possibly have denied it was that which had caused this potential cancer to vanish without trace?

Finally, two accounts from veterinary forums are reproduced below, with the kind permission of their original authors:

## Case 1:

I have been treating an 11 year old standard Schnauzer with an oral malignant melanoma confirmed by histology. This was removed from just behind the right lower canine with local margins of bone (the owners weren't keen on the more radical option of a hemi-mandibulectomy [*removal of part of the jaw bone*]). At this stage there was no sign of spread to the lymph nodes and a chest X-ray was clear. The mass sadly recurred though after a couple of months and grew three to four centimetres in size. This time the submandibular lymph node was enlarged, a sure sign it had spread. Four months after that however the tumour completely disappeared and the lymph node

41

had reduced to normal size. He lived another two years after that and when I finally put him to sleep there was still no sign of recurrence.

## *Case 2:*

I had a 9 to 10 year-old Dobermann cross with a lump on one toe on a front paw. The biopsy results came back as a malignant melanoma with a high risk of metastatic spread. I amputated the toe and gave a guarded prognosis. Sure enough the dog came back a few weeks later with a massively enlarged pre-scapular lymph node at the top of the leg. A biopsy confirmed this was metastatic melanoma – the cancer had spread up the limb. She went home for what we thought would be a maximum of a few weeks of tender loving care before the inevitable decision for euthanasia.

She didn't reappear until nearly twelve months later, when she presented with nothing more concerning than a mild case of diarrhoea and no sign of any enlarged lymph nodes or other lumps. As far as I know she is still alive and well three years later. She was a lovely dog with lovely owners – the sort of case that usually has a horrible outcome – so it was nice to have a miracle!

§

The veterinary profession has a well-deserved reputation for being a caring one. The vast majority of veterinary surgeons are deeply committed to their clients and patients, human and animal, and have a strong desire to do their best for them, not infrequently at considerable personal cost. Arguably the most important foundation of this positive reputation is trust. A veterinary surgeon could be the most highly qualified, best-informed practitioner of her generation, but if her judgement isn't trusted by those who turn to her for advice, that expertise is worthless.

There is nothing in this chapter that should come as a surprise to any veterinary surgeon, from self-limiting diseases, to those that wax and wane, to the possibility of misdiagnosis. One of the earliest things a veterinary surgeon learns is that it is not good enough to give medical advice based solely on a personal impression of what is wrong or whether or not a condition has improved. Veterinary surgeons know absolutely the need for objective evidence such as laboratory tests, X-rays and ultrasound examinations to temper their subjective views as to how well or otherwise the condition of an animal patient is progressing during treatment. They know that without impartial facts anything goes and it becomes possible to convince oneself of almost anything.

Yet there are still those in the veterinary profession who, despite all this, would have us believe that experience is all that matters when it comes to assessing treatment, no matter how far-fetched or implausible that treatment may be – whether it is the idea that somehow medicines become stronger the more they are diluted, or that the wave of a hand or the prick of a needle can manipulate mysterious, invisible and utterly undetectable energy streams and so treat disease.

Of course, we all have to judge by experience in this life, we'd never do anything if we waited for well-conducted research on every little decision that confronts us, but we also have to be on guard – experience can be a false friend, and if we're not careful it will lead us astray on the important things. If our 'experience' tells us something that doesn't fit with what we know about the real world then we need to be honest enough with ourselves to review exactly what it was we believed we saw happen and, to quote fictional pathologist, TV's Sam Ryan, when confronted with the possibility holy water may have cured cancer, 'question the original diagnosis'.

If the veterinary profession is to continue properly to serve its animal patients and justify the trust placed in it by owners and caregivers, what is required is honesty. A real-world, warts-and-all honesty grounded in open-mindedness and a willingness to believe the evidence, even if it means relinquishing a few dearly held personal convictions, even if it isn't what we would prefer to believe. Most of all, we need to be honest with ourselves.

This is not an easy thing. On the contrary, sometimes it is awkward and unpleasant and it can certainly make one unpopular. It is far more difficult than telling people what they want to hear. Such honesty though, is something to be defended – my patients have no say in the matter of medical dogma, they are 'dumb' animals and they trust us, their human masters, to make the right decisions for them and to act in their best interests. They deserve better than the easy answers and shallow assurances of the alternative practitioner; their trust must be echoed by our humility. We owe it to them to put pride and belief to one side, even if it means occasionally admitting, 'I'm just not sure'. Better honest uncertainty than false conviction.

CHAPTER THREE

# *What Is Science and Why Does it Matter?*

THIS book is not intended as an account of the philosophy of science. But since we've had a look in Chapter One at some of the ways CAM is defined and also that many of the arguments found in the rest of the book are closely tied up with how science works, it might be helpful to make a brief excursion into this somewhat rarefied field and say a few words about what we mean by science, how it underpins science-based medicine and what relevance it has to CAM. While not essential to an understanding of the rest of the book and not directly concerned with veterinary matters this section will go some way to explain the basis of some of the arguments directed at CAM, both human and veterinary.

The subject of the nature of science is important, since much of CAM is predicated on a distorted view of it. A recurring theme from those who practise CAM is that science is at best not up to the task of testing and validating CAM (in fact, as we shall see, nothing in the real world is outside the scope of science) and at worst is systematically seeking to undermine and marginalise it.

Paradoxically, given these reservations, CAM and its supporters also know full well the need for scientific respectability. While seeking to denigrate the science that has, time and again, exposed the flawed nature of the principles behind much of CAM, proponents are nevertheless happy to use science to their own ends when the opportunity arises.

Dr Harris Coulter, considered by some the leading homeopathic historian of the late twentieth century, typifies this one-sided view of science when he claims, 'the only reason for conducting clinical trials of homeopathic substances is to demonstrate the efficacy of the homeopathic system to allopathic observers', such results being 'a matter of indifference' to homeopaths themselves since 'poor results would be ascribed not to the inefficacy of the medicine but to the prescribers' imperfect knowledge of homeopathy, to the hopeless condition of the patient, or ... to the conditions of the trial'.[1]

Thus any research, no matter how flawed, that hints at an effect of CAM is held by its supporters as proof whereas any findings that confirm the ineffectiveness of CAM are ignored.

There is good science and bad science, of course, but the more one discovers of the attitude of those already convinced of the merits of CAM, the more it seems their preferred definition of good science is that which gives favourable results, irrespective of quality.

Science, to Dr Coulter and those like him, is a means for the enthusiast to prove CAM works; a mere propaganda tool. Real science, however, is not like that, it is agenda-free, unconcerned with supporting one position or another. It is a way of testing, not proving, hypotheses, and negative results are just as useful as positive ones. Arguably, science is not even interested in finding answers, only asking questions. When it comes to CAM, some of these questions are difficult for proponents to answer rationally and in the section below about other ways of thinking, the ways CAM attempts to sidestep such scrutiny are examined.

CAM is content to employ science as a blunt instrument to further its own agenda, yet is not itself scientific. In this way CAM is the antithesis of the spirit of free enquiry – not science but *pseudoscience*.

## What science is

Anyone looking for an exact definition of science is in for a bit of a disappointment; there are probably as many different ideas on the subject as there are philosophers of science. There are however, a few themes common to the various definitions that can help cut through some of the misconceptions and give us a feel for what science actually is and, more to the point, what it isn't.

## Science looks at the real world

Science is generally acknowledged to have originated with three philosopher–scientists – Thales, Anaximander and Anaximenes – who inhabited the Ancient Greek city of Miletus in Asia Minor in the sixth century BC at a time when it had maintained a privileged position with successive conquerors, allowing an affluent, tolerant society to develop and flourish that had a love of debate for its own sake.[2,3] The greatest of the three, Thales, is credited with predicting a solar eclipse in the year 585 BC and with laying the foundations of geometry. In the view of Aristotle he was the first natural philosopher.

Free of the oppression of state hierarchy and priestly castes that had so stifled previous civilisations, it was Anaximander who devised the unprecedented concept of the cosmos as an orderly place, running along rational, natural lines, independent of the whims of vengeful gods and capricious spirits. If the philosophers of Miletus believed in gods (Thales held that all things were full of gods, for example), they were well-behaved gods, who knew their place.

This radical idea, that theories for what lay behind earthly events could be devised and then tested, was a profound first step for humanity towards self-awareness and independence of thought that persisted long after the eventual sacking and destruction of Miletus in 494 BC. Science has viewed the world as a natural, rather than a supernatural, place ever since.

The concept – known as *metaphysical naturalism* – of a physical world fully open to inquiry continues to be central to science. In practical terms this means if a claim is made then it should be able to be proved, without the requirement for belief. Nowhere is off-limits for science, metaphysical naturalism maintains the world around us is real, independent of any observer, and can and should be scrutinised for the benefit of all. In this way science isn't a belief, nor is it a philosophy, rather it is a method, which has philosophical underpinnings. The scientific method is simply a way of finding out how things work, how the cosmos functions. If a god said 'let there be light' then the scientist would be the one asking where the switch was. More to the point, a homeopath can't claim the scientific process is fine for determining the effectiveness and safety of a conventional drug while at the same time claiming it is incapable of testing homeopathy. In science you can't have your cake and eat it.

This occasionally leads to the accusation that scientists are spoiling things. A Romantic view of the world holds that certain subjects should be beyond the pale for the scientist; that to subject them to scrutiny would ruin the glamour and the mystery. As John Keats, one of the best known of the Romantic poets wrote, 'Philosophy will clip an Angel's wings ...' meaning if something is studied too closely it will be diminished by that scrutiny. Scientists, say the Romantics, are on a par with the know-it-all sitting in the audience of a stage magician and announcing, 'he had it up his sleeve' at the conclusion of every trick, thereby ruining the illusion.

This point of view is echoed by many CAM practitioners, some of whom seem to take it as a personal affront when it is suggested their methods might be examined scientifically. Lawyer and ethicist Julie Stone makes this point in an article in the *British Medical Journal*. 'Many therapists are not prepared to sacrifice their therapeutic integrity to validate themselves within a scientific paradigm. To do so would, in the view of many therapists, be to create a medicalised version of the therapy, denying its philosophical underpinnings.'[4] It is not unreasonable to speculate whether there is an element of sour grapes here – as was noted above, when science occasionally does manage to produce results that appear to be in CAM's favour, practitioners are invariably happy to accept the results.

But this Romantic view of the world, with its insistence on unexplained mysteries and its dismissal of science as a mechanistic spoilsport, is not only disingenuous, it misses the point in its portrayal of science and scientists themselves. One only has to look to scientists who are popular in the media, who have presented popular science documentaries or written books on the subject, such as Brian Cox, Alice Roberts, Steven Hawking, Carl Sagan to name but a few, to see first-hand their enthusiasm for the subject and the sense of awe and wonder that positively shines from them when expounding on the real world. Geneticist Richard Dawkins, a high-profile campaigner for science, verges on the poetic when he talks of his passion for his subject, '... our DNA is a coded description of the worlds in which our ancestors survived. We are walking archives of the African Pliocene, even of Devonian seas, walking repositories of wisdom out of the old days. You could spend a lifetime reading such messages and die unsated by the wonder of it.'[5]

Far from doing away with mysteries, for every question science answers a dozen or so new ones arise – mysteries grow exponentially. Appreciating what lies behind some of the things we observe around us on a daily basis actually serves to increase, not diminish one's sense of wonder. It is perfectly possible to understand how something works and still be amazed by it. Knowing that different frequencies of light are scattered differently in the atmosphere depending on the distance of the sun from the horizon in no way reduces the appreciation of a magnificent sunset. And what could be more beautiful than the idea rainbows are created when sunlight shines through billions of raindrops, each one acting as a tiny prism in the sky.

Dawkins concludes his lecture with the suggestion to those who believe there must be something beyond our natural universe, that it wouldn't be a bad idea for those people '... to find out what is already here, in the material world, before concluding that you need something more. How much more do you want? Just study what is, and you'll find that it already is far more uplifting than anything you could imagine needing.'

Since the days of the Milesians we have come to realise what early scientists referred to as the Cosmos is an awesome place and investigating it, pushing back the boundaries of the mystery of it, is a large part of what makes us human. It is a matter of genuine regret that for some the real world with all its wonders is just not sufficient and their response to the unfolding majesty of nature is simply to demand 'is this all there is?' As Dawkins says, 'How much more do you want?'

## Science corrects for bias and the will to believe

While carrying out its investigations science has to be able to overcome the natural human tendency to see the results we want to see. This is a particular problem in medicine, where the results of clinical trials can be subtle or subjective. It is difficult to put a precise measurement on some things – just how quickly a cat recovers from cat flu for example, or exactly how itchy a dog's skin is. Which are, unfortunately, exactly the types of conditions CAVM claims most success with. This isn't to say that anyone has been deliberately deceitful or tried to mislead, rather, as British immunologist Peter Medawar points out, it is a sort of a 'kindly conspiracy' where everyone involved with the trial – doctor, patient, pharmaceutical company – all, with the best of intentions, want the trial to 'succeed' (i.e. to give positive results).[6] This determination is so strong we can convince ourselves of almost anything – the parents of autistic children who believe their symptoms are improved even when injected with plain salt water[7] and animal carers who believe there has been an improvement in their dog's arthritis, even when symptoms have actually worsened.[8]

For these reasons science has developed the Placebo Controlled Trial (PCT). To counter the possibility a patient or owner might be expecting a certain outcome following the administration of a drug, an identical-looking, but inactive placebo is given to some of the trial participants instead (the *control* group) and the true outcome determined by measuring the difference between the two groups. This basic model has been improved and refined over the years, arguably reaching its apotheosis in the Double-Blind Placebo Controlled Trial (DBPCT) where neither subject or experimenter is aware who received the placebo and who the drug under test (the *verum* group) until after the statistics have been analysed. Its essential purpose though remains the same; to compensate for our perfectly understandable tendency to see what we want to believe, rather than what is.

Of course, not every drug or medical intervention will need to be tested using the DBPCT. Some clinical outcomes are so obvious that it would be not only completely unnecessary but downright murderous to do so. The use of insulin to treat diabetes, for instance, the use of defibrillators in cardiac arrest, or intravenous fluids for shock are so clearly effective in everyday use that to withhold such treatment from the control group of a clinical trial would endanger the lives of the participants. In a tongue-in-cheek article illustrating this point, the authors of an analysis reviewing the evidence behind the use of parachutes as an aid during 'gravitational challenge' when falling from aircraft in flight concluded, 'We were unable to identify any randomised controlled trials of parachute intervention ... As with many interventions intended to prevent ill health, the effectiveness of parachutes has not been subjected to rigorous evaluation by using randomised controlled trials.'[9] Of course, the beneficial effects of wearing a parachute when falling thousands of feet is so patently obvious no controlled trials are needed, to suggest otherwise would be reckless in the extreme!

It is only necessary to go to the lengths required by the DBPCT when any alleged effects are subtle and consequently open to question. The results of treatment with CAVM, where the vast majority of positive claims are in minor or self-limiting conditions and mainly to be found within the pages of journals written, edited, peer-reviewed and sponsored by those who make a living from CAM, are certainly open to question. CAM treatments are far from being parachutes.

## Science looks at the evidence

The DBPCT isn't the only tool science has when considering the evidence behind a particular claim. In fact, there are a whole variety of ways of testing claims, some of which are more reliable than others. The study of how this is done has become a discipline in its own right with many books and papers being published on the various means of interpreting and scrutinising ... well, books and papers!

The different types of evidence are described as a hierarchy and presented in order of reliability, usually in the form of a pyramid. At the top of the pyramid are the two most robust types of evidence – meta-analyses and systematic reviews, both of which work by taking an overview of other forms of evidence. Meta-analyses look at the results of multiple trials that have used similar methodologies, and combines them to give a broad summary of the effect being studied. By effectively increasing the number of subjects studied, a meta-analysis is thereby able to increase the statistical power of the final result. A systematic review will use more diverse data as 'all relevant, valid studies are extracted and combined using standard, reproducible methods, in order to address a particular hypothesis.'[10]

Next in the hierarchy are randomised controlled trials (RCTs), which were introduced around the middle of the last century.[11] These are individual studies of a particular treatment or intervention using statistical methods to reduce the risk of bias as far as possible. Experimental subjects are selected for the different groups, or arms, of the study by means of a specific and pre-determined process of randomisation to ensure there has been no deliberate (albeit unconscious) selection for certain groups by the experimenters involved (it would be tempting, for instance, if an experimenter felt a participant was particularly unwell, to ensure they were included in the treatment, rather than the placebo group). The highest form of RCT is the DBPCT where, as we have seen, both experimenters and participants are unaware of which group is receiving the treatment under test and which group is receiving placebo. In the most rigorous RCTs even the statisticians are unaware of who is who until after the final analysis to avoid the risk of bias as a consequence of say, unexpected results being presumed to be errors and discarded.

Below RCTs come case-control or cohort studies. Case-control studies are a way at looking back at a group of individuals and studying their history in order to determine if they demonstrate the 'outcome of interest' and in turn discover whether they had been subject to the 'exposure of interest'. Cohort studies look at individuals that have been exposed to the item of interest and then study them from that event onwards. Both serve as useful starting points in the investigation of possible cause and effect but suffer from a lack of reliability, being observational or descriptive, rather than experimental studies,[12] usually having no true control group and being at risk of self-selection (owners with animals who have suffered apparent adverse effects are more likely to come forward than those whose animals have not experienced them).

The next step down in the hierarchy of evidence are case-reports that describe an intervention performed or treatment given in individual cases followed by an account of the outcome. Again, while these are of interest and occasionally serve as a starting point for more rigorous studies they carry little or no evidential weight. They are hardly more reliable than the next layer down in the pyramid, expert opinion, which in turn only just scrapes past simple anecdotes when it comes to reliability as evidence.

It is important to understand that when it is said that anecdotes and opinion are unreliable forms of evidence it does not mean anyone is doubting the word of those who are recounting their story. But while accepting that, yes, after giving treatment X, condition Y improved dramatically, what anecdotes cannot tell us is whether it was treatment X that *caused* the improvement in condition Y. This is a subtle but crucial distinction.

Another important consideration with all of the above is that of quality. The hierarchy of evidence depends on rigorous study design, the robust application and supervision of trial conditions and suitably large subject numbers to ensure a reliable result. It is all very well claiming one arm of a trial was given a placebo, but if members of the various groups aren't questioned afterwards and asked whether they thought they had received the placebo or the verum treatment, we can't be sure the placebo was an effective 'blank'. Also, even if a trial has been absolutely 100 per cent rigorous, blinded correctly, randomised properly and so on but only has three participants then we can hardly be expected to be able to generalise usefully from the results. And it should be obvious if a meta-analysis is carried out using RCTs of dubious quality then the results of that meta-analysis will also be similarly dubious – rubbish in, rubbish out, as the expression goes.

Space prohibits a full discussion of the details that underlie the art of considering evidence, study design and interpretation, as well as the other factors that have a major part to play such as statistical power, statistical significance and the peer review process. The reader is referred to the references in this section and also to Trisha Greenhalgh's definitive book on the subject, *How to Read a Paper: the Basics of Evidence-Based Medicine* for more information on this crucial subject.

## Science asks questions

Ever since its earliest beginnings, the major preoccupation of science has been to ask questions. This may come as a surprise to many of its critics, to whom the cliché 'science doesn't know everything' is a favourite trope, 'If science knows all the answers, who needs scientists?' as one homeopathic veterinary surgeon puts it.[13]

But such critics are, once again, missing the point (and, of course, it suits their position to do so). To quote comedian Dara Ó Briain, 'Science KNOWS it doesn't know everything, otherwise it would stop!' Physicist and philosopher of science, Mario Bunge expresses this paradoxical view most adroitly when he writes, '... the actual attainment of truth [is] less peculiar to science than the ability and willingness to detect error and correct it.'[14] Science isn't so much about knowing answers, as asking 'Why?' and in that sense, science will never stop.

And this delight in the asking of questions leads directly to the next defining aspect of science ...

## Science changes

Science and science-based medicine is in a state of perpetual change and enrichment, destruction and renewal. Every piece of research or new discovery will, in some small way, alter and improve the way we think about the world. This may be an imperceptible change such as with a single study on a subject already widely investigated, or it may be something ground-breaking such as the understanding of the structure of DNA by Watson and Crick in the 1950s, the discovery of insulin in 1921 or the finding, in 1982, that the majority of stomach ulcers in humans are actually caused by a simple bacteria, *Helicobacter pylori*.

CAM, by contrast, is fixed and unchanging, although perversely, CAM practitioners take pride in this. Dr Coulter, for instance, claims in the introduction to his book *Homeopathic Science and Modern Medicine*, 'that [homeopathy] should have remained unchanging for 180 years is seen ... as further evidence of its scientific nature, since a true science is cumulative'. This narrow, self-serving view of science completely omits the corollary that while science is indeed cumulative, building as it does on previous knowledge, it is also required to discard previous work or beliefs when they are found wanting in favour of newer, more robust findings. This can be a brutal process, particularly for individual scientists who may have invested much of their lives studying something now seen as obsolete, but it is absolutely essential if progress is to be made in the way we understand our world.

CAM may be 'cumulative' as Coulter states, but only in as much as new speculations or techniques are 'bolted on' to what has gone before – a new homeopathic remedy or acupuncture point is invented, electro-acupuncture or acupressure is used alongside traditional needling. With CAM though, there is never a serious scrutiny of the basic underlying principles: What is the *life-force*, what is *Qi*, can acupuncture meridians or chiropractic subluxations be demonstrated convincingly? None of these questions have ever been addressed to the satisfaction of the wider scientific community (rather than simply the chosen few). And nothing is ever discarded. There has not been one single example of a CAM technique that has been tested by the CAM community itself and been found wanting.

CAM has only every truly changed when forced to do so by outside pressures, mainly legislative, in situations where therapies have been discovered to be frankly dangerous or inhumane as with *laetrile*, a bogus cancer treatment containing cyanide and known to cause life-threatening toxicity that nevertheless had thousands of advocates for its unrestricted use,[15] or mega-doses of vitamins (some of which were discovered to cause cancer), never from the sheer challenge of investigating what exactly it is CAM practitioners do, how their various practices work and whether they can be improved upon. For this reason, this lack of a tradition of rational inquiry and honest self-analysis, CAM will always remain backward-looking and unchanging, it will only ever be cumulative in the sense that dust is cumulative as it collects on a neglected shelf. There will never be a homeopathic Watson and Crick; CAM will never have its *insulin moment*.

## Science thrives on innovation and new ideas

A common criticism of science by supporters of CAM is that science is unwilling or unable to embrace the ideas behind CAM. It suits the agenda of the pro-CAM lobby to portray science as a monolithic entity that acts as a unified whole to suppress dissent and silence doubters. In fact, nothing could be further from the truth. While science has at its core a number of axioms common to the way it functions, it is also run and organised by human beings. And, like any other collection of mere mortals, these people have ambition, are competitive and often strongly driven for a variety of reasons from improved funding to pure ego, to excel in their field, while beating their colleagues (or competitors) to the main prize. To be frank, scientists can be ruthlessly ambitious. To expect a group of disparate personalities like that – competing at a global level for the best research grants and the most prestigious prizes – to collaborate to suppress the existence of a universal life force, or a system of channels that transport a novel substance, *Qi*, around the body, or the mechanism by which a medicine can become stronger with increasing dilution, or even a 'cure for cancer', is patently absurd. Any true scientist who even suspected the existence of such things would be on a path to fame and fortune and would never have to worry about securing funding ever again.

## Science is simple

Well, anyone who has ever studied high school science knows science isn't simple – it can be pretty difficult in fact. While it is unquestionably true the processes and techniques that underpin science can appear complex, at its core science strives for simplicity. Its ultimate aim is to come up with the most economical, parsimonious explanation that fits the observed facts. This is highlighted in an essay by authors Scott Sehon and Donald Stanley on what they describe as the 'principle of simplicity'. In a measured and well-reasoned discussion of homeopathy they describe the principle thus: 'Given two theories, it is unreasonable to believe the one that leaves significantly more unexplained mysteries.' They further point out, far from being an obscure philosophical point, this principle is an integral part of our daily lives and prevents us from believing many clearly implausible things. For example, consider the possibility the world may have been created, in its entirety, just five minutes ago, with everything, from memories to fossils to the approaching light from stars billions of light years away positioned exactly as they are now. There is no logical contradiction to this view, in theory it could be true, but it leaves so many of what the authors describe as 'brute mysteries' – unanswerable questions about the nature of the five-minute universe – that in every practical sense the notion is ridiculous.[16]

By the same token, if a patient recovers after being given a homeopathic remedy it could, in theory, be that the patient was cured by the homeopathy. But that would leave us with the 'brute mysteries' of how homeopathy's unlikely ingredients could, at dilutions so enormous even homeopaths admit there is none of the base remedy remaining, somehow transfer an unidentified energy force to the body of a patient in such a way the (again unidentified) *life-force* of the patient is corrected and the body manages to heal itself (see Chapter Eleven for more detail). We have no evidence for any of these phenomena existing, still less how they are able to effect a cure. Another possibility is the patient has simply got better despite, not because of, the remedy. There is no difficulty with this explanation; we saw in the previous chapter how animals will from time to time, recover from a variety of sometimes quite serious conditions with minimal assistance, we know much about how the immune system works, how bones and soft tissues heal, we know that very many diseases are self-limiting. This latter explanation fulfils all the requirements of the principle of simplicity, it is more plausible and more economical, using as it does concepts already widely understood, than the first. The convoluted explanations of the homeopath are not needed to explain a perfectly natural event.

## What science is not – Changing attitudes to science

Although science, as we have seen, is a method for investigating and solving problems, its institutions are run and its discoveries put to use by fallible human beings. And the very human agendas behind some of these uses has led to an increasing disconnect, in certain quarters, from science and technology in the latter half of the last century.

During those years the science that had brought such profound social and medical benefits – the control of cholera and polio, the eradication of smallpox, the discovery of antiseptics and anaesthetics to name but a few – was becoming rather taken for granted. Some were starting to look more at the science that had brought us the atomic bomb, DDT, a series of devastating global conflicts, thalidomide and all the hardware and paranoia of the Cold War. And this was engendering a suspicion of 'the establishment' in general, increasingly perceived as authoritarian, faceless and materialistic, all at the expense of the 'self' and the 'spiritual dimension'.

This change in attitude within sections of Western society (mainly, it has to be said, among groups who had already reaped the benefits science had to provide) had its roots in various social movements and philosophies of the time. A loose melange of post-modernism, relativism, New Age spirituality and various counter-cultural movements, alongside a growing interest in altered states of consciousness, different cultures and in Eastern religions, all proved irresistibly attractive to a generation disillusioned by modernity. Old certainties and casual assumptions about the superiority of 'Western' culture and values were being questioned and found wanting. Unfortunately though, it didn't stop there.

## Science is not simply 'another way of knowing'

Relativism, a cornerstone of this new school of thought, regards all views, all opinions and all theories as to how the world works as equally valid and worthy of consideration. It began as a well-intentioned reaction against Western condescension and judgemental attitudes towards other cultures and, by challenging the *status quo,* arguably brought improvements – a greater tolerance of the diversity of customs and lifestyles, growing sexual equality, exciting developments in the arts and arguably, an erosion of elitism and privilege. But it is possible to have too much of a good thing. The desire of these cultural relativists to remove absolute values from a set of customs, languages or costume is one thing; taking other beliefs as to the way the world works seriously in literal and mechanistic terms is a step too far.

As it took hold, relativism became fashionable among academics (particularly non-scientists) and started to catch on in the popular imagination. Its sphere of influence expanded until it wasn't just prejudice and intolerance that were in the firing line, now everything was up for grabs – art, language and literature and eventually the fundamentals of science too, all fell under the critical gaze of philosophers who doubted the very existence of reality.

Relativism began to preach that science was no more than a Western cultural artefact, a contrivance with no more right to be taken seriously than the beliefs held by any other culture. Facts were dismissed as cosy convention, mere self-affirming platitudes. The concept of truth itself was challenged by *cognitive relativism.* As philosopher Paul Feyerabend famously declared, 'The only absolute truth is that there are no absolute truths.'

When applied to science-based medicine, such a stance allows proponents of alternative medicine and the philosophies and beliefs behind it to transform the failings and criticisms of CAM from simple questions of knowing and understanding (epistemology) into political ones. This philosophical contrivance reduces scientific investigation to mere empire building and facts to propaganda, with mainstream medicine accused of displaying '... an imperialist attitude towards healing practices from other cultures.'[17]

Thus, in the view of the relativists, the medical profession, by examining the claims of alternative medicine, isn't attempting to improve the totality of health care, or protect and inform patients, rather it is selfishly contriving to '[open] up new territory for the profession to colonise ...' in order that orthodox medicine '. . . maintained and/or increased its income, status and power.'[18] To its detractors, science-based medicine could now be considered simply as a *different way of knowing* from CAM, with no greater validity or right to be described as 'the truth'.

There is a flaw, however. In a twist of perspective worthy of the tale of the *Emperor's New Clothes*, when taken to its logical conclusion, relativism (and its co-conspirators, post-modernism and cultural constructivism) is ultimately self-defeating – if everything is true, then nothing is.

This inescapable paradox is evident even in its best known soundbite: 'The only absolute truth is that there are no absolute truths.' How can a statement denying absolute truth be an absolute truth?

If relativism's central concept tells us all truths are subjective, not objective or absolute, then it follows this central concept too is merely subjective and no more valid than any other, including the concept that there IS actually such a thing as absolute truth. To deny the idea of absolute truth the relativist has to deny the principles of relativism itself. It is not possible to hold as true the philosophical viewpoint that nothing is true by virtue of an argument that tells us how true it is that nothing is true!

And, whether or not we realise, or are prepared to admit it, we all know this to be the case. Ophelia Benson and Jeremy Stangroom, in their rapier-like deconstruction of relativism in its various forms, point out that while there are some 'fuzzy truths' concerned with beliefs and preferences, there are many other truths we consciously or unconsciously know to be absolute. They are 'true all the way down to the bottom', and we conduct our daily lives knowing them to be true.[19]

If we let a ball go it will fall, if we walk into a wall or burn our hand it will hurt, if we fall into a river we will get wet, a tree falling in a forest will make a noise whether anyone is there to hear it or not. And these truths hold wherever we are – whether it is in modern day New York City, or Bronze Age Delphi conversing with the Oracle – and regardless of which set of cultural beliefs we happen to hold. These are the 'truths' we live our lives by, we build bridges and fly aeroplanes using these fundamental concepts and if a wily guru tried to persuade us that, in his culture, humans have the ability to fly unaided we would be very unwise to jump off a high building on his advice (at least without insisting on a demonstration from him first). When it comes to the real world around us, we live and interact with it as if it is 'real', not an arbitrary social or philosophical construct, no matter how appealing it may be to our own particular *way of knowing* to believe otherwise.

The absurdity of the idea that individuals, cultures and belief systems can each have their own, individual version of truth, as relativism and many proponents of CAM would have us believe, is laid bare in one comic portrayal of what life might be like if alternative engineering was considered as real as alternative medicine is considered by some. In this account, the arguments and evasions of the postmodern thinker are neatly parodied as a fictional alternative engineer is described who claims to be able to build bridges 'unfettered by the annoying constraints of "reality" ...' and 'supported only by the ancient art of *Feng Shui*.'[20]

Although there is clearly much more to the concepts of truth and relativism than space allows here, the point is if we have no need for the irrational concepts of alternative engineering and wouldn't trust our persuasive guru when he told us to jump off that tall building, why then should we have any need for alternative medicine or trust its purveyors when they tell us they can heal us or our pets by manipulating invisible and undetectable energies supposedly suffusing our bodies, running in special channels, emerging from our skin surfaces or entering through equally insubstantial psychic or spiritual portals?

§

Like it or not, science is the only way we have of truly understanding the material world around us, its method frees us to think, to ask questions and to find out how things work for ourselves without risk of censure.

The view of much of CAM, that there are aspects of reality not amenable to scientific enquiry or undetectable by conventional means, is false and self-serving and in direct opposition to this view. It isn't good enough for those practitioners who want us to part with our hard-earned funds to claim CAM works because someone believes in it, or fails to perform in a test because someone failed to show sufficient faith, or due to 'negative energies', as happens so often when rational investigation has failed to confirm irrational preconceptions.

There is nothing about any of the claims of CAM that cannot be tested by science, despite proponents' efforts to cloud their arguments with romance and mystery, spirituality and belief. If homeopathy says it can cure cancer, if acupuncture claims to cure a bad back, if chiropractors say they can cure asthma, then all these are real claims and all can be tested, and it is the duty of all of us, in the interests of openness and honesty to demand they are.

Instead though, when the going gets tough, CAM prefers to simply opt out of the scientific process altogether. Regarding the use of Randomised Controlled Trials (RCTs) in homeopathic research, Dr Peter Fisher, one of the UK's most pre-eminent homeopaths, has this to say: 'RCTs are unlikely to capture the possible benefits of homeopathy'.[21] This remark, astonishing in one aspiring to scientific credibility, means in other words that while science is good enough for everything and everyone else, it is simply not required when it comes to telling CAM enthusiasts what they already know to be true.

CAM is a way of avoiding the need to think in favour of uncritical acceptance of what we are told. Every time we choose to believe a condition has improved because of an alteration in the flow of *Qi* without seriously asking what *Qi* actually is, or because of a restoring of *balance* without asking what exactly it is that is being balanced (in the real world that is, rather than according to simplistic explanations given by those with a vested interest), we are selling ourselves short and denying that which makes us human – our spirit of curiosity. We are, once again, back in that chaotic ancient world, at the whim of priestly castes, vengeful gods and capricious spirits.

§

## Why CAM and CAVM are not science – an illustration

One thing that distinguishes science from CAVM is the attitude of both authors and readers to written works on the subject. Part of the sheer joy in science is that it doesn't confirm our preconceptions, it challenges them. When reading about a subject, some of the most enlightening moments come as we encounter a remark that seems counter-intuitive or to dispute something we had previously believed true.

At which point, if the book or paper is written properly, we turn to the reference that should be there to give us more detail about where this remark originated. That way, we can judge for ourselves by looking at the evidence just how much weight we can place on it. We read the references, not to prove ourselves correct (although it's nice when occasionally that happens) but *to try to prove ourselves wrong*. This is how we develop new understanding and there is great satisfaction to be gained this way. This is what is meant by being a 'sceptic', the term simply refers to someone who questions the evidence and will admit they might be wrong and change their outlook if warranted.

Many books on the subject of CAM contain few if any references. Those that are to be found frequently refer to similar works by authors who have made the same, unsubstantiated claims or to sources handicapped by vested interest (mainly specialist journals whose continued existence depends on publishing results that put their speciality in a favourable light). This way all manner of unverifiable and fantastical claims are transcribed from text to text in an ever increasing spiral of circular reasoning and self-reference until they become – in the minds of those who wish to believe – incontrovertible truth, not by virtue of proper research but simply as a result of repetition.

This is one reason why many works on CAM, when written by enthusiasts, are actually rather boring to read. At the point where we are challenged by a remark that seems to contradict our everyday perceptions we are left high and dry. There is nowhere to go, references are either non-existent or inadequate and lacking in objectivity. We are simply expected to take the authors' word for it.

By way of example, consider the following remark, in this case from a radionics textbook, but typical of a great number of claims to be found in almost any CAM text one cares to mention:

> *'... the universe is an interconnected whole which operates in harmony. For instance, oysters, when taken inland, still change their feeding times to fit the changing times of the high tide ... It is this interconnection which makes radionic therapy possible.'*[22]

From the tone of the section that contains the excerpt, the authors apparently intend this remark to be almost a throwaway one, a nod and a wink for people already convinced of the benefits of radionics before moving on to the next section. But to those readers with scientific inclinations who take a more active interest in what they are reading, this sort of remark, with its extremely bold claim, is infuriating to the extreme.

The assertion being made (as explained in a nearby section of the text) is that radionics practitioners actually have Extra Sensory Perception (ESP), they can supposedly maintain psychic links with people and animals anywhere on the planet enabling them to accurately detect the supposed *electrodynamic energies* emitted by matter of all kind, and are thus privy to states of health and able to initiate cures in their patients. This is, literally, an incredible claim. If true, the implications for mankind would be enormous and for science it would mean there was a type of energy in existence that has been completely overlooked. Yet we are being asked to believe all this, in large part, because of the alleged behaviour of some oysters.

I say some oysters because, since there is no reference to back up the claim, we know nothing about how many oysters were involved in this apocryphal experiment or any other details about how it was done. We can speculate, however; and it turns out to be far from straightforward.

Adult oysters become permanently anchored to the sea bottom at a very early age and if torn from their rocky settings their health and levels of activity deteriorate rapidly. The only way an oyster could be removed from its natural home and survive long enough to perform a reliable study would be if it were part of a commercial enterprise and had been reared in bags or on racks that could then be moved en bloc.

So possibly a bag or two of oysters has been taken and moved inland. But oysters are sea creatures, they won't survive in fresh, inland waters. So they must have been moved to a marine aquarium of some description that would provide them with the levels of salinity and nutrients required to sustain them. On the subject of nutrients we can only guess how these were supplied – the most obvious solution would be to set up an artificial approximation of the natural ebb and flow of the tides, presenting algae and other morsels as a water-borne stream, moving over whatever passes for jaws in an oyster. If this technique were used it would affect the results in no small measure – would the subjects adapt to the artificial tides or obstinately stick to the intervals at their original location?

This initial, throwaway remark is turning into quite a complicated undertaking, albeit an interesting one. Frustration grows at not being able to read the original text from those who carried out the experiment.

So now we have an imaginary experimenter sitting beside a marine aquarium, clipboard and stopwatch in one hand, pen in the other, measuring and recording the times and duration each oyster is feeding. But a few oysters wouldn't give results accurate enough to satisfy us they weren't aberrations restricted to one or two individuals. Would one person be able to do this alone, in a large enough population of oysters and for the number of days needed to obtain useful results?

We have now to imagine a number of researchers, each assigned a manageable group of perhaps a few dozen oysters each to monitor, working on a shift system to ensure proper levels of concentration. Some way of ensuring consistency between observers now becomes essential – a standard set of parameters for what constitutes a feeding oyster as distinct from a non-feeding one. The complications are growing, and we don't even know if it is possible to maintain these unfortunate bivalves in such artificial conditions, no matter how carefully controlled.

Even if we overcome all these limitations and discover that a large enough group of oysters over a long enough period of time does indeed remain synchronised to the tide times at their point of origin, what would that mean? Our radionic enthusiasts have jumped to what seems to be the most unlikely of all possible explanations – an alleged telepathic connection with an inanimate object (the sea), using a form of energy unknown to science, whose only purpose in nature seems to be to allow human radionics practitioners to ply their trade since presumably there is no need for oysters to exploit this ability under normal circumstances when actually sitting in the tidal flow and not brought inland by enterprising psychics determined to prove a point.

Could there be other, less fanciful, mechanisms, already recognised, which might account for this supposed behaviour? We know animals possess an awesome array of senses that extend far beyond the traditional human five. Some creatures are able to detect gravity and motion, migratory birds navigate using the earth's electromagnetic field as a guide, certain species of fish hunt using their ability to detect the electrical activity generated by other living animals and dolphins and bats use sound in the way other species use vision. Could it be, instead of telepathy, our oysters are demonstrating an ability to detect something that would be apparent to them both in their inland location as well as their original one; the gravitational pull of the moon perhaps, which is responsible for the tides, rather than the tides themselves. Did our researchers take any steps to exclude this variable in their investigation (and how could this be done?) What about other things that might have an effect, were the rhythms of day and night considered, for example, or the phases of the moon?

And so it goes on. Once we start to consider the implications underlying this original, seemingly casual remark, the whole proposition becomes less and less plausible. This is not nit-picking, such considerations are exactly what will go through the mind of anyone used to a rational consideration of claims when reading this sort of thing. Neither is it a judgement on the authors' integrity, presumably they believe the tale of the oysters and see it as a genuine example of the 'interconnectedness' that they believe allows radionics to work. But there is always more than one way of looking at things, particularly if one doesn't have an agenda.

The experiment, if it was ever performed as such, is fraught with potential confounding factors and even then, if the results are as suggested, we have no end of already established possibilities to exclude before we need entertain the idea of ESP and 'electrodynamic energies'. As it stands, the statement in question tells us nothing whatsoever about the behaviour of oysters or the effectiveness or otherwise of radionics, we are simply being expected to believe what we are told, without asking awkward questions. From the tone of similar debates in the past, it is certain this is exactly how anyone making points outlined above would be regarded – awkward. But the entire scientific process is awkward and difficult, it is hard to master, often flying in the face of easy consensus, it requires dedication and study and a considerable amount of humility as we get used to the idea that our most strongly held beliefs and notions, that which we understood to be true, might be wrong. And then not only to acknowledge that, but to take great satisfaction from it as we realise we are actively learning, not passively taking someone's word for it.

CHAPTER FOUR

# *When Thinking Goes Wrong (Including Logical Fallacies, Cognitive Bias and False Arguments in CAVM)*

WHEN debating any subject, it is common for one or both sides to use logical fallacies in their arguments. A logical fallacy is an error in reasoning that renders an argument invalid. However, they are often delivered with such fervent belief that they sound as if they are fact. Although logical fallacies are rare in the scientific literature, they are common in writing aimed at more general consumption. They are particularly common wherever anyone has a belief, the validity of which they wish to persuade others. They are therefore commonly found in the blog posts and message board discussions dealing with subjects such as politics, conspiracy theories, and, of course, complementary and alternative medicine.

You may or may not have heard of logical fallacies, I didn't discover them myself until I became involved in debates about alternative medicine, and it was pointed out to me how common they were. Once you know about them, you start seeing them everywhere. The politician who dodges a question about his party's record on health care by pointing to the opposition's poor record when they were in power is indulging in a tu quoque fallacy. The climate change denier who refuses to believe the claims of a particular scientist because he has a history of sexist remarks is performing an ad hominem attack. The anti-vaccination campaigner who points out their child developed a medical condition after a vaccination is guilty of a post hoc error.

Logical fallacies have been understood since Aristotle listed thirteen examples in his *Sophistical Refutations*, and many more have been described since. Whole books have been written about the subject, with Bennett[1] describing

64

more than 300. A full discussion is beyond the scope of this chapter. However, I have listed some of the more common logical fallacies that are encountered in discussions regarding complementary and alternative medicine, in the worlds of advertising, politics or anywhere two people disagree.

## *Ad hominem*

This is one of the most depressing logical fallacies, which involves attacking the person making the argument, rather than the argument itself. Many people will be familiar with how quickly arguments on the internet degenerate into name-calling and abuse, and if you find yourself involved in this sort of debate, console yourself that the abusive trolls are committing the ad hominem logical fallacy. There are several subcategories of the ad hominem attack. The most straightforward is the abusive ad hominem. This takes the form: Person 1 claims X. Person 1 is an idiot, so X is untrue. As a hypothetical example: 'You say homeopathy is implausible, but you are fat. If you can't look after your body, why should we believe what you say about anything?'

Another is the circumstantial ad hominem attack, where it is suggested that a bias on the part of the person making the argument means the argument must be untrue. This takes the form, Person 1 claims X. Person 1 has a vested interest in X being true. Therefore X must be untrue. Clearly bias is a risk when making an argument, and the scientific process takes great pains to avoid bias. However, there is a known risk of publication bias, in which negative results tend not to be published, or journals promoting certain disciplines or treatments have a tendency to publish positive results. What makes this argument a fallacy though, is the supposition that the argument must necessarily be untrue because of the possible bias of the person making the argument. A hypothetical example from veterinary medicine would be to suggest that any claims made by a drug or vaccine company must be untrue because of their risk of bias.

Thirdly there is the guilty by association ad hominem, whereby an association by the person making an argument with another person or group is used to condemn their argument. The form is as follows: Person 1 states X is true. Person 2 also states X is true. Person 2 is unreliable, therefore Person 1 must be unreliable too. A hypothetical example from veterinary medicine would be to suggest that if a veterinary surgeon is a member of an anti-hunting group, and some of their number are hunt saboteurs who have harmed horses in their bid to stop fox hunting, then the arguments of that vet on hunting are invalid.

Finally there is the tu quoque ad hominem, often taken as a separate category of fallacy known simply as the tu quoque, or 'you too'. In this fallacy, it is claimed that the argument is false, because the one making the argument has committed the same offence they are arguing against. This takes the form that Person 1 claims X, but doesn't behave consistently with X, and so X cannot be true. A hypothetical example from veterinary medicine, and one that is frequently raised by proponents of complementary and alternative veterinary medicine, is that since not all conventional veterinary medicine is based on robust evidence, it is not necessary for CAVM to be based on evidence either. While this may seem fair on the face of things, it simply means that both sides should try harder. But where both possible treatments (conventional versus alternative) lack evidence, then other ways of considering possible efficacy, such as biological plausibility, can be taken into account. A comparison between the evidence for conventional and alternative veterinary medicine is discussed in more detail in the other chapters in Part One.

## Ambiguity fallacy

In this fallacy, a phrase with more than one meaning is employed, which can lead to an erroneous conclusion. One example is the old joke, 'Dog for sale, eats anything, fond of children.'

## Anonymous authority

Anonymous or non-existent authorities are often cited in arguments. This is often structured in the form, 'They say that …' or 'Studies show that …' and who 'they' are, or which study, is often unspecified.

## Appeal to faith

This fallacy is often invoked when a reasoned argument clearly disproves a position. This is most commonly used in veterinary medicine with arguments such as, 'Science doesn't have all the answers,' or, 'I don't need proof it works, I just know it.'

## Appeal to nature

Many think of alternative medicine as being more 'natural' than conventional medicine. How needles stuck into the skin (as in acupuncture), or poisons diluted tens or hundreds of times, while being shaken or banged against a book (as in homeopathy), are natural, is not usually explained. Regardless of this, the appeal to nature is a fallacy that takes the form that if X is natural it must be good, and Y is unnatural it must be bad. Although some 'natural' things may indeed be superior to 'unnatural' things, the mere fact of their naturalness or unnaturalness has no bearing on their quality.

There are numerous examples of things derived from nature that are bad for us, such as tobacco, ebola and lions. There are also things that are man-made that are beneficial to us, including antibiotics, vaccines, cars and the internet. The argument is often made with regard to pets, for example, asserting that a particular diet is superior because it is natural. Appeals to nature are also sometimes appeals to tradition as well, with the argument that people and pets were healthier before modern 'poisons' such as vaccines, drugs and regular nutrition. This clearly flies in the face of the facts, since life expectancy was lower in the past, childhood mortality was higher, and many diseases that were rife are now rare.

## Appeal to tradition

This is a commonly used fallacy in complementary and alternative medicine, and involves the argument that as this was how things were done in the past, this is how they should continue to be done. It is a seductive argument, since we always look into the past through rose-tinted spectacles. Even the Romans of the Late Republic and Empire looked back to earlier times (fallaciously) as days of moral rectitude and nobility. Common veterinary examples include the Chinese/Germans/Mayans have been using acupuncture/homeopathy/trephination for centuries, so if it has been used for all that time it must work. This clearly ignores all the other treatments that were used for centuries that are no longer recommended, such as the use of mercury as a cure for syphilis, which was popular from the Renaissance until the early twentieth century.

## Argument ad populum

Also known as the bandwagon argument, this fallacy is commonly encountered, though possibly less so in CAVM, since, almost by definition, CAVM is a minority belief, and so the 'They laughed at Einstein fallacy', described below, is often employed. Simply put, this argument relies on a majority, or at least a large number, of people believing or doing something. Sometimes a separate population is invoked, to imply a large number of other people are doing something better. For example, a recent internet meme originating from the US regarding genetically modified organisms stated, 'A million Europeans can't be wrong.' I'm not sure what it is they thought Europeans were doing better than them regarding GMOs, but the argument was neatly countered with a photograph of the Nuremberg rally.

Numerous other examples can be given to refute anyone who uses the argument, 'X number of people can't be wrong,' but a simple one is to respond, 'A million lemmings can't be wrong.' Note the fallacy does not imply that something must be wrong because a lot of people believe something, and indeed the more people believe something, the higher probability it is right. However, a large number of people believing a thing does not prove that thing to be correct.

## Argument by emotive language

In the absence of a strong rational argument, emotive language is often substituted. This device is commonly employed in arguments about veterinary medicine, often because the person making the argument truly believes that they are right, and that if their argument is accepted, it will reduce animal suffering. This can often stray into ad hominem attacks, changing from, 'If this isn't done, animals will suffer,' to, 'If you don't do this, animals will suffer.' However, emotive language alone does not prove an argument, though it can help clarify the import of an argument.

## Argument from authority

An authority figure can give a lot of credibility to an argument. An argument of this type should lead one to question the credentials of the authority. When I was a young vet, about a year out of college, I discussed diet with a disbelieving client. She did not accept my advice because her puppy's breeder had told her differently, and as she said, 'She has been a breeder for twenty years, and you have only been a vet for a year.' It was hard to argue against on the spur of the moment, but on reflection and with the aid of the back of an envelope, I calculated that I probably treated more dogs in a week than the breeder had bred in twenty years. There are many names quoted as authority figures in CAVM. Some will have performed genuine research in a subject, some will have merely practised the subject for some years. There are some who are not even vets or researchers, but have merely selectively read some articles and web pages, and hold themselves up as authorities. Even when the authority has impeccable credentials, such as an internationally recognised career in research, they are not necessarily correct simply because of their position, and one only has to follow the debates surrounding American College of Veterinary Medicine consensus statements to realise that since authorities often disagree with each other, they can't all be right. The position of expert opinion in the hierarchy of evidence-based medicine is discussed further in Chapter Three.

## Argument from ignorance

This fallacy is based on the argument that since something has not been proven to be wrong, it must be right. The argument in question may or may not be provable. In the case of a particular CAVM modality, it may be that sufficient research has not yet been done, but sometimes it may be something that is unprovable, and CAVM practitioners will often claim that their disciplines are not provable by scientific methods. As a hypothetical example, no one has proved that coffee enemas do not cure kennel cough, so why not try it?

## Begging the question

This is an argument in which the conclusion is derived from the premises. It is a form of circular reasoning. Note the phrase begging the question is commonly used to mean prompting one to ask the question, but this is not what it means in the context of logical fallacies. An example would be, 'We know homeopathy works, because it says so in Hahnemann's Organon.' Note that examples of begging the question often involve the Bible (we know the Bible is true because the Bible says so), but the Organon is an appropriate example since it is the homeopath's Bible.

## Biased sample fallacy

Sampling bias is a real problem in medical scientific studies, and there are various ways of designing trials to attempt to overcome this. Analysis of the treated group and the control group in a placebo-controlled trial to assess for biases in important factors such as breed, age and sex can help give confidence that the samples are not biased. The fallacy involves drawing a conclusion from a sample of a population that is not representative of the whole population. It is seldom possible to perform a study that involves the entire population of interest. Even in the 2015 UK general election, only 66 per cent of eligible voters actually voted. (Interestingly the polls before the elections, which typically involved asking 1,000 to 3,000 people how they would vote, got the results so completely wrong that the British Polling Council set up an independent inquiry into what happened. It will be interesting to know if there was a systematic error common to all the polling companies in their methods of data collection, but the answer is likely to be that some error in methodology caused a biased sample to be polled).

A hypothetical example from veterinary medicine would involve quoting as evidence a randomised, placebo-controlled trial in which there was a significant difference in age between the treated and non-treated groups, which could clearly impact on survival time.

## Cherry picking

In this fallacy, only evidence that supports a person's claim is presented in an argument, while evidence against the argument is excluded. This is a very common tactic in complementary and alternative medicine, in which one study is quoted providing support for a therapy, while the studies against it are ignored.

## Circular reasoning

In this fallacy, the conclusion is supported by the premises, but the premises in turn are supported by the conclusion. The classic example is, 'We know the Bible is the word of God, because it says so in the Bible.'

## Confusion of correlation and causation and the post hoc fallacy

'I used to confuse correlation and causation, but then I took a statistics class, and now I understand.'

'So the class helped?'

'Well, maybe.'

If you get that joke you probably don't need to read further about these two fallacies. Confusion of correlation and causation is also known as the cum hoc ergo propter hoc (with this, therefore because of this) fallacy, whereas post hoc is an abbreviation of post hoc ergo propter hoc (after this, because of this). The two fallacies are similar and involve an assumption that because something occurs at the same time as, or soon after another event, that the two occurrences are linked, and that one is the cause of the other. Clearly this is sometimes true, (if you prick us, do we not bleed?). But in other cases it is clear that there is no causative connection between two temporally associated events. For example, I go to bed when it is dark, but I do not cause it to be dark. Although these examples are clear, it is much more challenging in science and medicine to determine whether one event causes another. It is possible to give a statistical probability that two events are highly correlated, but this does not mean that one is the cause of the other. For example, osteoarthritis and mitral valve disease are often found together in the same animal, but one does not cause the other, they just happen to both occur frequently in older animals. The difficulties in medicine occur in areas such as pharmacovigilance, when trying to assess the incidence of adverse effects of a drug. Adverse effects reporting schemes require very large numbers to make statistical sense of whether a particular outcome is associated with a particular intervention. Anecdotes on the internet abound regarding various different demon drugs or vaccinations, along the lines of my pet had drug or vaccine X, and within a month it had developed kidney disease/cancer/ diabetes. To counter with an anecdote I recall being told by another vet, two puppies were brought in for vaccination. One of the puppies was vaccinated, and when the other was picked up for vaccination, it sadly died, before the injection had been given. If the vet had performed the vaccinations the other way round, the vaccine would likely, and not unreasonably, but wrongly, have been blamed for the poor puppy's death.

## Failure to elucidate

I hope I'm not guilty of this fallacy in this chapter, but this fallacy involves making the definition or conclusion more difficult to understand than the original concept. Most definitions of energy medicine, which invoke concepts such as life force, *Qi*, and other concepts that are poorly understood (or don't exist!), would fall into this category.

## False analogy

Analogy is an excellent way to help understand a concept. However, false analogies involve comparing two things that are not really comparable in all ways. For example, a mind is like a river. If it is broad it must be shallow. Weak analogy is a variation of this fallacy.

## *False dichotomy*

This is black and white thinking, in which it is argued that only two possibilities exist. For example, either all medicines are safe, or none of them are.

## *Half truths*

This is a deceptive statement that contains an element of truth. For example, the argument, 'we know we should use treatment X for condition Y, because we know it is safe', may miss out the fact that we know treatment X doesn't actually work.

## *Hasty generalisation*

This is similar to the biased sample fallacy, but involves making conclusions based on too small a sample size, rather than any inherent bias in the sample. For example, if you saw three red cars drive past in succession, it would be erroneous to conclude from this that all cars are red. An interesting example recently was a study into whether thimerosal-containing vaccines administered to rhesus monkeys caused autism-like signs or neuropathology[2] This was partly funded by an organisation called Safeminds, whose website states that, among other things, autism is caused by 'growing chemical exposures' and 'expansion of medical interventions'.[3] The study concluded that administration of thimerosal-containing vaccines or MMR vaccines did not cause aberrant behaviours or cause neuropathological changes similar to those found in autism. Safeminds said they found it 'disturbing' that this study contradicted smaller, earlier phases of the same study. This is likely an example of the hasty generalisation fallacy.

## *Magical thinking*

This fallacy involves connecting two events that are unlikely to be connected, using superstition. Superstitions surround us all the time and are largely harmless (unless the salt you throw over your shoulder hits someone in the eye). However, superstitious or magical thinking abounds in CAM, with homeopathy being a classic example. Although there is no logical reason to think that giving water or sugar pills that have none of the original active ingredient in would have any biological effect, homeopaths attribute any improvements seen to the magical effects of the pills or potions, and the succussion (banging of the container of water, originally against a leather-bound book, now done by machine) rather than the more plausible and well-recognised explanations such as regression to the mean or the placebo effect (see glossary).

## *Misuse of / misunderstanding of statistics*

This encompasses a large number of errors, but the misunderstanding of statistics can lead to inaccurate statistics being believed to support a case, and also because of the frequent misuse of statistics, there is often a general distrust of any fact derived from statistics. Statistics are vital in medicine, to distinguish real results from meaningless noise, and many if not most scientific papers will consult a statistician to help with the analysis of data. Politicians and other commentators will frequently quote statistics to bolster their positions, but cherry picking the data, biased samples, mis-reporting or misunderstanding of the estimated error, data dredging and outright data manipulation can all happen. Statistics are also frequently misunderstood, maybe because of their heavy reliance on maths. Even relatively straightforward concepts such as averages and percentages are often interpreted incorrectly, let alone more advanced and complex analysis. If someone tells you they are concerned at the fact that half the population is below average, they could benefit from a statistics lesson. If they are concerned that two-thirds of the population is below average they probably need a maths lesson. Sadly, after writing this paragraph in the first draft of this chapter, no less a person than the junior vice president of the British Veterinary Association (BVA) has been quoted in the *Veterinary Times* expressing concern that, 'More than a half of practices have below average profitability.'[4] Sigh.

One common misuse of statistics to highlight here is data dredging, where a large amount of data is analysed, often retrospectively, though sometimes intentionally and prospectively in the study design, to see if any associations can be found. Since it is common for a difference between two groups to be considered statistically different if the p value is $<0.05$, (meaning simplistically that there is a one in twenty probability of the association being due to chance), then clearly if twenty different variables are analysed, it wouldn't be surprising if a statistically significant difference in one of those variables was found, even if the effect was purely due to chance. Although this can occur in individual studies, where too many variables are examined, it is even more of a problem when looking at multiple studies. If twenty studies into a treatment are performed, it is likely that one would come out positive by pure chance. Systematic reviews and meta-analyses help clarify these statistical outliers, but given the tendency for both mainstream and CAM journals not to publish negative studies, there is a tendency for positive results to be over-interpreted. See also 'Proving non-existence' below.

## Moving the goalposts

It's the 2003 Rugby Union World Cup Final. Those great sporting rivals, England and Australia, are playing. Extra time, it's 17-17. Twenty-six seconds are left on the clock. Jonny Wilkinson receives the ball, kicks for a drop goal. The Australian team picks the goalposts up and runs 20 yards backwards with them. Jonny's kick falls short.

Moving the goalposts in an argument is similar to this scenario, in which the aims are changed after the argument has begun. Typically this would involve demanding proof of an argument, and when that was provided, demanding an even higher standard of proof. This can go on indefinitely, and with each proof of the lack of efficacy of homeopathy, or the lack of a link between autism and vaccine, new studies are demanded.

## No true Scotsman

This argument could be considered an example of moving the goalposts, and the classic example goes like this:

Fred: 'No Scotsman puts sugar on his porridge.'

Bill: 'My uncle is Scottish and he puts sugar on his porridge.'

Fred: 'Yes, but no true Scotsman would do such a thing.'

This is also a form of circular reasoning. Since Fred is defining Scotsmen as a group of men who do not put sugar on their porridge, by Fred's definition, Bill's uncle cannot be Scottish. Arguments invoking this fallacy would often begin along the lines of, 'No Christian would ...', 'No American would ...', 'No democracy would ...' or would include phrases like 'unBritish,' or even 'inhuman'. A more relevant example to this book would be:

Anne: 'No animal lover would eat meat.'

Brenda: 'My aunt rehomes abused cats, and travels to Eastern Europe to rescue homeless puppies. But she eats meat.'

Anne: 'Then she isn't a true animal lover.'

## *Poisoning the well*

This is another version of the ad hominem fallacy outlined above. In this case, negative material is presented about a person prior to their presenting their case. For example, 'I presented my evidence based on the latest research, but when Bill presents his case, just remember that it is a long time since he went to vet school and he is very out of date.'

## *Prejudicial language*

Loaded or emotive terms can be used to make an argument more persuasive, but that doesn't make the argument more true. For example, 'Don't you know that by vaccinating your pets, you are condemning them to a horrible death from autoimmune disease.'

## *Proving non-existence*

Sometimes an assertion will be made, and when challenged to provide evidence in favour of this assertion, the arguer will turn the argument round and demand evidence that the assertion is not true. There is a reason that when people make an argument, it is generally considered that the burden falls on them to prove the argument, not on someone else to disprove it, and that is because it is hard to prove a negative. Note that proving non-existence, i.e. evidence of absence, is different from absence of evidence. For example, if it was asserted there was a shark in a swimming pool, then seeing no shark would be evidence of absence, i.e. it would prove it was not there. However, if it was asserted that there was an amoeba in a pool, then merely failing to observe it would not prove it was absent, i.e. there is an absence of evidence. Although proving non-existence can be seen to be a tactic of alternative medicine proponents ('Prove that cranberry juice in your ear doesn't prevent flu!') it is also a common error in conventional medicine.

Many research studies test what is called the null hypothesis, which is the hypothesis that there is no difference between two populations. If a statistically significant difference between the populations is found (for example the treated group gets better quicker than the placebo group) then the null hypothesis is disproved. However, if no statistical difference is found, this is not the same as proving no difference exists, and a different calculation is needed to assess the likelihood that the two groups are actually the same.

Researchers who conclude that two groups are the same because they have failed to prove they are different are demonstrating an absence of evidence, not evidence of absence. This is known as a type II error in statistics. Many studies are underpowered to prove the null hypothesis, but by combining studies in meta-analyses and systematic reviews, it is possible to have stronger evidence for a position.

## Red herring

While the straw man fallacy (below) involves arguing against a distorted form of a person's argument, the red herring fallacy diverts attention to a different argument entirely, with the intention of abandoning the original argument that is harder to win. The new argument chosen may be another type of logical fallacy. For example, arguing that there are no placebo-controlled trials to prove the efficacy of chiropractic in elephants (yes, this is a thing!) may lead to the red herring argument that there are no placebo-controlled trials to prove the efficacy of cardiopulmonary resuscitation (which would clearly be unethical and unnecessary). This would be an example of a tu quoque ad hominem fallacy used as a red herring.

## Slippery slope

This fallacy implies that if something happens, then something else will happen as a consequence, and inevitably further down the line, something quite extreme. An example would be, if you ban vets from prescribing homeopathy, then non-vets will start prescribing it for animals, and soon clients will stop going to vets at all.

## Special pleading

This fallacy is commonly used in complementary and alternative medicine, using the argument that CAM should somehow be exempt from the usual rules of evidence. So as many forms of energy medicine and other CAM modalities cannot be proved by scientific methods, and their basic principles seem to disagree with known scientific fact, it is argued that science has not developed enough to test or understand the mechanism of the technique or treatment. If a treatment is proven to work, but no one knows how, then it is acceptable to use the treatment, and wait for the science to catch up. However, most CAM techniques are both scientifically improbable or impossible, and lack scientific proof of efficacy. CAM practitioners therefore often argue that they know a treatment works because they have seen the proof with their own eyes (although we know that observation and anecdote are poor ways of assessing treatment efficacy, see Chapter Two), and that if scientific studies don't agree, the studies must be wrong. They argue that their form of CAM (or all CAM) is a special case, and that it cannot be tested scientifically. For example, it is commonly argued that homeopathy cannot be tested by a blinded trial because of the need for individualisation, despite the fact that good blinded trials have been designed that allow individualisation, and also that many homeopathic treatments are sold in shops with no individualisation.

## Straw man

The straw man fallacy involves producing a distorted form of an argument, and attacking that, instead of attacking the actual argument, since the distorted argument is easier to knock down. For example, someone may say they favour evidence-based medicine. Their opponent may then claim that means the arguer is against anything that has not been proven by a randomised controlled trial (RCT), which would include many useful treatments that cannot ethically be studied with a RCT such as cardiopulmonary resuscitation (CPR). The opponent will then claim that the arguer should not perform CPR because it isn't evidence based.

## They laughed at Einstein

People who choose alternative medicine for themselves or their pets, often have deep mistrust of conventional authority figures, such as doctors, vets and scientists (especially those that work for drug companies). Perversely, they will often choose an alternative authority figure, whose opinions they will believe with almost religious fervour. When it is pointed out that this alternative figure's beliefs are out of line with mainstream thinking, it is often pointed out that 'They laughed at Einstein.' Carl Sagan refuted this line of reasoning with a wonderful quote. 'The fact that some geniuses were laughed at does not imply that all who are laughed at are geniuses. They laughed at Columbus, they laughed at Fulton, they laughed at the Wright brothers. But they also laughed at Bozo the clown.'

## *Wishful thinking*

I've put these fallacies in alphabetical order, but this one seems to crop up frequently in alternative medicine. Wouldn't it be nice if all drugs worked, and none of them had any side effects? This seems to be how alternative treatments are often presented. But this is just an example of wishful thinking. In the real world, if an intervention has an actual and beneficial effect on a biological system, then there is a chance that it will also cause an adverse effect. Drugs have what is called a therapeutic index, which relates the dose at which beneficial effects occur to doses at which adverse effects occur. A drug with a narrow therapeutic index such as digoxin is more likely to cause adverse effects, whereas a supplement with a high therapeutic index such as a vitamin is less likely to cause side effects. And yet even vitamins at high doses or taken over a prolonged period of time can have side effects or cause illness. Some alternative treatments have little to no biological side effects, but little to no efficacy. Other alternative treatments can have serious complications, for example pneumothorax following acupuncture.[5] It is wishful thinking to think that a magic treatment exists that cures everything and has no side effects, but this is what purveyors of snake oil in the Wild West claimed, and this is what some alternative medicine practitioners would like you to believe.

§

## Cognitive biases

If the logical fallacies are ways that people argue in favour of an erroneous position, used consciously or unconsciously, the cognitive biases are often reasons why people believe the erroneous position in the first place. We all like to think our beliefs and decision-making are born out of reason and logic, but we are all susceptible to biases in the way we think, which can lead to us believing things that are not true. Cognitive biases are separate from other biases such as cultural bias, or bias from self-interest. They arise not from an emotional or intellectual predisposition, but from inbuilt subconscious processes, and as such tend to be consistent and predictable.

Cognitive biases exist because of mental shortcuts that have evolved to speed up our reasoning and processing to give us the best chance of survival. For example, if there is a chance that that random collection of spots in the bushes is actually a leopard getting ready to pounce, it's better to run than just assume the pattern is random. For this reason we are very good at pattern recognition, but have a tendency to think we can spot patterns when in fact there is only random noise.

Cognitive biases frequently lead to erroneous and illogical conclusions, and so can lead people to hold incorrect beliefs. Faith in ineffective treatments by patients and pet owners can be induced by biases such as the Bandwagon effect or the Zero Risk bias and perpetuated by biases such as the Frequency Illusion, the Choice Supportive bias and the Hindsight bias.

Alternative medicine practitioners on the whole probably genuinely believe in their treatment practices, and though this is hard to prove, I personally believe there are few genuine fraudsters or charlatans in the CAVM world. It is more likely that practitioners of probably ineffective treatments are being fooled into believing their treatments are effective by a number of cognitive biases such as the observer-expectancy effect, optimism bias, anthropic bias, egocentric bias, clustering illusion, beneffectance, déformation professionnelle and even the Dunning–Kruger effect. Research by alternative practitioners into their preferred treatment modalities can be biased by the self-serving bias, selective reporting, the Texas sharpshooter fallacy and the observer expectancy effect.

Avoiding cognitive bias is clearly challenging, and beyond the scope of this book, but more detailed information about biases can be found in Dan Ariely's *Predictably Irrational*[6] and Daniel Kahneman's *Thinking Fast and Slow*.[7] For the purposes of this book, it is enough to be aware they exist, as they do help explain an individual's (perhaps even your own) fervently held faiths in certain types of treatment. Of course, conventional medicine is not immune to the same cognitive biases, but science-based medicine should attempt to eliminate bias from its conclusions, while alternative medicine tends to rely on faith in a practice rather than proof, the faith often created and perpetuated by cognitive biases. The existence of cognitive biases, and the dramatic effects they can have on people's beliefs, are why when an alternative practitioner states, 'I don't need proof, I have seen my treatment work with my own eyes,' this is insufficient justification for the treatment's use.

I have summarised some of the most common cognitive biases that are encountered in complementary and alternative medicine.

## Decision-making and behavioural biases

### *Bandwagon effect*

We generally have a tendency to want to conform. This doesn't necessarily mean we want to slavishly follow the rest of the population (alternative believers and conspiracy theorists love using the word sheeple to describe people who blindly follow authority and the majority opinion). However, we have a strong bias to want to conform to our peer group, and this can alter our beliefs.

In the 1950s, a psychologist called Solomon Asch performed a number of fascinating experiments, in which a group of people were given simple tests. When the rest of the group, who were actors, unanimously gave a clearly wrong answer, 75 per cent of the subjects of the experiment went along with the rest of the group in at least one test, and in total conformed to the wrong answer one-third of the time. I had my own experience of this as a young vet, when a lame dog had an X-ray taken of his shoulder by another, more senior vet in the practice. The vet was convinced he could see a lesion in the shoulder, and he pointed it out to the other vets and the vet student, who all nodded their agreement. I was inexperienced, and orthopaedics has never been my interest, yet I felt like the boy pointing out the Emperor was naked when I said I couldn't see the lesion. Fortunately, the senior partner who wasn't present that day had told the owners the radiographs would be sent away to a specialist orthopaedic surgeon for an opinion. The specialist opinion was that the radiograph of the shoulder was actually normal.

If a group of men in the pub or young mums at a National Childbirth Trust (NCT) meeting mostly agree that a particular therapy is wonderful and safe, then others without a strong opinion on the subject are likely to agree and share that belief. Similarly, a group of alternative medicine practitioners in a conference will tend to reinforce each other's beliefs, and in these situations sceptical voices tend to be mocked or frowned upon, in the same way that standing up in church and saying God does not exist would be considered rude.

### *Bias blind spot*

We all suffer from cognitive biases, and worse, we generally probably don't realise this. The bias blind spot is our inability to see our own cognitive biases.

## Certainty effect and pseudocertainty effect

People have a tendency to overweight certainty over uncertainty. So when given a hypothetical choice between a vaccine (the human papilloma virus vaccine) that was 100 per cent effective against 70 per cent of the causes of cervical cancer, or 70 per cent effective against 100 per cent of the causes of cervical cancer they preferred the former, since the first scenario involved elimination of a particular risk, whereas the second involved an overall risk reduction.[8] In the pseudocertainty effect, the certainty is only perceived. The pseudocertainty effect has also been defined as the tendency to make choices that limit risk if the expected outcome is positive, but make riskier choices if the expected outcome is negative.

## Choice supportive bias

We have a tendency to think our decisions in life are generally the best ones in the circumstances. Sometimes we are proven dramatically wrong, for example the Spanish couple recently whose child became seriously ill with the first case of diphtheria in the country for twenty-eight years, after they were persuaded by anti-vaccination campaigns not to have their child vaccinated. Most of the time however, our choices are neutral or have no bad consequences. Thus it is common in anti-vaccination circles to hear that a parent never vaccinated their child and their child is happier and healthier than they would have been if they had had 'those poisons' injected. The fact that the child has managed to avoid infectious disease, and is otherwise healthy, is taken as support of their choice, proving to them they were right.

## Confirmation bias

The seventeenth century polymath Francis Bacon stated that 'The human understanding when it has once adopted an opinion ... draws all things else to support and agree with it.' He was talking about confirmation bias, the tendency to seek out information and interpret it in a way that agrees with prior conceptions. Studies have proved that people attribute increased value to information that confirms their beliefs relative to those that contradict them. This may be because it is simply cognitively easier to process confirmatory than contradictory information. In medicine and veterinary medicine, confirmation bias can lead one to give too much weight to rare adverse outcomes such as a vaccination reaction, or too much weight to an example of success of a treatment that in fact may have been due to random chance.

## Congruence bias

A sequence of numbers starts 2, 4, 6, and there is a particular rule that the sequence must obey. You must find the rule, and you may produce other sets of numbers to test, to see whether they also obey the rule. Which numbers would you try? Most people think they can spot the rule already, and so will try numbers such as 3, 5, 7 to test their hypothesis that the rule is that the numbers ascend in steps of 2. So 3, 5, 7 would indeed be correct, as would 10, 12, 14. At this point, you may feel the point proved. But what if you tried 1, 4, 7 or 10, 11, 12 and were told these were correct as well? The rule is in fact simply that each number must be higher than the previous one. Most people test numbers that confirm their pre-existing theory, rather than testing numbers that attempt to disprove it.

Congruence bias is a reliance on testing a hypothesis in a way that will prove it (direct testing) rather than attempt to disprove it (indirect testing). The underlying problem is a tendency not to consider other hypotheses. Scientists are often accused of not being open-minded, when the reality is that a true scientist (with full awareness of the *no true Scotsman* fallacy here!) will consider all hypotheses, while alternative medicine practitioners are often unwilling to consider other hypotheses, for example as to why an ineffective therapy might seem effective.

## Déformation professionnelle

Timmy the dog collapses in the house when the postman rings the doorbell. He goes stiff and urinates. Afterwards he recovers, but looks disorientated for a while. This event could be syncope (a collapse due to reduced blood-flow to the brain, for example from a cardiac cause) or it could be a seizure. Timmy's owner takes him to his usual vet, who recognises that Timmy may need more expertise and equipment than he can provide in his primary care clinic, and decides to refer him to a specialist. But which one? If he sends him to a neurologist, there is a fair chance he will get a magnetic resonance imaging (MRI) scan, whereas if he sends him to a cardiologist, he will probably get an echocardiogram and electrocardiogram (ECG). Of course, specialists in these disciplines are skilled at recognising when a collapse is a seizure or a syncopal episode, but from medical history and observation it cannot always be conclusively determined into which category it falls, and so there is a tendency to see the case according to the bias of your own professional experience. This is not merely theoretical, I have been told by a cardiology specialist of a case of a dog with a serious arrhythmia that was seen first by a neurologist and put through a risky anaesthetic for an MRI scan of the brain, before it was realised the problem was actually cardiac in origin, and no doubt the reverse situation can also occur.

This situation is known as déformation professionnelle, the tendency to look at a patient only from a specialist's own perspective. How does this relate to alternative medicine? There is a tendency for alternative medicine practitioners to attempt to treat all conditions with their chosen specialism, or if they use a variety of alternative medicine treatments, to choose alternative medicine over traditional, possibly on the basis that this is what the client who has sought them out expects. If you look at the list of conditions that chiropractors, reflexologists and acupuncturists claim to be able to treat, it is hard to avoid the conclusion that they too are suffering from déformation professionelle bias.

## Framing

What's better, a 90 per cent survival rate, or a 10 per cent mortality rate? Of course, they are the same, but how a question is presented can affect decision-making, a process known as framing. This has been proven to be an issue for both patients and doctors in human medicine,[9] and as it is a widespread bias, it is likely to be an issue in veterinary medicine as well. So if an alternative practitioner discusses alternative treatments in terms such as survival rates, and conventional treatments in terms such as mortality rates, beware of the effect on your subconscious.

## Omission bias

This is the tendency to judge a bad outcome less favourably if it is the result of an action, compared to the result of an inaction. Is it morally worse to kill someone than to fail to save their life through your inaction? Most people would say yes, though the outcome is the same. Another way to think about this is to consider the scenario of a runaway train. A madman has tied two people to one railway track, and one person to another. The train is on the track to run over the two people. But you can switch the points by pulling a lever, and the train will divert to run over the one person. By doing so, only one will die instead of two. But you are the one pulling the lever, and it is a hard thing to do, to condemn that one person to death, rather than just stand back and say, whatever will be will be. People are worried they are more likely to regret a choice they make than one they don't make.

Omission bias is considered by some to be one of the reasons behind the decision of caregivers not to have their children or pets vaccinated. Though it is widely accepted that the risks of not vaccinating are much higher than the risk of vaccinating (see Chapter Nine), caregivers often feel a lot of conflict about making a positive choice to put their child or pet through a (perceived) risky procedure, and in many cases would prefer to fail to prevent the higher risk, rather than make that positive choice. Of course, inaction is still a choice, though it feels less like one.

### Outcome bias

This relates to the tendency to judge the quality of a decision by its ultimate outcome, rather than the quality of the decision making based on the information available at the time. Consider a game of Russian roulette. For those who don't know the rules, a single bullet is placed in a revolver that has chambers for six, and the barrel is spun so no one knows where the bullet is. Putting the gun to your head and firing will kill you with a one in six probability. Say someone offers you £10,000 to play this game. Most people would think this inadvisable. However, if you had already played and won, and now had £10,000 in your pocket, this might now seem like it was a great idea. The same bias can be seen in health and medicine choices. How many times has someone said something along the lines of my grandfather smoked twenty a day all his life and lived till he was 85 (and my grandfather really did this!)? This doesn't make smoking twenty a day the best choice. Similarly, someone choosing homeopathy over antibiotics to treat their pneumonia may think it was a good idea if they have lived to tell the tale, but it might not have been the best choice. See also survivorship bias and hindsight bias below.

### Reactance

Sometimes it feels like the more you present someone with evidence of a position, the more entrenched in their contrary position they become. This is reactance, the urge to do or think the opposite of what someone else wants you to do or think, because of a perceived threat to behavioural freedom. This seems to be an important factor in some people's reasons for using alternative medicine, or being anti-vaccination, that they don't want to do what they are told by an authority figure such as a doctor or vet, or government or a big corporation, and instead will react by refusing to vaccinate, or using alternative medicine.

## Selective perception

This bias involves us tending to ignore information that does not fit with our pre-existing beliefs, because of the emotional discomfort it causes us. It is exhibited when considering religion, politics, even sports. And, of course, there will be a tendency among believers in a certain treatment type, alternative or conventional, to select information supportive of their beliefs.

## Survivorship bias

A case report in a non-peer-reviewed veterinary journal a couple of years ago described the case of a dog that apparently had a prolonged survival after treatment with homeopathy for the usually fatal cancer, osteosarcoma. Apart from the other flaws in this case report this is a good example of survivorship bias. By concentrating on this one, unusual case, we are failing to take into account what happened in the cases of all the unsuccessfully treated cases, and this is one of the reasons individual case reports and anecdotes cannot be trusted as evidence for a treatment. Survivorship bias is an understandable consequence of our desire to hear and read about success – the author or sportsmen who made it big against the odds, for example. The many that failed don't make good stories. But this means we fail to learn the lessons of the failures, and why people or things fail, and how often, are just as important as why and how often they succeed.

## Von Restorff effect

Items that 'stand out like a sore thumb' are more likely to be remembered than those that don't. This can lead to outliers in a group being remembered when they are not typical of the average.

## Zero risk bias

This is related to the certainty effect, and involves a preference for reducing a certain risk to zero, rather than opting for an overall reduction in risk, which may be better. People tend to rate anything that has a risk above zero as risky, and can lead them to ignore other risks. For example, drinking caffeinated drinks can raise your blood pressure, which is considered a risk, but it can reduce your likelihood of death by improving your wakefulness and reducing your chance of a car accident. Yet many people would see the increase in risk by drinking the caffeine from zero to something as outweighing a relative reduction in having a car accident.

# Biases in probability and belief

## *Clustering illusion*

This is the tendency to see patterns where none exist, like the random pattern in the leaves that is perceived as a leopard, mentioned above. The clustering illusion helps us see faces in random rock patterns on Mars, or Jesus in the ultrasound scan of a baby. It can also fool us when a group of patients appear to behave in a particular way, and we attribute the response to a particular intervention, when in fact it is just random noise.

## *Frequency illusion*

This is the tendency, once you have learned about something, to see it everywhere.

## *Gambler's fallacy*

This is considered to be a logical fallacy, as well as a cognitive bias and involves a misconception that a random event is influenced by previous events that have no influence on that event. If you toss a coin and get six heads in a row, the probability of the next toss being a head is still 50 per cent, but many people will assume that run can't continue, and bet on a tail. Gamblers fall into this trap in roulette and card games, and even doctors can reason that as the last ten cases of chest pain have turned out to be myocardial infarctions, surely the next one will be something else.[10]

## *Primacy effect and recency effect*

More weight tends to be given to events at the start of a series (primacy effect) and at the end of a series (recency effect). Thus a vet may be more likely to remember their first and last patients of the day than all those in between, which may lead to a biased perception of a typical case (in my experience the first and last ones are more likely to be emergencies).

## Observer expectancy effect

'Clever Hans' was a German horse who seemed able to do simple arithmetic. When his owner read out sums, Hans could tap out the correct number with his hoof. He could even do the same when someone else read out the sums. However, it was discovered that he couldn't add up when he couldn't see his owner. Clever Hans was indeed clever, not because he could do maths, but because he could read his owner's body language as he performed the final tap in the sequence. This is an example of the observer expectancy effect, in which the observer or experimenter unconsciously influences the subjects of an experiment. One example of this from alternative medicine is the experiment performed by Jacques Benveniste and discussed in Chapter Ten, in which ultradilute samples of anti-IgE antibody seemed to have an effect on the degranulation of white blood cells called basophils, a result that seemed to support the concept of homeopathy, and which was published in the prestigious journal *Nature*. However, because the results were so unexpected and defied explanation, *Nature* requested the experiment was replicated. When this was done, but with the researchers no longer able to tell which samples were which, the results of the trial were negative. This suggests that the original positive results were due to the observer expectancy effect. This is why the 'double-blinded' trial, in which both the subject and the experimenter do not know whether an active ingredient or a placebo is given, is considered the gold standard in experiment design. It allows both the placebo effect and the observer expectancy effect to be taken into account.

## Optimism bias

Most of us know (or once were, or maybe still are) teenagers who believe they will live forever and are indestructible. Smoking, alcohol and drugs hold no dangers for them, because bad things happen to other people. Optimism bias is the cognitive bias that leads people to believe that their chances of experiencing a negative effect are less than their peers. It was first demonstrated among college students, who individually believed their chance of undergoing problems such as divorce or a getting a drinking problem was lower than the national average. Optimism bias leads to an underestimation of risk, and could have an implication in alternative medicine if a patient believes their chances of, for example, surviving cancer using homeopathy instead of chemotherapy are better than the statistics show.

## *Overconfidence effect*

This bias means that a person's confidence in their accuracy is higher than their accuracy actually is. Overconfidence can relate to overestimation of one's objective performance or performance relative to others or overestimation of the accuracy of one's beliefs. Many alternative medicine proponents believe strongly and wrongly in the accuracy of their beliefs. See also the Dunning–Kruger effect.

## *Texas sharpshooter fallacy*

A Texan blasts away at a barn with his six-shooter, and then draws a ring around the tightest cluster of shots and claims to be a sharpshooter. In the same way, it is common for people to ignore differences in data and stress the similarities, and is often seen where large groups of data are available. For example, cancer often occurs in clusters, but this is because by and large, cancer strikes at random, and a random pattern is not like the points of a grid, but like a starry sky, with some points randomly closer to others. In some cases, cancer clusters occur for reasons other than randomness, but complex statistics are required to differentiate this from random chance, and even then, proving cancer is non-randomly clustered tells us nothing about the cause.

When large groups of data are available, it is easy to single out the interesting and distinctive results, but the totality must be taken into account. It is easy in medicine and alternative medicine to take into account only successes and emphasise these, when to be meaningful, all cases in a group should be considered.

## Social biases

### *Dunning–Kruger effect*

Sometimes people are unaware of their incompetence. Dunning and Kruger showed that incompetent people overestimate their competence to a greater degree than competent people. This is clearly not a risk unique to alternative medicine, but should be taken into account when someone extols their own virtues.

## *Egocentric bias*

Fishermen's tales about the size of the fish they caught are notorious for their inaccuracy, but that doesn't mean the fishermen are outright lying. The memory is prone to distorting the past in a self-enhancing way. This is another bias that can lead clinicians to overemphasise their successes, and why scientific studies into treatments are required, rather than the assertions of clinicians and practitioners that they have seen a treatment work with their own eyes. The concept of beneffectance, the tendency to reinterpret events to put oneself in a more favourable light, which is known to be common, is related to this bias.

## *Self-serving bias (and modesty bias)*

Similar to the egocentric bias, the self-serving bias is any cognitive process that becomes distorted by a need to maintain or enhance a person's self-esteem, and leads to a tendency to attribute positive events to one's own interventions, and negative events to outside influence. Again, this can lead to clinicians and practitioners claiming their successes are due to their treatments, while their failures are due to factors outside their control. The modesty bias is the opposite effect, in which failures are blamed on oneself, and successes on external factors. Cultural factors are important here, with the Chinese and Japanese more likely to show a modesty bias, and males more likely to show a self-serving bias.

## Memory errors

### *Hindsight bias*

The outcome bias described above unfairly judges a decision based on information that was not available at the time the decision was made. By contrast, the hindsight bias overestimates one's predictive abilities, and is often summed up by the phrase 'I knew it all along'. The past is filtered in the memory with the benefit of current knowledge and makes those events look more predictable than they were. It is not uncommon for a veterinary client to be disgruntled because of an adverse outcome the veterinarian failed to predict. That adverse outcome may not have been easy to predict, but with hindsight may have seemed obvious, e.g. 'You know Davey is an unneutered male, and you know from your records that the next door's bitch is due in season, so you should have warned us not to let Davey in the garden after his stomach operation, because it should have been obvious he would try to jump the fence, and make the wound open up.' In alternative veterinary medicine, if an animal fails to make the desired recovery using traditional medicine, or makes a full recovery with alternative medicine, the cry will often be, 'I told you so.'

## Selective memory / reporting

Memory for health information can be biased by pre-existing beliefs. For example, in a study of patients presented with information about alcohol consumption, those that were more negative towards alcohol to begin with were more likely to retain anti-alcohol information, whereas those that were more positive towards alcohol were more likely to remember pro-alcohol information.[11] Thus, people's beliefs can be self-reinforcing.

This list of cognitive biases is not comprehensive. Nor is it meant to imply that only alternative medicine practitioners are prone to these biases. In fact we all are, to a greater or lesser extent (although medical experts have been shown to be less prone to confirmation bias than novices[12]). However, the existence of these biases can help explain why people hold incorrect, or even downright strange, beliefs. Scientists and sceptics should be aware of these strange mental quirks, both in others, and just as importantly in themselves. Sceptics should be always questioning the facts, and their interpretation of the facts, and examine their responses and arguments for fallacies and biases. Unfortunately, in the authors' personal interactions with alternative medicine practitioners, it seems to be uncommon for CAM practitioners to take a self-questioning approach to their disciplines, and in fact their practices are often defended aggressively against anyone presuming to ask questions.

Awareness of the cognitive biases in ourselves and others helps us to make sense of the conflicting interpretations of data from different sources. Above all it helps understand why it is vital that the scientific approach is used as the basis for medicine, in order to spare us our brains' inbuilt errors of reasoning.

§

## False arguments in CAVM

Having explored in the previous sections the most common logical fallacies that are encountered when debating CAM, let's take a look at some of the commonly encountered arguments in favour of CAM.

## The Big Pharma conspiracy

The term Big Pharma is a nickname for large pharmaceutical companies and an associated web of organisations and individuals such as doctors, regulators and politicians, usually used in a derogatory way in the context of implying or explicitly stating these large companies deliberately suppress information about alternative medicines in order to preserve their properties. The internet and social media abounds with conspiracy theories of all shapes and sizes, and the Big Pharma conspiracy theory is particularly pernicious, causing people to question the benefits of life-saving or quality-of-life-preserving drugs. This conspiracy involves such disparate characters as the British Royal Family (notwithstanding that Prince Charles is a big supporter of alternative medicine), Bill Gates, Mark Zuckerberg and Barack Obama, and makes a variety of claims. Some of the less outlandish ones include that Big Pharma invented a cure for cancer and then covered it up (which would involve thousands of people working in the pharmaceutical industry callously allowing the deaths of their own loved ones from one of the biggest killers in the Western world), that drugs and vaccines are part of a conspiracy to poison the population (it isn't clear who benefits from this, but population control is suggested as a rationale) and that Big Pharma invents diseases or exaggerates the prevalence or severity of diseases to justify their drug sales. A remarkably widespread belief exists that the US government is using 'chemtrails' (the vapour trails or contrails seen coming from aircraft that consist primarily of ice crystals formed from the water vapour in the engine exhaust) to spread toxins and/or vaccinations. In researching this section, I got diverted by one of the most bizarre pieces of writing I have found on the internet,[13] which contains such gems as the belief that cats are depopulating the skies to make room for CIA-controlled microchipped pigeons, and that the cat's purr is a way of communicating with their alien masters, and apparently explains the cat's wistful attitude to chemtrails. This may be satire, but a web search shows that many people aren't sure, and the comments below the article suggests that many people have taken it seriously.

Undoubtedly there are real problems with pharmaceutical companies, and Ben Goldacre's excellently researched book *Bad Pharma* goes into details regarding this.[14] To quote Dr Goldacre, though, 'Pharma being shit does not mean magic beans cure cancer.' Furthermore, there is no evidence or logical reason to believe that pharmaceutical companies suppress information on cures, or even that they possess this capability. It is also disingenuous to imply that pharmaceutical companies are only in it for the money, while alternative practitioners are purely working for altruistic purposes. Many alternative practitioners, especially those that sell their own brands of cures and supplements, often in conjunction with educational tours, are extremely rich, and the National Centre for Complementary and Integrative Health estimates that in 2007, Americans spent 34 billion dollars out of their own pockets on visits to CAM practitioners and purchasing CAM products. It should therefore be borne in mind that there is a profit motive for both 'Big Pharma' and 'Big CAM' to sell their products.

## Scientists are close-minded

Being close-minded can be defined as being unreceptive to new ideas or arguments. That scientists are close-minded to CAM treatments is a commonly levelled accusation. It is true that busy practitioners often dismiss claims that are implausible or unsupported by evidence with little consideration. This is not only understandable, but it is practical and inevitable. The number of alternative treatments is truly vast, and for one individual to evaluate them all would be an impossible task. Even for the medical profession as a whole, when using limited resources to evaluate treatments that might genuinely benefit patients, it makes sense to focus those resources on treatments more likely to yield a positive result, for example molecules that are known to act at previously identified cell receptors, rather than something with no prior likelihood of efficacy, such as homeopathy.

Generally, it is beholden on the proponent of a claim to provide evidence supporting that claim. Nevertheless, many scientists have engaged in open-minded study of CAM treatments. Occasionally, this will result in a positive result, as with certain supplements and herbs. In most cases, a CAM treatment will be found to be ineffective.

CAM practitioners often claim that there is no funding available to perform research, and if 'someone' would just pay for and do the research, all their claims would be found to be true. I have encountered this argument in debates with vets who are proponents of raw food diets. In fact, studies of longevity in animals fed raw versus commercial food would be simple to perform, retrospectively, or with more patience prospectively. Although more rigorous trials could incur costs and possibly some paperwork to get appropriate licences, for example if biochemical analysis was being performed, there are charitable sources of funding for practitioners to undergo research projects, and academics are often very helpful at assisting with study design and statistical analysis. To passionately argue in favour of a particular intervention, such as a specific diet, for decades, while failing to undertake research to back up these claims, seems to imply either an intellectual laziness, or a lack of confidence that one's claims are really verifiable.

When positive results of a well-controlled clinical trial are achieved for a CAM practice, and are repeatable and verified, then scientists will move to incorporate this information into mainstream practice. Ursodeoxycholic acid (to treat liver disease) from bear bile, silybin (to treat liver disease) from milk thistle and vinca alkaloids (to treat cancer) from research into the reputed therapeutic properties of the Madagascar Periwinkle are examples of alternative medicines that have made it into the mainstream. There are no doubt other as yet undiscovered or untested treatments in CAM that may be helpful, even ground-breaking. But as the numbers of potential treatments is so vast, without evidence, choosing a treatment that might be efficacious is as chancy as closing your eyes, walking down the cooking section of the supermarket and picking a herb at random in the hope it will cure a condition.

As the comedian Tim Minchin said, 'Do you know what they call alternative medicine that's been proven to work? Medicine.' Science is open-minded to using treatments previously thought to be ineffective, and to abandoning treatments proven to be ineffective, although scientists are only human, and inertia and cognitive biases can mean that new evidence does not make its way through to clinical practice as quickly as may be sometimes hoped. However, alternative practitioners, in contrast to scientists, are often remarkably close-minded. Homeopathy, for example has not changed for 200 years, even though it is based on a discredited paradigm of disease that was invented before Pasteur developed the germ theory of disease, or atomic theory had shown that ultra-diluted homeopathic preparations contain none of the original ingredient.

Note, this is not a tu quoque fallacy. CAM practitioners are remarkably close-minded to science, regardless of the evidence. Scientists are remarkably open-minded to CAM, and a good scientist is always prepared to re-evaluate their beliefs when new evidence is provided.

93

# Conventional medicines have side effects

A compound that has a biological activity would be expected to have the potential for side effects. This is quantified in a measurement called the therapeutic index, the dose at which toxic side effects are seen, divided by the dose at which beneficial effects are seen. For some drugs, such as phenobarbitone and digoxin, the therapeutic index is low, and monitoring of blood levels is often undertaken to ensure that the dose is sufficient to be having benefit and not too high to be causing harm. For other drugs, the therapeutic index is extremely wide, with large overdoses being required to cause toxic effects. However, a biological system is highly complex, and unpredictable side effects can occur. Drugs are tested for safety in a number of stages, including animal models, human volunteers and post-release monitoring. Trials and monitoring can lead to changes in recommendations or even withdrawals of some drugs. Thalidomide is often pointed to as an example of disastrous side effects associated with a conventional medicine. Thalidomide caused terrible birth defects when taken by pregnant mothers in the late 1950s and early 1960s. However, as a result of this, drug licensing laws were tightened, with the FDA requiring drug companies to publish all side effects of drugs encountered during testing.

Rare and idiosyncratic (i.e. peculiar to the individual) effects can occur with any drug. Every intervention, conventional or otherwise should be considered with regard to the ratio of risk and benefit to the individual. In many cases the risk:benefit ratio will clearly point towards the use or avoidance of an intervention. In other cases, the ratio is less certain, and requires an informed discussion between physician/vet and patient/client.

CAM interventions also have potential for side effects. Although it is often argued that CAM is 'natural' (even the decidedly unnatural practices such as homeopathy and acupuncture), the naturalistic fallacy that natural is safe is often used. Little thought is needed to list copious examples of things that exist in nature that are unsafe. (I enjoyed a recent thread on a Facebook page that recommended drinking lava, since it must be safe because it was natural, and Big Geology was trying to suppress knowledge of its benefits). Side effects are discussed in more detail in the individual sections on CAM therapies, but direct harm has been documented from herbal medicine (direct toxic effects and contaminants), acupuncture (pneumothorax), chiropractic (strokes) and raw food (pathogens and injuries from bones). Another potential harm from CAM practice is that it encourages people to neglect conventional medicines, which may be life-saving. In some cases this may be a philosophical belief on the part of the patient or owner towards CAM therapies, it may be due to limited financial resources meaning that investment in CAM therapies means fewer resources available to pursue conventional therapy, or it may involve an active discouragement on the part of the CAM practitioner for the patient or owner to pursue conventional therapy. Homeopaths, for example, often believe that conventional medicine will interfere with their practice, and will often withdraw conventional, effective medicines, in favour of their ineffective ones. Thus even something that has no biological effect, and so is unlikely to have direct physical side effects, can still lead to suboptimal or adverse outcomes.

## CAVM is holistic

Complementary and alternative medical practices are often referred to as holistic, but what does this actually mean? One definition in medicine is that it involves assessment and treatment of the whole patient, taking into account all factors, and not just the presenting symptoms. Many alternative disciplines proudly state that they are holistic, so much so that the term holistic medicine has almost become synonymous with alternative medicine. Homeopaths, for example, claim that they are holistic because the questions they ask during a homeopathic consultation will help to ascertain the cause of a condition and allow treatment to be tailored to the individual. Individualisation of homeopathic treatment is a vital part of the homeopathic philosophy, although this clearly hasn't been communicated to the high street chemists who sell over the counter homeopathic remedies for coughs, colds and allergies without a homeopathic consultation. The homeopathic consultation itself is a flawed and non-scientific process, however. The questions asked in the history taking (called case taking in homeopathy) often have no relevance to real diseases, and only make sense if you believe in the whole 'like cures like'/ provings philosophy (see Chapter Ten for more detail). Thus sensible questions regarding appetite and thirst may be included along with the irrelevant or downright bizarre, such as do you dislike being contradicted, or would you describe yourself as being easily offended? Similarly, while patients should receive physical examinations, if the basic concepts of disease and diagnosis are misunderstood or ignored by practitioners, it is no surprise that the examinations concentrate on the wrong factors, or completely neglect to perform an appropriate examination, substituting instead an irrelevant one. Thus, Traditional Chinese Medicine examinations will concentrate on the tongue and pulse quality, when a particular case may benefit more from an ophthalmic examination or auscultation of the heart. Chiropractic diagnosis is based on (non-existent) subluxations of the vertebra, so the examination will concentrate on the spine, even if the presenting condition is asthma, for which listening to the chest would provide much more information. And by concentrating on the wrong things, serious diagnoses can be missed, for example failing to spot spinal tumours while looking for subluxations.

So while CAM treatments claim to be holistic by not focussing solely on the presenting problem, they may in fact be worse that a non-holistic approach because of their potential for irrelevant and/or misleading findings. Furthermore, CAM advocates claim, often falsely, that their disciplines are holistic, and that conventional medicine is not. It may be true that if you go to your family vet or general practitioner for a five- or ten-minute consultation, a fully comprehensive history and physical examination may not be possible, unlike the hour or more often allowed for say a homeopathic consultation. But when a problem is more chronic, or more serious, or the diagnosis remains uncertain, then conventional medicine will often take a fully holistic approach.

The problem-oriented approach to veterinary medicine is described more fully in Gough & Murphy.[15] In brief though, when presented with a medical case, the vet takes a full medical history, performs a full physical examination, formulates a list of possible or differential diagnoses in order of likelihood, and then selects appropriate testing, e.g. blood tests, ultrasound scans, in order to narrow these possibilities down to a diagnosis. This to me seems a truly holistic approach, taking into account the owner or patient complaints, the physical findings and the results of scientific testing, wedded with the practitioner's knowledge and experience of disease.

## Scientific medicine only treats the symptoms of the disease, not the underlying cause

This is another common argument against scientific medicine, but again is false, and without wanting to indulge in a tu quoque fallacy, does seem rather like bricks in glass houses when coming from homeopaths. The homeopathic consultation involves a completely subjective assessment of the patient's symptoms, with treatments then selected based on the belief that 'like cures like', and that infinitesimally small doses of a substance that induces those symptoms will result in the alleviation of those symptoms. It is true that conventional medicine will sometimes aim to suppress symptoms (so-called symptomatic treatment), particularly where there is no cure for a disease, or where the cure may be more dangerous than the condition itself. So for example, there is no cure for asthma, but bronchodilators and steroids can allow the patient to breathe easily. While suppression of the symptoms is implied to be a bad thing by CAM practitioners, the asthmatic who can breathe properly because of his medication would likely disagree. Other scientific treatments still may not cure a disease, but do far more than suppress symptoms. Treatment with insulin or thyroxine are direct replacements for the lack of those hormones, and alleviate symptoms by restoring homeostasis in a real way, rather than by a vague concept of unblocking *Qi* channels, or rebalancing the life energy. And many treatments are in fact a cure of the underlying disease, such as antibiotic treatment for septicaemia (in the interests of full disclosure, as mentioned in the introduction, my vegan, alternative-minded aunt died of septicaemia after treating herself with homeopathy and refusing antibiotic treatment).

## Homeopathy is like vaccination

There is a passing similarity between the concepts of homeopathy and vaccination, in that small amounts of a disease-causing agent are administered in order to produce a response from the body against that agent. However, vaccination provides a finite, measurable quantity of the agent, which produces a measurable immune response, protecting against the disease, usually an infectious disease, although sometimes a cancer. Homeopathy on the other hand, involves infinitesimally small or non-existent doses of the agent, with no measurable effect on the body, and with no rational likelihood of effect, since the belief is not that the agent will induce a protection against future infections, but that by giving small amounts of a substance that causes similar symptoms to the disease, that somehow this will treat the disease. The flawed concept of 'like cures like' is discussed in more detail in Chapter Ten.

## Belief systems

It is argued that science and CAM are just belief systems. As the saying goes, it is true that everyone is entitled to their beliefs, but everyone is not entitled to their own facts. Science, while not perfect, attempts to describe the world as it really is, and if new evidence comes along to challenge the model, science will adjust to incorporate that evidence. CAM, on the other hand, has a tendency to be unchangeable, no matter how much evidence comes along to challenge it, and most CAM practices (e.g. traditional Chinese medicine (TCM), homeopathy) have barely changed since before the germ theory was discovered, and certainly before biochemistry, endocrinology and pharmacology were developed. CAM is very much a belief system, faith-based and resistant to evidence or change. Scientific medicine is constantly challenged by its own practitioners, and changes with new findings.

Some also argue, in a post-modernist way, that there is no absolute truth, and therefore my truth is as good as yours. This argument may be intellectually satisfying to philosophers, but is of scant use when it comes to choosing the most effective analgesia for the patient presented to you in agonising pain.

## Allopaths simply ridicule CAM

The term 'allopath' is used by homeopaths to differentiate everyone who is not a homeopath from themselves, and not a term that allopaths apply to themselves. Terms allopaths use to describe themselves include rational and scientific. But, sticking with the terminology, that allopaths 'simply' ridicule CAM is not true, as hopefully this book shows. We engage in debate and in research and attempt to educate. However, as the prizewinner of the Rhode Island Medical Society's competition said in his critique of homeopathy in 1851, 'When things are exceedingly laughable, it is a little unreasonable to demand of us an imperturbable gravity.'

## Royalty/celebrities use CAM

This is particularly egregious example of the appeal to authority fallacy. Because Prince Charles, a man with no medical training, recommends homeopathy, there is no more reason for anyone to take notice than when Gwyneth Paltrow recommends bee stings for anti-ageing, or rapper B.o.B claims the earth is flat.

## Science is incapable of explaining CAM

CAM practitioners like to co-opt the language of science when it suits them, for example claiming that homeopathy is explicable by quantum theory. At other times they will state that science is not yet sufficiently well-advanced to explain concepts such as vital force or *Qi*. These outdated concepts have been discredited scientifically, but even if they did exist, that would not be relevant, since science looks at both fundamental causes (i.e. biological plausibility) and tests whether treatments work (provability).

## Try it before you criticise

A common CAM argument is that you cannot criticise a treatment until you have tried it for yourself and seen the results. This is rather like saying you need to be a dairy farmer to know that the moon is not made of cheese. It is completely unnecessary and indeed potentially misleading to rely on personal experience to evaluate efficacy, not to mention completely impractical and unethical given the myriad of alternative medicine options. Homeopaths are convinced of their results, probably due to a range of cognitive biases described above. It is far more useful to assess the scientific evidence than to attempt to personally disentangle the confusion of experiences that comprises clinical practice. Nevertheless, some vocal critics of homeopathy have tried it, notably Edzard Ernst, Emeritus Professor of Complementary Medicine at the Peninsula School of Medicine, University of Exeter. In the veterinary world, Mike Jessop, past president of the British Small Animal Veterinary Association, used homeopathy in practice before becoming a critic and a founder member of the Campaign for Rational Veterinary Medicine.

## It works in animals

Really? Read on and find out if this is true.

# But We Just Know it Works! (A History of Unconventional Veterinary Treatments)

AT the time of writing there is, on the website of the British Association of Homeopathic Veterinary Surgeons (BAHVS) a story about Bedford, a dog who it is reported was diagnosed with a particularly nasty form of cancer, the squamous-cell carcinoma. This cancer affected the tissues of his head, causing distressing symptoms including facial deformity and pain. No one reading the account or looking at the photographs could fail to be moved by this dreadful case. The story continues, explaining that Bedford's owner, feeling conventional medicine had reached its limits, went on to seek homeopathic help, which was duly given, and to which he reportedly responded, eventually returning to his old self and able to enjoy life again, with no more problems.

Taken at face value, although the word 'cure' while persisting in the web address has been removed from the account itself, this story appears strongly to support the position that homeopathy can have profound, positive effects on one of the most dreaded of diseases, cancer. From the photographs it is clear the mass was initially large and painful, yet after treatment, although the second photograph provided is from a different angle, Bedford appears almost back to normal, the distortion of his brow and eyes seems to have gone and there is a keen look in his eyes.[1]

And what could be simpler – dog gets cancer, dog is given homeopathy, dog recovers. Surely this must be convincing proof of the power of homeopathy? Well, not necessarily, as I hope will be clear by the end of this chapter.

Stories, or anecdotes, such as that of Bedford, are not all they appear to be. They are fickle friends, purporting to convey real information in convincing form but in actual fact often misleading us in the search for the truth. In this chapter we will discover why there is a need to be cautious by looking for examples in the history and development of the veterinary profession itself and its changing attitudes to the evidence behind novel treatments and the nature of disease.

In the final analysis we believe simple stories at our peril and we are wrong to trust those who try to use them as evidence to convince us that Complementary and Alternative Veterinary Medicine (CAVM) is effective – anecdotes can mean anything we, or anyone else, want them to.

§

## The 'we just know it works' fallacy

In the end, a great number of debates with CAVM enthusiasts comes down to one impassioned cry, 'But we just know it works!' Practitioners of alternative medicine, unable to provide impartial proof and frustrated at critics unwilling to accept their claims at face value will, after giving the rhetorical equivalent of a deep sigh, come out with remarks such as, 'People bring their animals, we treat them and they get better – job done',[2] 'No amount of placebo-controlled crossover trials is going to convince me that the effects of homoeopathy, which I observe daily in practice, are a delusion',[3] or 'As a veterinarian now practising homeopathy and chiropractic almost exclusively, I have all the proof I need every day in my practice to justify these modalities'.[4]

What is being said is, in effect, never mind the science, just look at the results.

## CAVM and story-telling

These observations and alleged proofs come in the form of stories; hundreds of them – case reports, testimonials, personal anecdotes, from owner and therapist alike – in books, popular magazines and on websites. Life-affirming miracle cures, against all odds, involving real people and animals with which the reader can identify and empathise; they all reinforce the message that CAVM is good and effective, and will triumph where science-based medicine has failed.

The subjects range from the commonplace – homeopathy calming a skittish cat,[5] or zero-balancing curing constipation,[6] to the far-fetched (a farmer claiming to have calved a cow using homeopathy[7]) to downright irresponsible accounts of supposed cancer cures using CAVM (a claim that would be illegal in many parts of the world if it were made in the context of human medicine). The more one reads of these stories, the more it seems there is hardly a disease in existence that can't be cured by one form or another of CAVM. From womb infection (pyometra) to impacted anal glands in the dog; from an itchy cat to an egg-bound chicken; from aggression in pets to depression in baby elephants,[8] they are all relieved, gently and harmoniously, by the alternative therapist. At least, that's what we are led to believe.

## Just what is wrong with a good story?

Everyone loves a good story; they are one of the best, most vivid ways of getting a point across, and encouraging supporters. By simplifying things and making complicated issues seem easy to understand they illuminate and bring to life mundane facts and figures by giving us something familiar, something close to home. They win hearts and minds, as any propagandist or spin doctor will tell you.

It's hardly surprising, after all the human race was sitting round campfires swapping stories, millennia before some bright spark thought it might be a good idea to put one slab of sun-dried mud on top of another and call it a city. Tales, sagas, fables – oral history – allowed our ancestors to educate their children, swap hunting techniques and keep their past alive, all the time enhancing group cohesion and tribal identity. Stories are in our blood, we respond to them at a visceral level scientists can only dream of achieving with logic and reason.

But their power is illusory; in bypassing the brain and going straight to the emotions, stories also eliminate the need for rational thought and hard facts. Stories are no way to win an argument or debate the merits of a particular form of treatment. There will always be an equal and opposite story and if they are all we have to go on, then it is just one person's word against another.

Stories aren't all bad, of course, some have played an important role in medicine. William McBride's 1961 letter to *The Lancet* expressing his concerns about the apparent link between the use of the anti-morning sickness drug *thalidomide* and multiple, severe abnormalities in newborn babies was, at a mere 112 words, a master class in brevity.[9] In the same way, Dr J. M. Preston's brief letter to *The Veterinary Record* in 1983 warning practitioners about increasing reports of illness in certain breeds of dog following the use of the drug *ivermectin* served as the first indication of what proved to be a serious genetic problem in collies.[10]

Both these accounts however, were simply starting points, not proof-positive but precautionary advice only, until a scientific investigation was carried out to look into the anecdotal evidence that was accumulating. It is when anecdotes are used on their own, in the absence of rigorous scientific study, or even in an attempt to contradict research findings, that we run into problems – anecdotes are not a substitute for firm evidence.

## Why stories can't be trusted

With such great numbers of dramatic testimonials to support CAVM around though, wouldn't it be reasonable to question why scientists and practitioners of science-based medicine still insist there is no proper evidence to support the idea that CAVM is effective? Do cold-hearted scientists really believe the owners of animals treated homeopathically are incapable of judging whether or not that animal has improved? Veterinary practitioners of alternative medicine have completed long and difficult university courses; just the same as any other veterinary surgeon currently in practice; how can it be claimed those few, unlike their non-CAVM colleagues, are uniquely incapable of properly assessing a response to treatment?

Individual accounts used to illustrate the alleged benefits of CAVM have specific problems that may or may not be obvious on first reading. Errors, biases, omissions and partial truths all serve to cloud the issue and hide the full facts. In his book *How We Know What Isn't So*,[11] social psychologist Thomas Gilovich lists numerous ways by which such stories are, often unconsciously, 'improved' by those telling them as they attempt to make a story more appealing to the listener. These include the way some details are enhanced, or 'sharpened', while others are reduced, or 'levelled'. He also describes the story-teller's need to deliver a message in a way that is entertaining, for instance by placing themselves more centre-stage in events thus making the story more vivid and giving it more impact. This is done with the best of intentions – for clarity and to ensure the point the teller is making is properly illustrated – but it inevitably leads to a distortion in what we can truly 'know' from second-hand information.

On the same theme, Gilovich discusses the tendency for people to see what they want to see. He describes a predisposition to see certain events as 'one-sided', where the outcome (in this context, following treatment with CAVM) is perceived as an event only when it comes out one way (i.e. when the results appear to be 'successful'). Any outcome which conflicts with a person's world-view will be more likely to be dismissed as a mistake, the result of unavoidable external factors: the wrong remedy was chosen perhaps, or not administered for long enough, or for too long, or some outside influence blocked the effectiveness of the cure. This asymmetry, says Gilovich, will 'tend to accentuate information that is consistent with a person's expectations and pre-existing beliefs. As a result, people tend to see in a body of evidence what they expect to see'.

This inclination, while entirely understandable in those with such beliefs, means the CAVM success stories that we hear about are inherently partisan as we will inevitably hear about the 'positive' ones – the hits – while the rest are ignored. Someone whose ailing animal companion appears to have benefited from a 'miracle cure' will not only have their own beliefs reinforced but will be sure to tell their friends and neighbours all about it, while those whose pets have recovered from a minor ailment on their own, or after science-based treatment, are unlikely to want to shout this, rather unexceptional, fact from the rooftops.

The popularity of some stories and the means by which they come to our attention virtually guarantees they will be unreliable as evidence. Their very appeal makes them biased. How widely a story is disseminated depends on many factors, but it has distressingly little to do with the facts of the claim being made. Stories featuring alternative medicine, 'baffled scientists', appealing pets and an evangelical owner are a tempting prize for a media industry driven by an overriding commercial imperative that, of necessity, values entertainment and amusement more highly than truth and balance. In short, such attention-grabbing stories sell, in a way more mundane accounts can never hope to do in the popular press. After all, when did you last see a headline that read 'Elvis Still Dead'?

Popular appeal and literary merit, however, no matter how profitable, are no way to conduct a scientific debate and have no bearing on whether such stories reflect real life.

## The good old days?

Even if we recognise the inevitable spin imparted to accounts of supposed cures following CAVM treatment by enthusiastic and sincere proponents, that still leaves us with a number of cases where animals appear to have recovered from a variety of conditions following treatment that is regarded by the scientific community as implausible and ineffective. So doesn't that still mean those positive cases show CAVM works, even if only occasionally?

Unfortunately, like a lot of things in life, it's not that simple.

There is a well-known phenomenon, known as the caregiver placebo effect, where there is a powerful tendency in those looking after animals and who have an emotional attachment to them, to see what is expected or wished for following treatment, even in the absence of a genuine effect, or even to report an improvement when, to an objective observer there has been a deterioration.[12] There are plenty of real-world examples of this (most veterinary surgeons in practice will see examples every day), but for some of the most dramatic, we need look no further than the history of the veterinary profession itself. The story of how the profession has developed is replete with treatment regimes and diagnostic techniques long since discredited by science as useless, even harmful, but which were at the time regarded as highly effective, so much so they were considered mainstream and discussed and promoted in countless journals and texts of the day. Examining these archaic practices give us a means to hold a mirror up to the current claims of those who promote CAVM.

Although people have been treating illness and injury in animals for millennia, the veterinary profession as we know it today is said to date from 1761, when the first veterinary school was founded in Lyon, France by Claude Bourgelat.[13] In the same way that practitioners of human surgery were originally humble *Barber Surgeons*, veterinary surgeons were then known as *Surgeon Farriers*; the original horse doctors. Unsurprisingly there has been considerable change and an amount of reinvention since those early days as the profession grew and matured into its current form.

For a considerable period veterinary surgeons had great freedom to use non-evidence-based, idiosyncratic treatments and have done so until much more recently than was the case with human physicians. Not that long ago many treatments that would be regarded now as uncomfortably unorthodox were employed liberally and with vigour. Many veterinary surgeons qualifying as recently as the latter half of the last century will remember seeing collapsed cows being injected intravenously with methylene blue[14] (normally employed as a laboratory stain) to rouse them and get them up and walking again, coal-tar capsules – pungent smelling, green and shiny – used for the treatment of *Orf* (a viral disease of sheep), sulphur capsules for skin conditions and vitamin E for heart disease. Many veterinary practices, even today will have a dusty storeroom or basement somewhere, still containing the ingredients for long-forgotten medicines: enormous boxes full of ginger or kaolin powder, or demijohns labelled *Tincture of Heroin*, *The Red Drench*, the sinister-sounding *Black Drench* (a drench is a liquid medicine given by mouth to a horse or other livestock), or simply *Strychnine* (this last used as an appetite stimulant, needless to say in extremely small quantities). There were all manner of eccentric, often home-made (to secret recipes) tonics and restoratives, rubs and liniments (red or white: containing mercury or turpentine respectively). A form of folk medicine was also practised from time to time, with junior colleagues being admonished that if a cow or a pig was so ill it couldn't be induced to eat poison ivy (also considered to be an appetite stimulant) then its chances of recovery were limited and its days numbered.

Few, if any, of this eclectic range of treatments had anything approaching scientific proof behind them and virtually none of them are used today. Yet despite this, like many CAVM therapies today, people swore by them. Farmers and horse owners would insist on having them and vets would happily dispense them in the sure and certain knowledge they must work, otherwise people wouldn't keep coming back for more. It stands to reason, vets would tell themselves – in the same way that modern CAVM practitioners still convince themselves about their remedies – these products cost money to buy and were often fiddly to administer (as anyone who has ever tried giving a capsule to a sheep will testify), so why else would thrifty farmers and sensible stable-owners continue using them? Popular acclaim was seen as irrefutable proof of efficacy; 'results' were what mattered.

Going further back in time, two centuries or more ago, we come to a much darker and more harsh period in the history of the nascent veterinary profession, and treatments that most veterinary surgeons of today would scarcely recognise as true veterinary practice.

The age of *heroic medicine* was a painful and brutal world of phleams and blood-sticks, the rowelling bistoury, Seton needles, purgatives, cathartics and emetics, hot irons, blisters and irritants. In addition to the principal practices of the day – firing, cautery and blood-letting – the newcomer and darling of its age, phrenology, was also extended to animals as practitioners made great claims for its capacity to judge the characteristics and behavioural traits of animals.

## Cautery and firing

The first mainstay of the heroic age was cautery – attempting to promote healing by the application of what were euphemistically known as 'irritants' to the flesh of diseased patients. In practice this involved taking a horse with a particular condition and smearing the skin over the affected area with various compounds, often corrosive glacial acids, or alkalis, or substances derived from the plant or animal kingdom such as cantharides, mustard or oil of turpentine. Depending on their strength, these compounds would produce anything from a slight redness (the *rubefacients*) to full-blown blistering with actual destruction of tissue (the *pustulants* and *caustics*). If this wasn't considered adequate then these substances could be introduced directly into the deeper tissues by means of probes and tapes (Setons) inserted under the skin.

Even more dramatically, firing (also referred to as 'The Actual Cautery') used, not chemicals, but red-hot irons or pins that were applied to the affected area in order to create burns at different depths depending on the heat of the iron or how far the firing pin was driven through the skin.

Such procedures were performed by the surgeon and endured by the patient without the benefit of anaesthesia or analgesia with the (completely untested) assurance that ' … the higher the temperature, the less the pain attending its application …'[15]

## Bloodletting

The second mainstay of heroic medicine was bloodletting, or phlebotomising. This included local and general forms. Local bloodletting, not much practised by veterinary surgeons, usually involved the scarification of tissues to release blood; but could include either cupping or the application of leeches to an affected part of the body.

General bloodletting was however, greatly favoured by the veterinary surgeon and involved the drawing out of often prodigious amounts of blood from major blood vessels (usually the jugular) using a phleam (a sharp blade propelled into the vein by a spring or a blow from a wooden blood-stick) to open the vein, then pinning the vessel closed once finished. According to Finlay Dun, in the 1901 volume *Veterinary Medicines*:

*'Blood may generally be taken from full-grown horses or cattle to the extent of three or four quarts [a quart is two pints]. The amount drawn should be accurately measured. The circumstances of the case materially affect the amount of blood to be drawn. It should flow freely until its abstraction has made a decided impression on the volume and strength of the pulse, or until the earliest symptoms of nausea and fainting are apparent.'*

The truly heroic (and brutal) nature of this form of treatment is illustrated in this excerpt from William Youatt's 1843 work *The Horse*, describing the treatment of phrenitis (an arcane condition associated with over-excitation of the nervous system):

'*... now is the surgeon's golden time, and his courage and adroitness will be put to the test. He must open, if he can, both the jugulars: but let him be on his guard, for the paroxysm will return with its former violence and without the slightest warning ...*

'*The treatment of phrenitis has been very shortly hinted at. The first – the indispensable proceeding – is to bleed; to abstract as much blood as can be obtained; to let the animal bleed on after he is down; and indeed not to pin up [close] the vein of the phrenetic horse at all. The patient will never be lost by this decisive proceeding, but the inflammation may be subdued, and here the first blow is the whole of the battle.*'

## Phrenology

A relative newcomer to the veterinary medicine of the heroic age was *phrenology*. Widespread, respected and highly influential in the Western world, phrenology – the art of divining patients' personality traits by feeling bumps (presumed to reflect the relative development of different regions of the brain) on their heads – was employed by every strata of society.

The art of phrenology was taken to increasingly far-fetched heights when applied to animals, the external contours of whose heads conform even more loosely to those of the brain than is the case with humans. Yet authors in veterinary journals, such as Bracy Clark's 1828 *Farrier and Naturalist*, made great claims for its usefulness in improving breeding stock, and featured elegant engravings of the skulls of horses and dogs, portraying somewhat contrived-looking lumps that it was claimed demonstrated characteristics such as courage, meekness, temper (good or vicious) and 'love of offspring'.

In one account, veterinary phrenologists took the step of confronting the inventor of the phrenological art, the renowned Dr Spurzheim himself, with the skull of the late *Eclipse*, 'the celebrated race-horse'. The great doctor was allegedly able to pronounce as to the personality of this internationally famous animal by the sole means of examining the skull, so much so the article concluded, rather optimistically 'the Dr's observations may serve to show that this science will hereafter prove eminently useful in judging of the living animal'.[16]

It is said there is nothing new under the sun and while modern CAVM clearly has nothing approaching the barbarism of the ancient practices of bleeding and firing there are a lot of parallels between it and the defunct practices of antiquity in the way both claim to be effective and useful methodologies.

## Ancient roots

Like many current manifestations of CAVM, these heroic and now discredited techniques boasted an ancient provenance. The virtue of continued use over time prompts the claim that a technique wouldn't have been used for centuries or even millennia if it were not effective. While acupuncture today claims (with questionable justification) to have ancient Chinese roots dating back thousands of years, the origins of bleeding as a treatment for both human and animal disease has been reliably traced as far back as 3,000 years or more, to the Ancient Egyptians, the Ancient Greeks and Hippocrates in the fourth century BC.[17]

The origins of using fire to treat disease are so ancient as to be lost in the mists of antiquity but it is certainly mentioned in ancient Chinese writings,[18] and the Roman author, Vegetius, recorded its use during the fifth century AD.[19] In Europe its use was widespread; as far back as 1565 the author Blundeville was cautioning against its excessive use. This plea evidently fell on deaf ears as in 1796 John Hunter, in his *Dictionary of Farriery and Horsemanship*, gives us the first written recommendation, in the English-speaking world, of firing for the treatment of injured tendons in the horse.[20]

## A flash of genius

As we will see in Part Two, some types of CAVM claim more recent origins with homeopathy, chiropractic and the flower remedies having been created *ex nihilo* by inventive and charismatic individuals. In the same way, phrenology first emerged as the *Skull Doctrine* of German anatomist Franz Joseph Gall around 1790. Gall reasoned, purely on the basis of personal observation, that since the brain was the seat of intelligence, artistic endeavour, agility, maternal instinct and other traits, then naturally the parts of the brain connected with such traits must be larger in individuals with particular strengths in these areas and this, logically, must be reflected in the contours of the surrounding skull. The fact that none of this is true in any way didn't stop the doctrine later being consolidated by Gall's more influential and canny co-worker, Johan Spurzheim. Spurzheim invented the more scientific-sounding term *phrenology* and marketed it across the developed world until it became an apparently unstoppable, and highly lucrative, phenomenon, questioned only by a few isolated 'non-conformists' who were regularly derided in phrenological publications.

One of the main arguments of supporters of phrenology in the face of criticism could almost have been taken from any standard CAVM text today: 'test it and see.'[21]

## Plausible modes of action

Neither is there anything to distinguish modern CAVM from the ancient practices of the heroic age when it comes to how these treatments were imagined to work. For each technique there is, or was, a convincing-sounding explanation, from the patently pseudoscientific to the spiritual or metaphysical.

CAVM claims to be able to correct 'imbalances' or 'boost the immune system', or to help the body heal itself, or correct the flow of so-called natural energies. If pressed for a more scientific explanation practitioners of acupuncture will refer to pain-relieving endorphins, homeopaths will describe how quantum physics is just about to reveal its inner workings and chiropractors will point to spinal subluxations, visible only to chiropractors themselves.

Equally implausibly, cautery was thought by some to encourage the drawing back into the body of the harmful products of inflammation. English veterinary surgeon William Youatt advised, in the 1831 edition of his text, *The Horse,* that in the case of sprained ligaments in the horse, 'no stimulus short of the heated iron will be sufficient to rouse the absorbents' in order that 'injurious deposits' be removed and thickened tissues return to normal.

James Irvine Lupton, editor of the 1890 revision of *Mayhew's Illustrated Horse Doctor*, describes how some proponents of firing asserted the process created 'excited vital action' and allowed the absorption of diseased tissues. Finlay Dun's 1901 *Veterinary Medicines*[22] reported, without any justification in science, the similar idea that the direct application of corrosive chemicals to the skin were effective because 'they stimulate the trophic nerves and blood-vessels, promote healthy nutrition, and thus hasten healing'. In the same volume firing, it was claimed, '... modifies the nutrition of the diseased part' and '... increases the activity of the inflammatory process and hastens consolidation'.

Youatt also describes the concept of the *counter-irritant* whereby the (quite arbitrary) view was held that two forms of irritation could not exist in the same area of the body at the same time, so the application of an elective irritation (firing or cautery) would, by unspecified means, drive out a more harmful, disease-causing inflammation that was already present, thus resulting in a cure.

Further back in history, ancient societies, like modern proponents of CAVM, had more spiritual explanations and believed that fire imparted its healing effect by virtue of its cleansing properties and ability to drive out evil spirits.[23]

Bloodletting was claimed to have, as its mode of action, a more spiritual, 'restoring of balance', a mantra that has lasted until today, there being very few modern modes of CAVM that do *not* claim to restore balance in some way or other. This idea betrays strong links with the ancient so-called humoural medicine of Hippocrates and Galen, which maintained that, in a healthy body, the four humours (blood, phlegm, black bile and yellow bile) were in balance, with disease representing a disturbance of this balance that the physician's role was to correct, for instance by abstracting blood from a patient whose red, flushed countenance suggested a surfeit.[24]

And, as with CAVM, results were assured. In the 1843 edition of Youatt's *The Horse*, the author describes the radical degree of bleeding employed in the treatment of tetanus, assuring the reader, who is advised to 'bleed until the horse falters or falls', that the practitioner 'never had occasion to repent of the course which he pursued'.

## A loyal following

Popularity too, is a thing that heroic medicine had in common with CAVM; a popular mantra of the CAVM practitioner being to the effect that it must work, otherwise why would millions of people use it.

Throughout the Middle Ages in Europe bloodletting was one of the principal ways of treating illness and infirmity in animals.[25] The popularity of firing too, is evident from the multiple references to its use in virtually every veterinary textbook, particularly those dealing with the treatment of horses, until well into the twentieth century. Indeed as recently as the 1980s firing was still practised in the Saharan regions of Africa, in Central Asia and the Arabian Peninsula for the treatment of both man and animals.[26]

Phrenology had an extraordinary following in Victorian Europe and the USA. In its heyday it had millions of converts. There were thirty different phrenological societies in the early 1800s, including the British Phrenological Society, which even had its own library; eighty-five different phrenological journals were in publication during the period 1801–1889, and 4,000 books and pamphlets were published prior to 1928.[27] This level of popularity and literary activity, in an age without the benefits of electronic communication and mass media, must at least equal that of modern day CAVM practices such as homeopathy and acupuncture. Small wonder phrenologists believed, in the same way CAVM practitioners now believe, their art would endure forever and eventually come to stand as an equal with other branches of medical science.

With the seemingly sure foundations of ancient provenance, convincing modes of action and great popularity, proponents of firing, bleeding, cautery, phrenology and the like were more than able to convince themselves of the effectiveness of their preferred method of treatment or diagnosis. Their advocates – from eminent and impressively whiskered veterinary surgeons and surgeon-farriers, to horse owners, lowly grooms and stable boys – 'just knew' these methods of treatment and diagnosis worked because they believed the evidence of their own eyes and the stories of their contemporaries.

After all, they would have reasoned, if it doesn't work, why would my patients keep coming back time and again despite all the inconvenience and expense. Surely, if pressed about the truth behind their convictions, practitioners of heroic medicine would very likely have responded in the same way then, as practitioners of CAVM do now, 'People bring their animals, we treat them and they get better – job done,' or possibly, 'As a veterinarian now practising firing and bloodletting almost exclusively, I have all the proof I need every day in my practice to justify these modalities.' Just look at the results.

Yet, despite the firm, unshakable convictions of practitioners of the age, none of the practices of the heroic age of medicine survive in any meaningful way today. As time passed and scientific knowledge developed, careful, methodical research was slowly but surely able to disperse the obscuring smoke of the firing iron and the cloying stench of the blood pot. Now genuine, reliable evidence allows us to see the fallacy of using medical practices based solely on tradition, habit and dogma.

§

Today, firing and bloodletting are rightly regarded as pointless barbarism, while phrenology has been reduced to an amusing Victorian pastime and a source of novelty ornaments, literally relics of a bygone age.

The lesson we have learned from those 'bad old days' is that, no matter how tempting or obvious it may seem, it is simply not good enough to believe the evidence of our own eyes. We humans, however much we may wish to believe otherwise, are past masters of self-deception; not through any particular failing or desire to deceive, but simply because it is in our nature to be this way. We are hard-wired to find patterns and assume cause-and-effect, even where none exists. Such behaviour was saving our lives long before science came along to suggest there might be other ways of looking at things, ways more suited to life in a modern world. The ancestral hominid who stopped to rationally consider the options and weigh up the possible causes of the sound of a twig snapping behind him on a jungle path would have been highly likely to end his days expiring noisily in the jaws of an apex predator, while his companion; who just thought 'LION!' and immediately leaped for cover; would be the one more likely to live to produce similarly minded offspring for many years.

This type of evolutionary programming is extremely hard to overcome, and perhaps hoping we have learned lessons from the age of heroic medicine is being somewhat optimistic. Judging by the continuing success of the non-science-based medical practices discussed in this book, there is some way to go. Jumping to conclusions; seizing on one explanation of events on the basis of preference alone, while questioning or even ignoring others that are at odds with the way we like to imagine the world; is still the favoured option for many even in modern times when the likelihood of being attacked by that lion is infinitely lower than being deceived or even directly harmed by a plausible-sounding CAVM salesman.

§

Which brings us back to where we started this chapter, with the uplifting story of Bedford, treated homeopathically for his cancer.

I was curious to say the least when I first heard Bedford's story. My first thought, given what is known about homeopathy, was this story was unlikely to be true. Rather than dismiss it out of hand however, I wrote to the BAHVS, which was kind enough to send me an anonymised copy of Bedford's clinical history as far as November 2012, roughly five months after homeopathic treatment was started. On reading the notes I discovered there had been a significant omission from the BAHVS's version of Bedford's story. It transpires at the same time Bedford was receiving homeopathic treatment, he was also being treated with a drug of the non-steroidal anti-inflammatory (NSAID) group. This class of drugs, related to aspirin, is well researched and is widely known to have sometimes very dramatic anti-cancer properties, occasionally even on a par with chemotherapy,[28] particularly in the type Bedford had.[29]

Which treatment – homeopathy or NSAID – one believes contributed to the improvement in Bedford's condition will clearly depend on a number of factors, not least one's own 'belief', or lack of it, in homeopathy, and this case would certainly be worthy of debate in the light of the full facts, if only they had been given in the original story.

On the balance of probability it is almost certain Bedford's cancer was ameliorated by conventional medicine, not by homeopathy. Anyone reading the account as it stands and accepting it at face value however, could be forgiven for assuming the changes in Bedford's cancer were solely the result of homeopathic treatment and there was no such debate to be had. The BAHVS has been advised of this discrepancy in its account and, although the term NSAID now appears, there is still no explanation as to the significance of this treatment or how effective it is known to be in the treatment of cancers such as Bedford's.

Bedford's case makes the perfect illustration of why simple anecdotes can never be taken at face value or used as serious evidence. There is always an angle, whether it is selling newspapers or promoting CAVM – something to bear in mind the next time you hear the phrase 'I tried it and it worked!', no matter how plausible the story may sound, or who is telling it.

§

# PART TWO

## *Types of CAM, CAVM and related thinking – a critique*

# Herbs and Supplements (Including TCM, Ayurveda, Essential Oils and Zoopharmacgnosy)

## Herbal medicine

HERBAL medicines are defined by the NHS Choices website as 'those with active ingredients made from plant parts, such as leaves, roots or flowers'. Herbal medicine (or herbalism) is one of the oldest forms of medicine. As noted below in the section on zoopharmacognosy, even non–human primates (and other species) are observed to self-medicate in order for example to treat parasitism. A Neanderthal burial site yielded a number of pollens, seven out of eight of which were from species that were considered to have 'herbal and medicinal properties'.[1] Herbal medicines are important parts of the ancient arts of Ayurvedic and Traditional Chinese Medicine (TCM) (both of which are discussed in more detail below), and were used extensively in Ancient Egypt and classical antiquity.

Before the ability to synthesise compounds or to extract and purify medicines from plants was developed, herbal medicine, along with other ingredients found in nature, was the mainstay of the healer's toolbox. Efficacy of herbs in specific conditions would have been discovered by trial and error, and then passed along by word of mouth. Unfortunately, before controlled clinical trials were started, it is likely that many of the supposed effects of herbal medicines could be attributed to placebo, regression to the mean and so forth (see Chapter Four).

Some of the ancient recommendations for medical treatments have scientific merit. For example, Pliny the Elder included *Atropa belladonna*, which contains atropine, and *Urginea maritima*, which contains cardiac glycosides, in his list of cardiovascular remedies.[2] However, some of his suggested remedies are clearly absurd, such as a suggestion that to cure headaches, tie fox genitals to your head, or to cure incontinence, urinate in your dog's bed.

It is interesting to ask the question: why should ingestion of plants have any biological effect on mammals? In order for a herbal medicine to have an effect on the body, it must in some way interact with it, for example by binding to a pain receptor site, or blocking the action of a hormone, or alternatively interacting with a pathogen. Although there are some common biochemical pathways, the physiology of plants and mammals is vastly different, for example in areas such as enzymes, hormones and neurotransmitters. There are three main reasons why a compound found in a plant should have an effect on a mammal.

The first is pure coincidence. There are a vast number of chemical compounds within even the simplest plants, and some of these may interact with the mammalian physiology, in a beneficial or detrimental way, by chance. The toxic effects of lilies on cats and grapes on dogs are likely to be examples of this.

The second is due to an anti-pathogen effect against a common foe. For example, penicillin produced by fungi to destroy bacteria are also useful to mammals to fight those same bacteria.

The third is an evolutionary strategy on the part of the plant to deter consumption by mammals. In other words, plants have evolved mammalian toxins to prevent them being eaten. Plants and herbivores have co-evolved over millions of years in something of an arms race, plants developing toxins and other defences, herbivores developing resistance to those defences.[3] Mammals that have not evolved resistance to those defences, for example species that live in geographically separate areas, or carnivores, will still be susceptible to the toxic effects of those defences.

There is an aphorism in toxicology that states that the toxin makes the dose. This means that sublethal doses of a toxin will have an effect on the body system that may still be harmful but in other cases may have a beneficial effect. For example, atropine in belladonna is fatal in high doses, but in lower doses can treat bradycardia (low heart rate). Cardiac glycosides in digitalis are also fatal in high doses, but in lower doses improve cardiac contractility and reduce heart rate.

It follows from this last point that herbal remedies have the potential to be both efficacious and harmful (the exact opposite of homeopathy). It is therefore important to evaluate each herbal remedy individually for efficacy and safety.

Systematic reviews and meta-analyses are often considered the gold standard when it comes to evaluating the efficacy for medicines and interventions. There are a number of these, including Cochrane reviews, of herbal medicine. Many of these reviews draw similar conclusions, that there is some evidence of variable quality for the use of herbal medicines in certain diseases. For example, Liu et al[4] concluded that some herbal medicines may improve the symptoms of irritable bowel syndrome, but caution should be exercised due to small sample sizes and inadequate methodology. Liu et al[5] also concluded that herbal medicines may be of use in the treatment of fatty liver disease as assessed by biochemistry, ultrasonography and computed tomography, but that the findings were not conclusive because of the high risk of bias and the limited number of studies of individual herbal medicines. Cameron et al[6] concluded that although there is a rational basis for the use of topical herbal medicines in the treatment of osteoarthritis, that there was insufficient quality and quantity of studies to prove effectiveness. Nevertheless, topical Arnica gel was probably as effective as topical non-steroidal anti-inflammatory, although it probably was no safer. In a systematic review of herbal medicines in the treatment of childhood and adult asthma, Arnold et al[7] concluded that the evidence base was hampered by lack of available data and poor reporting. It should be noted that Cochrane reviews on herbal medicine have been criticised for not taking into account the lack of characterisation in many studies of the herbal medicines involved (e.g. which plant parts were in the medication prescribed).

A number of herbal medicines have made the transition from alternative medicine to veterinary medicine (i.e. have been proven to likely work) in the veterinary field. A recent example of this is the milk thistle extract silybin. Milk thistle has been extensively studied for its use in liver disease. Silymarin is a complex of milk thistle extracts, with silybin being the most biologically active.[8] Silybin has become accepted as a treatment of liver disease in dogs, and in a placebo-controlled trial, dogs undergoing treatment with the chemotherapy drug CCNU that were given a silybin-containing liver supplement suffered less liver damage than controls.[9] The effects are due to a combination of anti-oxidant and anti-inflammatory effects.[10] It is less clear whether whole milk thistle is more or less effective than the extracts. However, it is probable that if the active ingredients have been correctly identified, as the clinical trials indicate, then the purified form will be more concentrated than the whole milk thistle, and so can produce higher biological effects. Similarly, aspirin is more effective as an analgesic than the willow bark from which it is derived.

Another example is *Boswellia*, which is being incorporated into some nutraceuticals for the treatment of osteoarthritis. There is some evidence that this herbal extract is effective in reducing the signs of osteoarthritis such as intermittent lameness and stiff gait.[11]

However, a large number of other herbal treatments are recommended by alternative veterinary practitioners for which evidence of efficacy is much less, non-existent, or even suggests lack of efficacy. A search of 'herbal remedies' in the Veterinary Information Network (VIN) Message Board's alternative folder quickly revealed:

- a recommendation for treatment of nasal carcinoma with Essiac tea, for which there are no controlled clinical trials to demonstrate efficacy in people or animals, though it does appear to be associated with nausea and vomiting in people.
- a recommendation for use of tea tree oil as a topical anti-bacterial. There is weak evidence that tea tree oil has antibacterial and antifungal activity,[12] but is also commonly associated with side effects, mainly skin irritation, although these are usually mild and self-limiting.[13]
- a recommendation to use cranberry in the treatment of a case of feline lower urinary tract disease. Although initial studies of cranberry in humans for the treatment of idiopathic cystitis were promising, more recent, larger studies have cast doubt on this.[14]

The consultants on VIN are broadly very good at highlighting lack of evidence and potential for adverse effects. Nevertheless, herbal remedies with weak or no evidence of efficacy and some evidence of side effects are being recommended in the alternative medicines folder, and prescribed to pets on a regular basis.

Paul Pion, founder of VIN, when asked for comment, noted: 'You can find these recommendations on VIN if you seek them, but they are not the overwhelming message and the mass of more conventional recommendations are there in orders of magnitude greater volume. The discerning and mature colleague can easily find the conventional and evidence-based recommendations while being aware of alternatives which clients might bring up. Seems a reasonable balance to me.'

## Risks

Risks associated with the use of herbal medicines include side effects, lack of efficacy, inconsistency of formulation, drug interactions, contamination and non-adherence to medication. Edzard Ernst[15] wrote that the 'notion of herbal medicinal products being inherently safe is naive at best and dangerous at worst'. Historical use is no evidence of safety – although this may mean that the herb is safe in the short term, long-term side effects may be dangerous, as was discovered with tobacco, which as well as having recreational uses, was previously recommended for conditions such as colds, fever, digestive problems, strangulated hernia and malaria.[16]

## Side effects

In a review of cardiovascular side effects of herbal medicines Edzard Ernst listed adverse events including arrhythmias, congestive heart failure, pericarditis and death, though he noted that because of the anecdotal nature of the reports, it was hard to assess frequency of these events.[17] Herbal medicine is thought to be a cause of hepatotoxicity, although it is hard to attribute causality, especially because of the poor methodology of reporting.[18] It is probable that the incidence of toxicity from herbal medicine is lower than that from drugs, but the lack of regulation of the safety of herbal medicines and the poor reporting of adverse events make it hard to know how safe these treatments are. What is certain however, is that herbal medicine can be associated with serious adverse reactions, and that the fact that it is natural does not mean it is necessarily safe (see also the Mother Nature fallacy in Chapter Four).

## Lack of efficacy

There is some evidence for the efficacy of certain herbal preparations. In a systematic review of herbal medicines in cancer, Chaudhary et al found a significant reduction in mortality when herbal medicine was used alongside conventional treatments, compared to conventional treatments alone, and that adverse events were also lower.[19] Another overview of systematic reviews found evidence in favour of a few herbal medicines such as ginger for pregnancy-induced nausea and feverfew for migraine prevention.[20] However, the authors note that firm conclusions of efficacy cannot generally be drawn, and highlight inconclusive or contradictory evidence for the efficacy of echinacea for prevention of the common cold, gingko for tinnitus and *Aloe vera* for psoriasis.

## *Inconsistency of formulation*

As herbal medicines are unregulated, they often contain active ingredients in different proportions making it hard to generalise the effects. As whole plants are often used, there can be many active ingredients. Although multiple drug use is minimised in conventional medicine because of the risk of interactions and unpredictable side effects, herbal medicine advocates claim that the multiple ingredients reduce toxicity, a concept known as buffering. There is some limited evidence of this effect, but it is not known how much it can be generalised.[21]

## *Drug interactions*

Herbal medicines often contain biologically active ingredients, and this means there is the potential for unexpected interactions with other biologically active chemicals such as drugs. One well-known example of this is grapefruit juice extract, which is recommended by some as an anti-microbial, as well as in flea control. Grapefruit juice extract inhibits the intracellular enzymes known as cytochrome P450, which function to metabolise some drugs. Grapefruit juice extract administered at the same time as many drugs can elevate the amount in the blood from safe to toxic levels. Veterinary relevant drugs that can dangerously interact with grapefruit juice include diazepam,[22] sildenafil, amiodarone[23] and cyclosporine.[24]

## *Contaminants*

Contamination of herbal medicines with toxins is commonly reported in the scientific literature. Chan[25] reports anticholinergic poisoning from herbal medicines, due to contamination or erroneous substitution of non-toxic for toxic herbs. Chan[26] also describes aconitum alkaloid poisoning because of contamination of herbs with aconite roots. Zamir et al report contamination of herbal medicines with pathogenic bacteria.[27] In an overview of systematic reviews about the contamination and adulteration of herbal medicinal products, Posadzki et al[28] found contamination of herbal medicines with 'dust, pollens, insects, rodents, parasites, microbes, fungi, mould, toxins, pesticides, toxic heavy metals and/or prescription drugs'. Adverse effects of these adulterations included 'agranulocytosis, meningitis, multi-organ failure, perinatal stroke, arsenic, lead or mercury poisoning, malignancies or carcinomas, hepatic encephalopathy, hepatorenal syndrome, nephrotoxicity, rhabdomyolysis, metabolic acidosis, renal or liver failure, cerebral edema, coma, intracerebral haemorrhage, and death'.

## *Non-adherence to medications*

Patients taking herbal medicines (and other alternative medicines) seem less likely to adhere to the regime of prescribed conventional medicines and this has been demonstrated by Martins et al, which showed that medication non-adherence in elderly people increased with increasing use of herbal medicines.[29]

Another potential problem with herbal medicines is the approach of herbal practitioners to diagnosis and prescription. Diagnosis is considered in more detail in Chapter Twelve. Also, in many cases, once a 'diagnosis' is made, a combination of herbal medicines are prescribed, individualised to the patient based on unscientific diagnostic procedures. This makes it hard to assess the efficacy of a preparation, when so many herbs are given together, and patients suffering from the same medical condition are prescribed different medications.

§

# Nutraceuticals

The term nutraceutical was coined by Dr Stephen L. DeFelice, the head of the Foundation for Innovation in Medicine (FIM), to mean 'a food or part of a food that has a medical or health benefit, including the prevention and treatment of disease'. Specific nutrients such as vitamins and minerals are not usually considered to be nutraceuticals. The word was derived from a combination of nutrition and pharmaceutical, but Dr DeFelice notes that spelling 'nutra' rather than 'nutri' came about because he was drinking grappa in Rome when he came up with the word, and felt that nutra simply sounded better than nutri.[30]

A nutraceutical is an attractive sounding concept. At its simplest, it involves eating foods deemed to be beneficial to health (known as a functional food). However, more commonly, a nutraceutical is an active ingredient isolated from food in a more purified form, termed a dietary supplement.

The term nutraceutical has no meaning in US or European Law, and so these products are regulated as a drug or a food depending on their ingredients and their health claims. The UK Advisory Committee on Borderline

Substances (which advises on the prescribing of foodstuffs and toiletries) notes that while the European Commission states 'health claims for foods should only be authorised for use in the Community after a scientific assessment of the highest possible standard' (Regulation (EC) No.1924 / 2006), this is not always met by companies wishing to bring nutraceutical products to market. Specific health claims are therefore not usually made for nutraceuticals, and they are marketed in terms of health promotion and disease prevention rather than disease management, which the committee notes often makes them attractive to the 'worried well'.[31]

When nutraceuticals are considered to be foodstuffs, they do not have to conform to the same level of safety and efficacy rules that apply to prescription drugs, although they have to comply with food safety legislation. They are more readily available than conventional medicines, since they don't need a prescription from a doctor or veterinary surgeon to purchase them, and many people choose to medicate themselves or their pets with these products, with or without medical or veterinary advice.

It is beyond the scope of this chapter to examine the claims for all the available veterinary nutraceuticals. However, there are many cases where the use of a nutraceutical is grounded in good research and is considered the standard of care. One example is S-adenosyl methionine (SAM-e). This chemical is produced and used in the liver for various biochemical reactions, and decreased SAM-e production occurs in all forms of chronic liver disease.[32] It has been shown in meta-analyses to have a role in the treatment of chronic liver disease in humans, although maybe without as much effect as was previously thought to be the case.[33] It is important to use caution when extrapolating the results of human trials to the veterinary field. There is some (albeit slightly mixed) evidence from human meta-analyses that SAM-e may have a role in the treatment of osteoarthritis[34] but a veterinary trial did not find a beneficial effect of SAM-e on the same condition in dogs.[35] Nevertheless, SAM-e is generally considered a safe and efficacious treatment for chronic liver disease in dogs.

One of the biggest selling nutraceuticals in the veterinary field is glucosamine, often given in combination with chondroitin and other supplements. As it is not marketed as a pharmaceutical it does not come under the control of the Veterinary Medicine Directorate (VMD) in the UK, and as with other nutraceuticals, health claims have to be made cautiously. It is therefore often marketed as maintaining healthy cartilage and supporting joint function, rather than claiming to treat osteoarthritis specifically. Glucosamine is produced naturally by the body, and is important in the manufacture of cartilage. In vitro studies show it to be mildly anti-inflammatory and able to stimulate proteoglycan synthesis by chondrocytes – the cells that produce cartilage.[36]

Initial trials of glucosamine in the human fields showed promise. For example, a 1994 randomised trial of glucosamine sulphate in knee osteoarthritis in humans showed the supplement to be as effective as ibuprofen, with fewer adverse effects,[37] and a 2000 meta-analysis was cautiously positive.[38] However, the more trials that were performed, the weaker the evidence in favour of glucosamine became. Osteoarthritis is a problematic condition to study because it has a natural variation in severity, and the placebo effect may be quite powerful in this disease. Many patients therefore see an initial improvement when taking any intervention for osteoarthritis, due to either placebo effect or regression to the mean (see Chapter Four). One useful study examined patients who had shown an initial improvement after starting glucosamine treatment. In a placebo-controlled trial, patients were swapped on to a placebo instead of glucosamine, and were monitored for a flare up of symptoms. There was no evidence of a decreased rate of symptom flare up in the patients continuing to receive glucosamine compared to placebo, nor any other secondary measurements, such as use of other analgesic drugs and changes in pain, function, stiffness and quality of life.[39] A 2005 Cochrane review showed no benefit of glucosamine over placebo for pain or a standardised arthritis index, except with a specific brand from the Rotta company, which did show some superiority over placebo.[40] However, it has been noted that the Rotta trials were older, and also tended to come from non-English speaking countries where the percentage of positive trials published is higher,[41] and also that since this review further negative evidence for glucosamine has emerged, such as a large trial by Clegg et al.[42]

In veterinary trials, the evidence is mixed. D'Altilio et al showed in a small trial that glucosamine and chondroitin appeared to alleviate some pain in dogs with osteoarthritis, especially when used in combination with glycosylated undenatured type II collagen, and withdrawal led to a relapse of pain.[43] It is important to note in veterinary osteoarthritis trials that both owners and vets are very bad at subjectively assessing the pain levels of dogs,[44] and that trials using force platform gait analysis are required to measure improvements in osteoarthritis-associated clinical signs. A systematic review of treatments of osteoarthritis in dogs concluded there was a high level of comfort for the evidence that meloxicam is efficacious, but that there is only a moderate level of comfort for the evidence backing a combination of glucosamine, chondroitin and manganese. A review of glucosamine-based nutraceuticals in the treatment of equine joint disease was even less positive, concluding that the quality of the scientific evidence was too low to make meaningful conclusions about the use of these nutraceuticals in horses. A study of pharmacokinetics of glucosamine and synovial fluid analysis in horses also concluded that the levels of glucosamine in the joint fluid after oral administration was 500 times lower than the concentration at which glucosamine modifies chondroitin (an important component of cartilage) in tissue culture studies.[45] The authors speculate that the apparent improvement in pain with the use of the drug may be due to effects on non-articular tissues, but of course this study was produced before the larger scale studies questioning whether there is genuinely an improvement in pain with the use of glucosamine. More recently, a three-month trial of a glucosamine-based nutraceutical in twenty-four geriatric horses using objective treadmill measurements of gait found no improvement over placebo.[46]

The use of glucosamine in human and veterinary medicine remains controversial. With a perceived improvement in humans, and a very low adverse effect rate, many guidelines still recommend a place for glucosamine-based treatments in the management of osteoarthritis. However, as pets probably don't receive the benefits of the placebo effect, and since we know from the caregiver placebo effect that vets and owners are bad at recognising pain in pets, glucosamine for the painful and common condition of osteoarthritis should be used with caution, and probably not in place of a proven effective treatment such as non-steroidal anti-inflammatory drugs.

Nutraceuticals are dietary supplements and as such, and in common with many complementary and alternative medicines, do not and should not make specific medical treatment claims. This means, however, that they are not required to show scientific evidence of efficacy prior to marketing. If considering using a nutraceutical in the management of a health condition, a careful examination of the available published evidence is sensible, and if the conclusion is that the dietary supplement or nutraceutical is safe and efficacious, then it should be purchased from a reputable manufacturer who guarantees the formulation of the product.

§

## Traditional Chinese Medicine

Traditional Chinese Medicine (TCM) refers to the practice of medicine based on ancient Chinese practices, including herbal medicine, acupuncture, dietary therapy and massage. Herbal medicine is considered in the first section of this chapter, acupuncture is considered in Chapter Eight, and manipulative therapies are considered in Chapter Eleven. However, TCM has an ethos and philosophy that differs from the Western approach to herbal medicine and acupuncture and Western medicine in general, from its theories on the causes of disease, to its approach to diagnosis, as well as treatment.

Evidence for medical practices in China dates back to the Shang Dynasty, which ruled in the fourteenth to eleventh centuries BC. Documentation of Chinese Materia Medica (the collected knowledge about a therapeutic product) dates back to 1100 BC and by the end of the sixteenth century AD almost 1,900 different medicines had been documented.[47]

TCM was given a huge boost in China by Chairman Mao. His barefoot doctor idea attempted to take health care to the masses in the countryside, where urban-trained doctors would not settle. They were to provide basic preventative health care and treatment. Dr Alan Levinovitz, in an article in Slate.com,[48] asserts that Mao did not believe in TCM and did not use it himself but as there were few Western-trained doctors who could provide modern health care, many people relied on traditional methods. From necessity therefore, Mao invented the concept of One Medicine, a unification of western and Chinese medical theories. As romantic Westerners with idealised notions of Chinese mysticism showed an interest in TCM, knowledge of TCM became a valuable export, improving Chinese–Western relations. Unfortunately, there wasn't really any one thing that constituted TCM, since local practitioners tended to use an individualistic mix of astrology, demonology, yin-yang, folk wisdom and personal experience. Mao brought about the standardisation of practices, with new textbooks being written to codify these practices, as well as marketing TCM to Westerners with sensational reports of efficacy. It has been reported that one reason for TCM's popularity in the West is its promotion by the amazing propaganda machine of Maoist China.

The philosophy behind 'modern' TCM (if you will excuse the oxymoron) is complex and beyond the scope of this book to examine in any detail, although Chapter Eight is devoted to the development of acupuncture, a branch of TCM. TCM incorporates the concepts of *Qi*, the body's vital energy, which flows through channels called meridians, and the concepts of yin-yang, two forces that act in balance to form a dynamic whole, and are present in all things. *Qi* has similarities to the concept of vitalism, the discredited notion that living and non-living tissues can be distinguished by the presence of some non-physical element. Imbalances in yin–yang supposedly result in diseases. TCM also believes that everything in the universe can be broken down into one of five phases or elements – water, fire, earth, wood and metal. Although these concepts may seem like historical oddities, with no place in the real world, they are considered important when it comes to TCM diagnosis and treatment.

The art of TCM diagnosis is also covered in Chapter Twelve, but in brief, involves history taking, observing, listening, palpating and smelling. Emphasis is placed on the pulse and the tongue, and will lead to a diagnosis, not of a disease, but of imbalances in yin/yang and *Qi*, which allow the TCM practitioner to select the correct herbs.

The evidence for the effectiveness of TCM in health conditions is generally low. A study in the *Journal of Complementary and Alternative Medicine* looked at the evidence from seventy Cochrane systematic reviews of TCM, twenty-six involving acupuncture and forty-two involving Chinese herbal medicine.[49] In nineteen of the acupuncture reviews and twenty-two of the herbal medicine reviews it was decided there was not enough good quality evidence to draw any firm conclusions. The rest suggested a possibility of benefit, while pointing out the quality of evidence was poor. It should be noted, however, that systematic reviews of TCM have been criticised, for reasons such as including studies that did not have TCM practitioner involvement, or not searching Chinese databases.[50]

As well as concerns about the diagnostic procedure, and a dearth of high-quality evidence for efficacy of TCM therapies, two other concerns exist about the practice of TCM. One is safety. Chinese medicines are poorly regulated and as such often contain undeclared ingredients, many of which may be toxic. One recent study used mass spectrometry and DNA sequencing to audit twenty-six TCMs. Fifty per cent of the samples contained DNA from undeclared plant or animal species, and in 50 per cent an undeclared drug was discovered, such as warfarin, steroids and non-steroidal anti-inflammatory drugs. Arsenic, lead and cadmium were also discovered, with one sample containing ten times the acceptable level of arsenic. Ninety-two per cent of the medicines tested had at least one contaminant.[51] Even for the declared ingredients, toxicity studies are uncommon, and although the ancient texts give information on toxicity based on observation over the years,[52] to truly assess the long-term effects of products requires sophisticated large-scale epidemiological studies.

The other concern about TCM regards conservation and animal welfare. TCM often involves the use of endangered species. Recent textbooks advocate the use of rhino horns, tiger bones and bear or snake bile.[53] One study in China revealed that consumers of TCM believe that medicines made from wild animals are more effective than those from farm-raised animals.[54] The Coghlan DNA study mentioned above revealed the presence of an endangered species of Snow Leopard in one sample. The demand for TCM and other forms of traditional medicine is having a real impact on the survival of certain species. For example, the rhino is being illegally hunted by poachers for its horn, which is used as an aphrodisiac, a medicine and a status symbol, according to the charity Save The Rhino.[55] The problem is summarised succinctly by Richard Ellis, author of *Tiger Bone and Rhino Horn: The Destruction of Wildlife for Traditional Chinese Medicine*. He stated, 'It is heartbreaking to realise that the world's rhinos are being eliminated from the face of the earth in the name of medications that probably don't work.'[56]

One of the few therapies to make the transition from TCM to the mainstream is ursodeoxycholic acid (UCDA), a derivative of bear bile. UCDA has important properties that aid in a variety of liver diseases. Unfortunately, unlike conventional pharmaceutical companies that use a synthesised version, TCM prefers the use of bear bile in its natural state. As hunting for bears to extract the bile was causing their numbers to decline, it became common practice to farm bears for their bile.

Various methods exist to extract the bile from living bears, including repeated needle extraction under ultrasound guidance, temporary or permanent catheterisation, and creating a fistula, i.e. a permanent hole into the gall bladder allowing bile to drip out. Bears are caught when they are cubs, kept in cages that are too small for them to turn around or sit up, and bile is extracted from the age of about three for up to twenty years. More than 50 per cent of the bears die from complications associated with bile extraction. There are currently around 7,000 bears undergoing this inhumane procedure in China.[57]

In conclusion, TCM relies on a non-scientific philosophy of ill health, promoted for political reasons by Mao. Its diagnostic methods are unsafe, its evidence base is poor, there are significant risks of toxins both from the medicines used and contaminants, and there are major ecological and welfare issues involved in the production of TCM remedies. The downsides of TCM overall seem to greatly outweigh its benefits.

§

# Ayurveda

Ayurveda is Sanskrit for 'life knowledge' and is an alternative medicine system with its origins in India as long ago as 5000 BC. As with Traditional Chinese Medicine, Ayurveda has its own diagnostic system using the practitioner's five senses, plus evaluation of faeces, urine and pulse. Similar to the beliefs of classical antiquity, Ayurveda believes physical matter is made up of the elements of fire, water, air, earth and ether. Seven basic tissues are described: blood; semen; bone; marrow; muscle; fat; plasma. Ayurvedic practitioners take a holistic approach to wellness, believing that the physical and mental existence and the personality are linked and influence each other. Reminiscent of chiropractic, Ayurveda believes the body has fluid-containing channels, which if unhealthy can cause disease, and which can be opened up by massage and fomentation.

Many Ayurvedic treatments are derived from plants such as roots, leaves, bark and seeds, although animal extracts such as bones and gallstones, and minerals such as sulphur, arsenic and lead are also used.

There are very few studies of Ayurveda in veterinary medicine. One paper appeared to show a protective effect in an experimental model of acute pancreatitis in dogs from the plant *Emblica officinalis* which is prescribed in Ayurvedic medicine.[58] Another showed that extract of the bark of *Terminalia arjuna* could induce hypotension in anaesthetised dogs, consistent with its use in cardiovascular disease in Ayurveda.[59] Another showed evidence of improvement of quality of life and no evidence of toxicity in a mercury preparation given to geriatric dogs.[60] In the human literature, various reviews have shown some evidence of efficacy for Ayurvedic treatments. For example, Gupta et al concluded that there is evidence for efficacy in the treatment of oral disease in a review of Ayurveda in dentistry, although the search terms of the review included all mentions of herbal treatments.[61] In a systematic review and meta-analysis of Ayurveda in the treatment of osteoarthritis, some evidence for the efficacy of certain herbs was found, but not for therapies such as massage, steam therapy and enema.[62]

Ayurvedic has some risks associated with it. Like other types of herbal medicine, there is some risk of toxin contamination, but unlike Western herbal medicine heavy metals are included deliberately as a treatment. One fifth of US-manufactured and Indian-manufactured Ayurvedic preparations in one study had detectable lead, mercury or arsenic levels,[63] with cases of lead poisoning from Ayurvedic medicines being reported in pregnant women,[64] and a cluster of lead poisoning cases in a community using Ayurvedic medicines has also been identified.[65]

Ayurveda does not currently appear to be in widespread use in the treatment of pets, but it is offered by some vets with an interest in herbal medicine.

The herbal aspects of Ayurveda, as with other types of herbal medicine, have some scientific plausibility and some evidence of efficacy. There are also significant risks of some forms of Ayurvedic, particularly those containing heavy metals.

§

# Essential oils (see also aromatherapy)

The term essential oils refers to the concept that these chemicals contain the 'essence' of the plant's fragrance. It does not mean the oil is essential to the body, unlike essential amino acids or essential fatty acids that are absolute nutritional requirements for an individual. Essential oils are hydrophobic chemicals derived from plants by processes such as steam distillation, solvent extraction and cold pressing. They can have various uses, including in oil paints (linseed oil), perfumes, cosmetics, household fragrances and for medicinal purposes. One website selling essential oils lists products to be used as household cleaners, shampoos, moisturisers and fragrances for religious and spiritual purposes. Modern medicinal use of essential oils tends to involve aromatherapy, since the oils may be toxic if ingested. Aromatherapy is discussed in more detail in Chapter Thirteen. This section will discuss the non-aromatherapy medicinal uses of essential oils, which include lavender, cinnamon, clove, eucalyptus, peppermint and tea tree oils.

In human medicine, essential oils are not well studied. This is partly due to the difficulty of experimental design. Because of the fragrances of essential oils, it is hard to blind a study, making controlled trials problematic. Without blinding, it is hard to know if any observed effect is due to the oil itself. For example, some oils are applied by massage, and any improvement may be due to the relaxing effects of the massage itself. Also, as was noted in the herbal medicine section, essential oil treatments are not standardised, and the constituent of a preparation may vary with factors such as where and when the parent plant was harvested, how it was prepared and how it was packed and stored.

Nevertheless, some studies appear to show beneficial effects from essential oils. Tea tree oil (TTO) is one of the more popular essential oils, used for its reported antimicrobial and anti-inflammatory effects. One review of the use of TTO reports that the evidence shows that TTO has anti-bacterial, anti-viral, anti-protozoal and anti-fungal properties.[66] TTO has been shown to be effective in vitro against methicillin resistant *Staphyloccocus aureus* or MRSA[67] and its antibacterial mode of action has even been elucidated – it inhibits respiration and increases bacterial and yeast membrane permeability.[68] In vitro work has also demonstrated inhibition of inflammatory mediators[69] although it is important to recognise that success in vitro does not always translate into a successful in vivo treatment (see glossary). There is some evidence of in vivo efficacy, for example Dryden et al showed that TTO can be as effective in clearing MRSA colonisation as a standard antibiotic regimen.[70]

However, tea tree oil can be associated with significant toxic side effects. If ingested it can cause lethargy and ataxia, and the LD50 (the dose at which 50 per cent of a population will die from toxic effects) is 1.9 to 2.6ml/kg.[71] There are reports of oral poisoning in children and adults, although no human deaths have been reported. Topical application has been associated with allergic reactions, and with irritant reactions when TTO is applied at higher concentrations. Packaging of TTO preparations can be problematic, since the oils can be absorbed into plastic packaging. Also there is evidence that the antimicrobial activity can be reduced in the presence of organic matter leading to concerns as to how effective TTO is in the presence of pus and blood.[72] Nevertheless, in an age of increasing worries about antibiotic resistance, TTO may have a role in human medicine, although further work with large-scale controlled trials is needed to confirm safety and efficacy.

The veterinary literature on TTO is sparse. One small, non-controlled study describes the treatment of prostatic abscesses in six dogs by aspiration of pus followed by injection of TTO into the abscess cavities, with disappearance of the purulent material and reduction in volume of the cavities being noted on follow up.[73] A topical TTO cream has been shown to be effective in the treatment of acute and chronic dermatitis in dogs in a controlled trial.[74] TTO has also been shown to be effective in vitro against *Malassezia* isolated from dogs with skin disease.[75] However, there have been reports of toxicity in animals. Villar et al reported findings from the National Animal Poison Center in the USA in which signs of depression, weakness, inco-ordination and muscle tremors were noted as the main presenting signs of TTO toxicity, although the authors noted that most cases were associated with inappropriately high doses.[76] A more recent study of 443 cases of 100 per cent TTO toxicity in dogs and cats reported signs of salivation, central nervous system depression, tremors, ataxia and paresis.[77] Doses ranged from 0.1ml to 85ml. Fifty per cent of the cases involved topical cutaneous application and 15 per cent oral, the rest being both oral and cutaneous. Eighty-nine per cent of cases were treated deliberately. Younger and smaller cats were more likely to be more severely ill.

Another essential oil that is recommended for its anti-inflammatory properties is wintergreen oil, which contains methyl salicylate. When topical oil of wintergreen was compared to oral aspirin (acetyl salicylic acid), it was found that anti-platelet effects were similar, maybe unsurprisingly given their chemical similarity.[78] However, this is a potential use for patients requiring anti-platelet treatment who cannot tolerate oral aspirin.

Other studies of essential oils in veterinary use include an in vitro study showing efficacy of extracts of the Peruvian pepper tree, *Schinus molle*, against the flea *Ctenocephalides felis felis*.[79] Manuka oil has been demonstrated in vitro to be effective against canine *Staphylococcus pseudintermedius*.[80] A spot on of fatty acids and essential oils has been shown to have been safe and effective in a controlled study of the treatment of atopic dermatitis.[81] In a blinded crossover trial of twenty dogs, a topical gel containing essential oils and antioxidants was shown to reduce oral malodour.[82] However, Genovese et al[83] reported adverse reactions in dogs and cats from essential oil-containing natural flea products, with three out of forty-eight cases resulting in death or euthanasia of the pets.

Other reports of toxic effects of essential oils in humans include a possible cause of gynecomastia (development of breasts) in three prepubescent boys.[84] Use of essential oils in pregnancy is controversial, with many women self-medicating with essential oils when pregnant, despite a lack of safety information at this time.

In conclusion, as with other natural and herbal medicines, some essential oils show promise in the treatment of certain conditions. However, as with all biologically active treatments, adverse reactions are reported, and domestic pets are potentially vulnerable to serious adverse effects associated with the use of essential oils.

§

## Zoopharmacognosy

Zoopharmacognosy is a particular type of herbal medicine that involves the animal itself choosing its own cure. The word zoopharmacognosy is derived from the Greek words zoo (animal) pharma (drug) and gnosy (knowing). The term was coined in 1993 to describe observations that wild animals sometimes appear to have the ability to self-medicate using naturally occurring remedies, in order to treat certain diseases.[85] A number of scientific reports demonstrate this behaviour in a wide range of animals, from insects to primates. In many cases, this behaviour is anti-parasitic in nature. For example, fruit flies seek out ethanol-containing foods when infected with the larvae of endoparasitoid wasps.[86] Bees have been shown to increase resin collection, which they incorporate into their nest architecture as an anti-fungal treatment.[87] There is even some evidence to suggest that urban birds incorporate cigarette butts into their nests as the nicotine is anti-parasitic.[88] Chimpanzees, bonobos and gorillas have all been shown to swallow whole leaves that are excreted undigested, thought to be an anti-parasitic treatment.

Most dog owners will have seen their dogs eat grass. It has often been stated they do this when they are ill in order to make themselves vomit. My personal observations are that many dogs eat grass regardless of their health, although I believe that a nauseous dog will seek out grass more than a non-nauseous one. One study showed that 68 per cent of dogs ate plants on a regular basis, and that only 9 per cent were ill before eating grass, and only 22 per cent vomited frequently afterwards.[89] Plant eating is therefore thought to be normal dog behaviour, and may be another anti-parasite strategy.

It is not surprising that animals have developed anti-parasite behaviour. Parasites are a major threat in the wild, reducing fitness, survival and ability to reproduce. There is therefore a strong evolutionary imperative to reduce parasite burden, and an animal that evolves a successful anti-parasite strategy, for example making use of phytochemicals or physical cures (e.g. grooming or purging) will have an advantage in the struggle to pass on genes.

Zoopharmacognosy therefore has a basis in scientific fact. However, recently, the concept of Applied Zoopharmacognosy, or AZ, has been coined to describe self-medication in pets and other animals for behavioural and medical issues. Animals are offered essential oils, clays, algae and dried plants in order to self-select cures. The cures may be inhaled, ingested or applied topically. AZ practitioners assess the facial and body language of the animal to decide which remedies it is showing a preference or a dislike for. Success has been claimed in the treatment of behavioural problems, dermatological problems, liver tumours and even skin wounds.

It may come as no surprise that analysis of case studies on the internet provide little or no evidence for the efficacy of AZ. A 'liver tumour' case study was not in fact a confirmed liver tumour, but a cat with ascites and jaundice. The cat improved over seven months of AZ. Concurrent medical treatment is not described. These findings however, could easily be explained by a case of cholangiohepatitis, responding to conventional medical therapy, or even being self-limiting. A skin wound case study involved a superficial laceration approximately 2cm in length that the dog 'self-selected' to treat with yarrow and green clay. In this case, a more detailed case history, including photographs, allows a better assessment of the course of the condition. Despite the AZ practitioner expressing surprise at the speed of healing, the photographs simply show the progress of a wound healing by second intention over a two-week period. This is the normal time course for a wound of this nature to heal.

Numerous criticisms can be levelled at Applied Zoopharmacognosy. First, there is to my knowledge not a single peer-reviewed paper regarding the use of AZ. A search of PubMed and the Veterinary Information Network (VIN) using the terms 'Applied Zoopharmacognosy' and 'Self-medication dogs, cats' gave no examples of controlled clinical trials, case series, or even a single case report of the use of AZ. This makes AZ a biologically plausible treatment, with no evidence of efficacy.

Second, the limited range of options that the animal is offered to treat itself with does not replicate the situation in the wild, and the reliance on essential oils, concentrated chemicals extracted from plants by processes such as steam distillation, solvent extraction or cold pressing (which themselves have limited evidence for efficacy and involve some risks) seems at odds with the concept of allowing the animal to select cures that are available in nature.

Third, the choice of treatment does not involve the animal ingesting the product voluntarily. Rather, it relies on the AZ practitioner interpreting the animal's wishes via its body language and facial expressions, something that must be extremely subjective and subject to misinterpretation.

Fourth, some of the treatments selected may be toxic. It is well known to all vets that dogs and cats voluntarily ingest toxins on a regular basis, be they drugs, chemicals such as anti-freeze or natural products such as chocolate. AZ practitioners argue that pets only ingest toxins that come from geographical areas that those pets did not evolve in, and so have not evolved an aversion to the substance. For example, cocoa comes from the New World while dogs evolved in the Old World. However, this is clearly not the case for other substances. Onions can cause haemolytic anaemia in dogs, and have been cultivated in the Old World since Bronze Age times, with wild onion native to the same areas as dogs. Grapes can cause acute kidney injury in dogs, and are found throughout the old world. Lilies can cause acute kidney injury in cats, and have a wide geographical distribution across Europe and Asia.

Finally, it needs to be considered whether AZ practitioners, most of whom are currently not vets, are performing acts of veterinary diagnosis and treatment, something that is illegal under the UK's Veterinary Surgeons Act 1966 Section 19.

The bottom line regarding Applied Zoopharmacognosy is that while the discipline is not as scientifically irrational as say homeopathy or crystal therapy, it is still a method of treatment that has no supporting evidence, and has potential risks to the animals.

# CHAPTER SEVEN

# *Raw Feeding*

IN 70 BC in Ancient Rome, Columella wrote in his treatise, *On Agriculture*, that barley meal mixed with whey was a convenient food for dogs, or alternatively wheat bread with the liquid from cooked beans. Various other commentators over subsequent centuries advised on how best to feed dogs, but dogs were predominantly fed table scraps and whatever was left over from human consumption. It was not until the mid-1800s that James Spratt, an American electrician visiting London, noticed that dogs at the dock were being fed on leftover hard tack (flour, water and salt, baked till it was hard). He had the idea of creating a similar food that was convenient and cheap for the growing numbers of urban dog owners, and eventually marketed a biscuit of baked wheat, beetroot, vegetables and beef blood.

Canned horsemeat as petfood was introduced in America after the First World War as a way of disposing of dead horses. Canned dog food became increasingly popular, but rationing in the Second World War led to an increase in feeding of dry food.

The pet food industry expanded massively in the middle of the twentieth century and in the 1960s university-led research began to analyse the nutrient requirements of dogs and cats, with diets being adjusted accordingly. The US Food and Drug Administration (FDA) federal agency now oversees pet food quality in the States, and any pet food that is labelled balanced and complete must meet nutrient guidelines developed by the Association of American Feed Control Officials (AAFCO), either by a feeding trial or a nutrient analysis.

There are many criticisms of the pet food industry, some of which are more valid than others. The fact that pet food was once seen as a convenient way of selling ingredients not fit for human consumption was seen as a major benefit, and to be fair to the industry in its early days, most pets were likely being fed in this way before the development of commercial pet food anyway, with dogs being given the leftovers, the spoiled vegetables, the mouldy bread and the bones that had been stripped of the best cuts. It is a testament to the adaptability of dogs that they can survive on such a variety of diets, a point I will come back to.

While the fact that ingredients can include offal, meat and bone meal, and 'animal digest' (clean animal tissue that has undergone chemical or enzymatic hydrolysis, usually used as a flavouring) may be distasteful to humans, it doesn't necessarily affect the nutrient quality of the food, nor are dogs sensitive to the niceties of the origin of an ingredient.

Over the years, mistakes have been made in the formulation of pet foods, which have in some cases had catastrophic consequences. In 2007, hundreds of deaths from renal failure were linked to contamination of pet food with the toxin melamine, most of which was traced to wheat gluten from a single source in China. The discovery of this problem in animals also led to concerns about the safety of the human food chain.

One of the worst, however, is the problem with taurine deficiency in cats. Taurine is an amino acid, which humans and dogs can synthesise from combinations of other amino acids, and so is considered a non-essential amino acid in these species. Cats, though, being obligate carnivores, have always had a plentiful amount of taurine in their diet, and so have lost the ability to synthesise it for themselves. In the 1970s, it was noticed that a lot of cats were developing dilated cardiomyopathy, a fatal heart disease that had previously been uncommon. In 1987, Paul Pion, founder of the Veterinary Information Network (VIN), discovered the link between dilated cardiomyopathy and taurine deficiency in pet food.[1] Taurine deficiency also causes retinal degeneration, altered white cell function and abnormal growth and development in cats. Since this was discovered, cat foods are supplemented with taurine in order to prevent the problems associated with deficiency.

The FDA website lists other pet food recalls.[2] Recent reasons for withdrawals include contamination with salmonella, listeria and mould. Both raw and cooked feeds had problems reported, although the only dietary deficiency was reported in a frozen raw cat food, which had low levels of thiamine, lack of which can lead to serious neurological problems.

Pet foods have undoubtedly had problems in the past, and in rare cases problems may still arise, as they do in the human food chain. But statutory monitoring of safety and nutritional value allows a high degree of confidence when feeding commercial pet foods. Furthermore, pet food companies invest considerable resources researching improvements to diets to optimise health, and many diets are now tailored much more individually, e.g. by breed, age, activity levels. In addition to this there is a range of commercial prescription diets that are formulated to accord with veterinary recommendations for conditions such as pancreatitis (low fat), renal disease (low phosphate) and allergies (hypoallergenic or anallergenic foods). For some conditions diet is the primary treatment, and restricted phosphate diets are the only medical intervention proven to significantly increase life expectancy in animals suffering from chronic kidney disease.

So over the years, commercial pet foods have moved from being a cheap, convenient, and nutritionally questionable way of feeding our pets, to a highly researched and highly regulated industry, still offering convenience and a reasonable price, while now giving reassurance of safety and nutritional completeness. It could be argued that if humans ate a scientifically balanced complete diet, that was regulated in levels of saturated fats, sugars, fibre and vitamins and minerals, we would likely see a significant drop in dietary-related health problems such as type II diabetes and coronary artery disease.

Despite this, there are vocal minorities among pet owners and vets who consider pet foods to be dangerous to animals' health, and advocate home-cooked diets.

Creating a nutritionally complete diet is challenging in the home environment. Dogs are resilient, and can survive, and even thrive, on a variety of diets. Cats are less able to adapt their requirements to varied dietary conditions because of their obligate carnivore status. Both dogs and cats can suffer nutritional deficiencies from home-cooked diets, and the disease nutritional secondary hyperparathyroidism, a condition that can cause weakened bones and fractures, occurs because of too much meat in the diet and too little bone or other sources of calcium. For this reason the condition is also known as Butcher's Dog Disease, for this reason whenever I hear the phrase 'fit as a butcher's dog', I always raise my eyebrows.

Undoubtedly home-cooked diets can provide adequate nutrition to dogs and cats, provided nutritionally complete formulae are followed. However, some vets and other vocal factions recommend that home-cooked diets are fed raw, and the rest of this chapter will concentrate on the evidence and the pros and cons of this approach.

§

In the 1930s, Francis M. Pottenger Jr conducted an experiment involving 900 cats over a ten-year period. Cats that were fed a diet of raw meat, raw milk and raw cod liver oil were compared to cats that were fed the same diet cooked. The cooked diet cohort suffered more health problems than the raw diet, with problems reported including reproductive, skeletal and cardiac disease. Since cooking is known to reduce taurine levels, it may be that these cats were suffering from taurine deficiency, but the importance of taurine to cats was not known at that time, so diet and blood levels were not tested. Nevertheless, this experiment is often quoted by the raw food lobby as evidence of the benefits of raw over cooked food, and certainly it raises interesting questions.

Maybe the problems with taurine dented confidence in the pet food industry, or maybe an increased consciousness of the importance of diet to health in humans and concerns over junk food caused people to question the diets of their pets. Whatever the underlying reason, in the 1980s and 1990s, people began to question the wisdom of feeding pet foods, and the concept of feeding raw began to be recommended.

One of the first raw food advocates was Ian Billinghurst, an Australian vet with a background in complementary medicine. He describes how seeing his own pet's health improve after feeding raw food led him to develop the Bones and Raw Food Diet,[3] better known as the BARF diet (BARF is a registered trademark). According to Dr Billinghurst's biography in his book, *Give Your Dog a Bone*,[4] he does not have any postgraduate qualifications in nutrition, nor any related subject, although he has an undergraduate degree in agriculture that included some farm animal nutrition. As with many advocates of raw food, Dr Billinghurst also has an interest in alternative medicine, and has passed examinations in Traditional Chinese Medicine (TCM, see Chapters Six and Eight). In his own short biography on the above website he notes that his attempts to persuade the veterinary profession that poor nutrition was the cause of most diseases in dogs and cats was met with disbelief.

Rather than proving his case via published research, he decided to take his theory straight to the public, writing the successful book, *Give Your Dog a Bone*, which he says is based on talking to clients about their dogs' feeding habits, reading, attending lectures and conducting feeding trials (which do not appear to have been peer-reviewed). Dr Billinghurst claims this book has improved the health of tens of thousands of pet dogs, and that many people look to him as an authority on feeding pets an evolutionary diet.

Another vocal raw food advocate is Tom Lonsdale. A graduate of the Royal Vet College (RVC) in London, Dr Lonsdale has practised most of his life in Australia. Despite this, for twenty consecutive years he has sat as a candidate for election to the Royal College of Veterinary Surgeons (RCVS) council, the governing body of UK vets, on a platform of attacking commercial pet food. The RCVS website (www.rcvs.org.uk) lists the election results back to 2004 (with the exception of a detailed breakdown of 2005), and in every year documented, Dr Lonsdale has come last in the elections, typically with around one-third of the votes of the second to last candidate. His candidate biography on the RCVS website for the RCVS council election in 2016 starts by saying that in the 1980s he woke from a 'vet-school induced stupor to realisation that the junk pet-food industry relies on bogus science and negligent vet "profession".' His manifesto begins, 'Pompous, arrogant, mouthing incantations, the vet high priests worship at the altar of bogus science. Founded on fallacy, they oversee the junk food poisoning of pets, betrayal of consumers and brainwashing of vet students.' He claims that, 'Vet schools deliver industry-funded propaganda on diabetes, periodontal disease and obesity.'

Dr Lonsdale published a paper in the prestigious *Journal of Small Animal Practice*[5] in which he noted that white cell counts were low in eight out of fourteen animals undergoing dental procedures for periodontitis, and that these cell counts improved after treatment. From this small study, Dr Lonsdale coined the term 'Foul-mouthed AIDS' to describe what he believes to be an immunodeficiency caused by periodontitis secondary to poor nutrition. He then sent out a press release, reproduced in his book, *Raw Meaty Bones*,[6] headlined 'Many pets not old but stricken with diet-induced AIDS'. An article subsequently appeared in *The Australian* newspaper under the headline, 'AIDS-like disease threatens family pets'.

Dr Lonsdale published his book, *Raw Meaty Bones* in 2001. The main thrust of the book is that modern pet food (junk food as he calls it) promotes periodontal disease, which in turn leads on to a variety of chronic systemic diseases. His Raw Meaty Bones (RMB) diet is claimed to reduce the build-up of plaque and tartar, contributing to improved animal health. In contrast, Dr Billinghurst's BARF diet is aimed at improving the overall nutrient content of food in comparison to pet food.

Dr Billinghurst and Dr Lonsdale were initially allies in their anti-pet food crusade and promotion of raw feeding. However, they disagreed on certain fundamental issues, most importantly as to whether dogs should be classed as carnivores or omnivores. This in turn led to a disagreement on whether the diet should include fruit and vegetables. Dr Lonsdale describes BARF as 'pap' and a 'scam.'[7] The schism confuses pet owners who are hoping to feed raw. Helping them make a decision between these two 'denominations' is not easy since, as we shall see, the evidence supporting either side, or the concept of feeding raw at all, is weak.

A third model, that differs from both Drs Lonsdale and Billinghurst is the prey model, in which whole animals are fed. There is a similar movement in humans known as the paleo diet (or Paleolithic or caveman diet, since paleo diet, like BARF, has been trademarked), which advocates feeding only foods that were available to hunter gatherers, prior to the farming revolution of the Neolithic period (i.e. any food only available from the New Stone Age onwards is considered too modern for humans to have adapted to), and consists primarily of nuts, fruits, vegetables and lean meats. A detailed analysis of this diet is beyond the scope of this book, but critics point out that the true diet of Paleolithic man is unknown, and also that 10,000 years of evolution is plenty of time in which adaptations to changes in diet can be made.

What Lonsdale and Billinghurst retain in common is a hatred of the pet food industry, an assertion that most disease in animals is due to pet food, and that feeding raw will prevent most diseases of dogs and cats.[8, 9] While the first point is opinion, the second two can be analysed for evidence.

§

## The claims

Let's examine some specific claims of raw feeding proponents. The following are some of the claims regarding raw food and commercial food made by Dr Billinghurst (in *Give Your Dog a Bone*) and Lonsdale (in *Raw Meaty Bones*) and also Dr Pitcairn (in his *New Complete Guide to Natural Health for Dogs and Cats*).[10]

**The key ingredient missing in processed pet foods which can only be found in uncooked whole foods is 'life energy.' (Pitcairn)**

Pitcairn goes on to describe life energy as a force that permeates all living things (a concept familiar to many as The Force from *Star Wars*), which is supposedly responsible for the healing powers of acupuncture and homeopathy. A belief in life energy is essentially a form of vitalism, a discredited scientific hypothesis dating back to the Ancient Greeks' belief in the four humours. Many vitalistic theories have been falsified, but vitalism is often framed in a way that makes it unfalsifiable. A claim that is unfalsifiable is not considered to be scientifically valid, and belongs only in the realm of faith and religion.

**Commercial diets contain toxic or unpalatable ingredients such as drug residues, artificial colours, flavours and preservatives which cause diseases such as cancer and even the remains of euthanased pets.** (Pitcairn)

The disgusting myth about euthanased pets being made into pet food may have come about because of the discovery of pentobarbitone, which is used to put dogs and cats to sleep, in some pet foods. The FDA investigated this claim by testing pet foods for dog and cat DNA and found none present.[11] The pentobarbitone was found in levels too low to cause ill health, likely as a result of the euthanasia of bovines and horses. Ingredients such as artificial colours, flavourings and preservatives used in pet foods are similar to those used in human foods, which are passed as fit for human consumption, and are generally considered safe. Antioxidants are added to food to prevent toxin formation during processing, and to preserve vitamin levels, and synthetic antioxidants are better at doing this than naturally derived anti-oxidants.[12] Two reviews of commercial pet food recalls using Freedom of Information Act requests from the FDA describe episodes of chemical adulteration of pet foods, but note that the incidence is low and that pet foods overall are safe.[13, 14]

**Most sick dogs are fed either commercial dog food or badly designed home cooked food, while the really health dogs eat raw meat bones, plus healthy food scraps.** (Billinghurst)

There are no published studies that compare dogs or cats fed raw food to dogs that are fed commercial food. Companies producing commercial diets perform studies to assess the nutritional adequacy of their own products, but it is generally considered that the burden of proof lies with the person making an assertion. Raw food advocates should consider publishing controlled clinical trials themselves. If Drs Billinghurst and Lonsdale had over the last thirty years performed a prospective clinical study comparing raw fed pets to commercially fed pets in a properly designed trial, we would have a wealth of data to prove one way or the other whether raw food diets were a benefit or a harm to our pets.

Unfortunately, we mainly have to rely on anecdotes and testimonials on the benefits of raw food diets, which as we saw in Chapter Five are unreliable evidence. When I have debated with raw food advocates and suggested that they back up their claims with scientific studies, I have been told that to do so would be too expensive. In fact, it would cost next to nothing. A simple study comparing life expectancy, for example, would have no costs associated with it. Other studies of value, for example monitoring biochemical parameters, would incur some costs, but funding is available for research by vets in general practice, and given the controversy, any scientific research into the subject would likely be looked at favourably. If a raw food advocate was interested in running a clinical trial, but felt they did not have the right research training to design the trial, university academics are often extremely helpful in providing advice on these matters.

But for whatever reason, the will of raw food advocates to perform scientifically valid studies is not present, and until these studies are performed, we won't know whether raw fed pets are more or less healthy than commercial diet fed pets.

**Dogs fed cooked and processed food and no bones will always develop a weakened immune system and poor dental health.** (Billinghurst)

There is no evidence for this sweeping assertion, especially with regards to the immune system, and the use of the word 'always'. However, it is true that dietary texture has an effect on oral health.[15] It has also been shown by research that feeding raw beef bones reduces calculus,[16] and no complications such as tooth fractures or intestinal obstructions were found in that study. However, this only involved eight dogs and the duration of the trial was short, so does not give any useful information regarding risks of feeding raw bones.

Furthermore, feeding bones is not the only way of improving dental health. Daily toothbrushing has been shown to be safe and effective at reducing pre-existing gingivitis and retarding the build-up of plaque and calculus in kibble-fed dogs.[17] Similarly, feeding a daily dental chew reduced plaque and calculus accumulation and improved gingivitis and oral malodour.[18]

The small study by veterinary surgeon Dr Lonsdale and published in the *Journal of Small Animal Practice* mentioned above does link poor dental health with reduced white cell count, so it is possible that dental disease can affect the immune system. This is not the same as saying that a raw food diet will improve the immune system, however.

Improving dental health is one of the main purported benefits of the raw food diet, but there are risks associated with feeding raw, so using a safer method to improve dental health may be desirable. In a systematic review of home care for prevention of periodontal disease in dogs and cats in the *Journal of Veterinary Dentistry*, the authors specifically consider raw, meaty bones for dental care, and conclude that only the poorest quality evidence exists for the benefits of this diet for dental care. They consider the known risks, including of dental fracture, outweigh the benefits of raw meaty bones.[19]

Additionally, there is evidence that wild carnivores are far from immune to dental problems, including periodontal disease, decay and tooth fractures, as illustrated in a study of the skulls of thirty-four Croatian wolves[20] and in Figure One, showing a male lion, photographed in the Serengeti National Park in 2016 and affected with a marked degree of dental disease.

**Cooking destroys enzymes which are important nutrients, aiding digestion and slowing the ageing process. The destruction of enzymes in food forces the pancreas to work harder, resulting in pancreatitis, pancreatic insufficiency and diabetes mellitus. Enzymes in the food are absorbed whole into the blood stream.** (Billinghurst)

This is just plain wrong and demonstrates a lack of understanding of the workings of the digestive system. Enzymes are proteins, and most are digested by proteases in the stomach and small intestine in order to be absorbed. They are large molecules, and so cannot be absorbed by the healthy gut until they

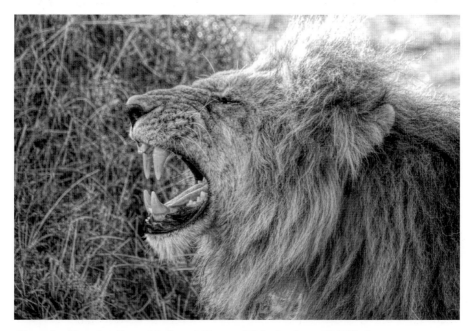

*Figure 1*   Yawning lion with dental disease. With thanks to Phil Hyde

145

have been broken down into their constituent amino acids. The function of most enzymes is also destroyed by stomach acid. Furthermore, all the enzymes needed to digest food are produced by the healthy gastrointestinal tract and pancreas. No benefit of preserved enzyme action from feeding raw food to dogs and cats has ever been proven.

**Anti-oxidants are destroyed by cooking.** (Billinghurst)

A comprehensive database of the antioxidant contents of more than 3,100 foods, beverages, spices, herbs and supplements has been compiled.[21] The authors of this study found that while in some cases processing of food reduced anti-oxidant content, in other cases processing released anti-oxidants that in the unprocessed food would be less available or unavailable for absorption by the body. However, it is true that certain nutrients are reduced in certain cooking processes, for example taurine.[22] Taurine is supplemented in cat food in order to meet the nutritional requirements, as discussed above.

**Cooked food is responsible for most ill health including cancer, kidney disease, heart disease, arthritis and pancreatic disease. 'Dogs fed cooked foods live shorter, less healthy, more miserable lives.'** (Billinghurst)

The ultimate causes of many diseases are incompletely understood, but scientists have made excellent progress over recent decades in fields such as cardiology and oncology. Many diseases are multi-factorial, with genetic influences, diet and other environmental factors involved. Cancer, for example, is ultimately a disease of the DNA, and many cases have hereditary factors involved. For example, flat-coated retrievers are prone to developing tumours called sarcomas, likely because of a genetic tendency. However, the transformation of a healthy cell into a cancer cell involves several stages in which the DNA mutates, and factors that can cause these mutations can include viruses (especially the feline leukaemia virus), environmental pollutants, cosmic radiation, radon gas, secondary smoking and ultraviolet light from the sun. Although diet is implicated as a factor for many diseases in humans, there is no evidence in humans or animals that feeding raw reduces the incidence of disease.

**Most dry dog foods are deficient in zinc and essential fatty acids and have an excess of calcium.** (Billinghurst)

The calcium:phosphate ratio in a diet is very important in the health of pets, especially in juveniles in which the skeleton is rapidly growing. The AAFCO guidelines for calcium content of foods is (expressed as percentage of dry matter) a minimum of 1.2 for growth and reproduction and a minimum of 0.5 for adults, with a maximum of 1.8. For phosphate, the minimum recommendation for growth and reproduction is 1.0, 0.4 for adult maintenance, and a maximum of 1.6. The ratio of calcium:phosphate should be 1:1 minimum and 2:1 maximum. Diets outside this range risk causing skeletal and potentially renal abnormalities.

In a recent study, thirty-nine out of forty-five commercial diets analysed were in compliance with the AAFCO guidelines on calcium and phosphate for all life stages. Four had an excess of calcium and two were zinc deficient.[23] The authors of this study recommended feeding life stage-specific foods to ensure correct mineral levels. It is therefore incorrect to say that most dry dog foods have excess calcium and deficient zinc, but some do have a problem.

Essential fatty acid (EFA) deficiency can cause problems in skin, liver and kidneys in cats. The type and ratios of different types of essential fatty acids has an influence on how beneficial they are. One study in dogs showed that EFA levels, types and ratios varies considerably but that all commercial diets studied showed they were above recommended levels of EFAs.[24]

Is raw any better? One study of four raw meat diets for captive exotic and domestic carnivores revealed that all were deficient in essential fatty acids.[25] Another study of a raw diet showed excesses of copper and manganese and deficiencies in zinc and iron compared to the recommendations for adult cats.[26] A further study showed that many bone and raw food diets fed to dogs in Germany were deficient in calcium, zinc and copper.[27]

Getting calcium and phosphate levels wrong can have serious consequences. Five German Shepherd puppies fed a diet of raw meat and rice were found to have developed nutritional secondary hyperparathyroidism, a rickets-like condition causing limb deformities. The diet was found to be primarily to blame, although genetic factors may also have been involved.[28] Nutritional osteodystrophy has been reported in two litters of puppies fed a bones and raw food diet.[29] A German review of raw meat diets also noted that: 'Additionally, raw-meat diets often show nutritional imbalances. Over-supplementation and deficiencies of nutrients are frequently found, especially regarding calcium, the trace elements copper, zinc and iodine, vitamins A and D and the calcium:phosphorus ratio.'[30]

**Dog foods have low vitamin levels e.g. vitamin A, B complex, C and D. When dogs are fed processed dog foods, they make much less vitamin C than dogs fed a properly balanced raw diet.** (Billinghurst)

Vitamin C is not an essential vitamin for dogs, since they make their own, and dietary supplementation is unnecessary. I could find no evidence in literature searches to support the assertion that raw-fed dogs make more vitamin C than dogs on a diet of processed dog food. Interestingly, critically ill cats are found to have higher than expected levels of Vitamin C, which may be a natural antioxidant response to stress.[31]

The AAFCO guidelines dictate minimum and maximum levels of vitamins A, B complex, D and E, so pet foods complying with AAFCO guidelines are not deficient in vitamins. One study compared the blood levels of vitamin B12 as well as urine methylmalonic acid and total homocysteine concentrations (both markers for B12 deficiency) in dogs fed raw and commercial diets and found no difference.[32]

Again we can look at the nutritional composition of raw foods by comparison. Roasting and grilling has been shown to have no effect on vitamin B12 levels, although frying did reduce them by about one third.[33] A German study of bones and raw food diets showed many were deficient in vitamins A and D.[34]

**Bones are only dangerous if they are cooked.** (Billinghurst)

As a young vet I had the misfortune to be presented with a small breed dog that was suffocating on a pork bone stuck in its throat. The bone was uncooked, which made it hard to get hold of with forceps, and although I eventually successfully removed the bone, we were unable to resuscitate him. Veterinary dental specialists on vet forums report that teeth fractures are commonly caused by chewing bones, and at least one case report has been published.[35] Gastrointestinal obstructions, perforation of the stomach and oesophagus and impaction of the colon are all common problems associated with eating bones. While raw food advocates claim this only occurs with cooked bones, there are no studies to confirm this.[36]

**Salmonella and Campylobacter are of no consequence to the healthy dog.** (Billinghurst)

Salmonella is a known pathogen of dogs and cats. However, healthy dogs can be asymptomatic carriers of the bacteria, and there are similar rates of isolation of the bacteria in healthy and ill animals in some studies. In a review of enteropathogenic bacteria that comprises a consensus statement from the American College of Veterinary Internal Medicine (ACVIM), Marks et al note that while salmonella is pathogenic, its ability to cause disease depends on infective dose and strain, as well as the host immunity.[37] The authors believe that prolonged shedding in healthy dogs is likely to be at least part of the reason for the similar isolation rates in the sick and healthy.

Salmonellosis is primarily a disease causing acute gastroenteritis, but can also be associated with chronic diarrhoea. Signs of acute salmonellosis include vomiting, diarrhoea, which is often bloody, and abdominal pain. Sepsis may also occur, and other signs associated with salmonellosis include nasal discharge, hindlimb weakness and abortion. A case of discospondylitis and spinal empyaema has been reported to be associated with salmonellosis.[38]

Philbey et al reviewed cases of salmonellosis in cats between 1955 and 2005 isolated at Glasgow Vet School.[39] They note that several strains were associated with gastrointestinal disease and at least one fatal example was noted. Another study reports the death of two kittens fed a raw food diet from septicaemic salmonellosis.[40] It is interesting that one website encouraging raw feeding suggested the study must be a fraud or hoax.

There are also similar rates of isolation of campylobacter species from healthy and sick dogs. It is known from experimental studies that the bacteria have pathogenic potential, but the disease is often mild.[41]

It is important to note that both salmonella and campylobacter are zoonotic, i.e. they can be transmitted to humans, in which they can cause serious disease and death, especially in the young, the old and the immunosuppressed.

**Raisins and sultanas are a good source of iron.** (Billinghurst)

This is one of Dr Billinghurst's most dangerous assertions. When *Give Your Dog a Bone* was first published, it was not known that grapes, raisins and sultanas can cause a fatal acute renal failure in some dogs. Many reports in scientific journals have since described this problem though, with a paper in the *Veterinary Record* in 2003 highlighting the issue,[42] which makes it surprising that the 2012 edition of *Give Your Dog a Bone* continues to recommend feeding these canine toxins.

**Grain is not a food the dog has evolved to eat in large quantities.** (Billinghurst)

Dogs diverged from wolves tens of thousands of years ago, time enough for genetic drift to occur. One of the interesting findings of the canine genome project that sequenced the whole of the DNA in a dog was that ten genes involved in starch and fat metabolism had shown signs of adaptation in dogs compared to wolves. According to this study in the prestigious journal, *Nature*, novel adaptations in early dogs allowed them to thrive on a starch-rich diet, compared to the carnivorous wolves, which may have been a crucial step in the domestication of the dog.[43] It is fascinating to find that the assertion that dogs have not evolved to eat grain is completely wrong, and in fact dogs have evolved specifically to digest starch-rich diets. This highlights one of the issues of the 'evolutionary diet' concept, that in fact the diet of early dogs is not clearly known.

**The heart disease responsible for iliac thrombosis is likely to be caused by toxins and bacteria from a foul mouth, which is usually diet-related.** (Lonsdale)

Iliac thrombosis is a blood clot that forms in the heart (mainly in cats), which then breaks away and lodges in the far end of the aorta or the iliac arteries, causing hindlimb paralysis. It is a painful and life-threatening condition, with a high mortality rate. The blood clot forms because of an enlargement in the left atrium (one of the chambers of the heart), almost always a sequel to one of the cardiomyopathies to which cats are prone (dilated cardiomyopathy, restrictive cardiomyopathy, hypertrophic cardio-myopathy). Genetic factors are suspected to be a cause in many of these cases and are proven in others (for example hypertrophic cardiomyopathy is inherited in the Maine Coone cat). Certain metabolic conditions such as hyperthyroidism can also lead to thickening of the heart walls. Most of the time, an underlying cause cannot be identified for the development of these heart muscle conditions.

However, it is unlikely that dental disease plays a role. Blood-borne bacterial infections, sometimes dental-related, can lead to an infection of the heart valves known as bacterial endocarditis, but this is a very rare condition.

Dietary deficiencies in taurine can also lead to dilated cardiomyopathy, but since this problem was corrected in pet foods, dilated cardiomyopathy in cats has also become rare, and in those cases where it is found, blood tests usually reveal normal taurine levels, suggesting there is some other factor causing most of the cases that are seen nowadays.

Interestingly, dietary history has been implicated in heart disease in cats, with a study showing that 57 per cent of cats with heart disease had their diet supplemented by treats and table scraps, and tended to have eaten more fat, protein, sodium, potassium and magnesium than the minimum recommended amounts.[44]

**Liver diseases seem to be artificial diet related.** (Lonsdale)

There are a large number of known causes of liver disease. These include infections (e.g. leptospirosis, canine infectious hepatitis), toxins (e.g. aflatoxin, hepatoxic mushrooms, xylitol), drugs (e.g. phenobarbitone, lomustine, glucocorticoids) and abnormal copper accumulation due to a genetic abnormality of copper metabolism. In dogs many cases of chronic hepatitis are seen, a slowly progressive inflammatory disease of the liver. The cause of this is unknown, but as it runs in certain breeds there are likely to be genetic factors. There is no evidence that diet causes this condition in dogs.

In cats the situation is different. Cholangiohepatitis (inflammation of the liver and biliary tree) is common in cats, and often associated with pancreatitis and inflammatory bowel disease. This can be caused by infections ascending into the liver from the gut, or may be immune-mediated, e.g. a food allergy. Fatty liver disease can also occur in obese cats, especially obese cats that have become ill and stopped eating. This is reportedly more common in the USA than the UK. Neither of these diseases are the fault of pet foods per se, but in obese or allergic individuals, diet may play a role.

There is no evidence that feeding raw food would treat or prevent these conditions. If evidence was to emerge that a raw food diet for cats helped with weight control, then this would be an argument for its use, given the role of obesity in a variety of disorders including liver disease and diabetes mellitus. However, there appears to be no evidence that raw diets help maintain optimum body weight.

§

# The risks

If those were the claims of benefits of Raw Meaty Bones and BARF diets touted by their proponents, what are the risks of feeding these diets?

There are a number of peer-reviewed studies that assess this issue. Risks of raw feeding fall into four main categories: risk to animals of contracting disease from pathogens; risk to animals from malnutrition (over- or under-supplementation); risk to animals from physical factors, e.g. obstruction and dental damage; risk to humans from zoonotic disease.

# Risk to animals from pathogens

A number of pathogens have been associated with feeding raw food. Several studies have shown an increased risk of salmonella infection from feeding raw.

A preliminary study by Joffe and Schlesinger found that salmonella was isolated from 80 per cent of samples of a bones and raw food (BARF) diet, and from the faeces of 30 per cent of dogs fed this diet.[45] Weese et al studied samples from twenty-five commercial raw food diets and found salmonella spp in 20 per cent.[46] They also found coliforms in 100 per cent of samples, *E. coli* in 64 per cent and *Clostridium perfringens* in 20 per cent. No campylobacter were isolated in this survey.

Strohmeyer et al, in a study involving 240 samples of twenty raw meat diets, twenty-four samples from two dry dog food diets and twenty-four samples from two canned food diets, found that salmonella was recovered from 5.9 per cent of raw samples and none of the cooked samples.[47] *E. coli* was recovered from all diets, and campylobacter from none. Morley et al investigated salmonella infections at a greyhound breeding facility where the dogs were being fed primarily raw food.[48] Salmonella was isolated from 93 per cent of faecal samples, and the authors concluded that the raw food was the likely source of the pathogen.

Leonard et al examined the risk factors for salmonella carriage in dogs, and they found that increased risk was associated with feeding a commercial or home-made raw diet, although a home-cooked diet was also a risk factor.[49] In an experimental study sixteen research dogs were fed a salmonella-containing raw food, and twelve were fed a non-salmonella-containing raw food.[50] Seven of the dogs fed salmonella-contaminated diets shed salmonella in faeces, five of which had serotypes the same as that recovered from the food. None of the dogs fed salmonella-free diets shed salmonella in their faeces.

Finley et al assessed the occurrence of salmonella in 166 commercial raw food samples purchased randomly.[51] The prevalence of salmonella was 67 per cent. Many of these isolates demonstrated antibiotic resistance. Lefebvre et al evaluated the risk of shedding of salmonella and other pathogens in therapy dogs.[52] They found that dogs fed raw food were twenty-two times more likely to shed salmonella than dogs that were not fed raw food. Raw fed dogs were also seventeen times more likely to test positive for *E. coli* than dogs that weren't fed raw food.

Lenz et al found salmonella in 14 per cent of raw fed dogs' faeces but in none of the non-raw fed dogs' faeces.[53] They also found salmonella in 10.5 per cent of samples taken from vacuum cleaners in the households of raw fed dogs compared to 4.5 per cent of households where dogs weren't fed raw (this difference was not statistically significant, however).

Interestingly, this last study also looked at the attitudes of raw feeders and found that although owners who fed raw had similar levels of concern regarding their choice of diet's impact on their pet's health, raw feeders tended to worry more about the environmental impact of feeding, and were more likely to choose organic food for themselves. The authors note that raw feeders seem to make rational choices about feeding choices based on information they believe to be true, but unfortunately the evidence is lacking for the benefits of raw foods. The authors also speculate that some of the choices of raw feeders may be based on anthropomorphic principles, i.e. the mistaken belief that what is good for humans must be good for animals.

Pathogens other than salmonella that have been associated with raw feeding include the tapeworm *Echinococcus granulosus*,[54] campylobacter,[55] (although this study did not reach statistical significance), and *E. coli*.[56, 57]

One study from Brazil showed that antibodies to the parasite *Toxoplasma gondii* were more common in dogs fed kitchen food, especially ones with raw ingredients, with neurological signs being observed in affected dogs.[58]

Consumption of raw food was also implicated in a recent report of tongue worm in stray dogs imported to the UK.[59]

## Risk to animals from malnutrition

Dietary hyperthyroidism has been reported in dogs fed a raw food diet that included necks. Twelve dogs fed this diet were found to have elevated thyroxine levels (the neck is where the thyroid gland, containing high levels of thyroxine, is located), and six of these dogs showed clinical signs of hyperthyroidism.[60] Another study showed hyperthyroidism in seven dogs fed raw meat.[61] Primary anestrus, a condition where the normal reproductive seasons cease, was reported in a bitch fed raw food, with high levels of thyroxine being found in both the dog's blood and its food.[62] Note, however, that there have been reports of hyperthyroidism in dogs fed meat-based commercial diets.[63] Other reports of nutritional deficiencies such as nutritional osteodystrophy and nutritional secondary hyperparathytoidism have been discussed above.

It is also important to realise that preparing a balanced home-made diet is difficult, and malnutrition may arise because of non-adherence to recommendations.

## Risk to animals from physical factors

Oral fractures are reported in dental journals following bone chewing.[64] This review did suggest that pre-existing periodontal disease may be a factor in tooth fracturing from bone chewing.

Many vets are concerned about the possibility of dental fractures from bone chewing, and specialist veterinary dentists on veterinary forums such as the Veterinary Information Network (VIN) do report tooth fracture being commonly caused by bones. However, rawhide chews, elk antlers and other dental chews have also been discussed on the forums as causes of tooth fractures.

## Risk to humans

One of the most comprehensive reviews of raw food diets was published by Schlesinger and Joffe in the *Canadian Veterinary Journal*.[65] After reviewing the published literature, the authors concluded that despite top level evidence for human health risk not being present (nor any good evidence for health benefits to pets from feeding raw), there was compelling evidence that there was an at least theoretical risk to human health from feeding raw food. The authors of the review believe that vets should be obligated to discuss the human health implications of feeding raw food. All the consensus statements below discuss the human health risks of feeding raw food to pets, and the risk is noted to be particularly large in vulnerable sectors – including the young, the old and the immunosuppressed.

Even pro-raw food organisations acknowledge the risks. An uncontrolled survey of 1,870 owners feeding raw diets, produced by an organisation promoting raw feeding, Raw Fit Pet, found an 11 per cent complication rate with feeding raw.[66] Of these 11 per cent, 65 per cent reported broken or fractured teeth, and 4.7 per cent reported a foreign body requiring surgery.[67]

§

## Consensus statements of professional veterinary bodies

The AVMA consensus statement on raw foods was produced after an inquiry on their stance from Pet Partners, the USA-based charity for animal-assisted interventions in vulnerable people such as those with post-traumatic stress disorder (PTSD), Alzheimer's, and intellectual disabilities and those approaching the end of their life. Pet Partners did not request the review or input into the review. After reviewing the evidence the AVMA stated: 'The AVMA discourages the feeding to cats and dogs of any animal-source protein that has not first been subjected to a process to eliminate pathogens because of the risk of illness to cats and dogs as well as humans.'[68]

The American Animal Hospital Association (AAHA) also has a position statement on raw food. It states, 'based on overwhelming scientific evidence, AAHA does not advocate or endorse feeding pets any raw or dehydrated non-sterilised foods, including treats that are of animal origin'. Their statement has been endorsed by the American Association of Feline Practitioners and the National Association of State Public health Veterinarians.[69]

The British Small Animal Veterinary Association (BSAVA) has a weaker position on raw feeding, stating, 'Where raw food (especially that containing meat and meat products) is fed the BSAVA strongly recommends that hygiene measures are in place to minimise the risk of the transmission of communicable disease. Where there are children or immune compromised adults in the household medical advice should be sought, before considering whether to prepare, handle and store raw food.'[70]

The Canadian Veterinary Medical Association takes a more robust line and in a joint statement with the Public Health Agency of Canada, they state that, 'The CVMA holds that the documented scientific evidence of potential animal and public health risks in feeding raw meats outweigh any perceived benefits of this feeding practice.'[71]

The World Small Animal Veterinary Association nutritional assessment guidelines also discuss the risks of pathogens from raw food and dental damage and oesophageal/gastro-intestinal obstruction from raw bones.[72]

§

## Conclusions

Commercial pet food is clearly not perfect. Early pet foods were able to sustain life, without being anywhere near optimum nutrition. In recent decades though, pet nutrition has become a scientifically validated discipline, with large amounts of peer-reviewed data based on feeding trials to back up the nutrient content of commercial diets. Mistakes have been made along the way, with taurine-deficient diets being one of the most serious. Contamination of ingredients can also occur, which can lead to serious problems. This can also occur in the human food chain as well, with contaminants being discovered periodically. However, in comparison to the volume of commercial pet food consumed worldwide, the risks of pet food from chemical and microbiological contamination is very low.

This contrasts with the situation in raw food diets. There is a marked lack of scientific data regarding the safety of raw foods, and most of the studies that have been published highlight the risks, particularly regarding the high levels of pathogens, and the fact that these pathogens are passed on to the pets, as demonstrated by finding the bacteria in the faeces. Other risks of raw food diets are anecdotally reported, such as choking, gastro-intestinal obstruction and perforation and tooth fractures.

There are theoretical benefits of feeding raw food. The two main ones are increased nutrient content (which is controversial, and not borne out by the current evidence), and improved dental health, which can be achieved in other ways.

Every intervention, medical or nutritional, has a risk:benefit ratio. With a treatment such as homeopathy, the risks are low, but the benefit is zero. With the intervention of feeding raw food, there are plausible but unproven benefits, and known risks. The risk:benefit ratio is therefore high, i.e. high risk and low proven benefit.

Many proponents of raw food appeal to the Mother Nature fallacy (see Chapter Four). The belief is that what animals evolved to eat in the wild is the optimum way of nourishing them. Analyses of wild cat and wolf diets suggest that there are differences between the diets of the closest wild relatives of dogs and cats, and the commercial food that is fed to pets. However, it is acknowledged that dogs have evolved to have different nutrient requirements from wolves[73] to the extent that wolves could be considered carnivores while dogs should be considered omnivores.[74]

Furthermore, just because an animal has adapted to an environment, it doesn't mean that that environment is optimal. From a biological and evolutionary point of view, nature is only concerned with survival of the individual for long enough to reproduce and ensure the passing on of genes. Once an animal has finished reproducing and rearing its young to independence, there is no evolutionary benefit to longer survival. So 'nature' has no interest in nurturing our middle aged and old pets, or optimising their nutrition for their age. The average life expectancy of a wolf is estimated to be around five to six years, though they can survive to the age of 15 in captivity. Claiming 'natural is best' is clearly not borne out by the facts, whatever the reason for the early age of mortality in the wild (starvation/malnutrition, parasitism, trauma, inability to fend for itself once older age begins).

It is likely that dogs, as highly successful scavengers and opportunists, can survive on a wide variety of diets. Cats have narrower nutritional requirements. In neither species though, is there good evidence that commercial diets or raw food diets are superior nutritionally. What is clear is that pets survive much longer in domestic settings than in the wild, with the average life expectancy of dogs in a Japanese study of 13.7 years.[75] Whether this is due to protection from predation and other injuries, preventative and remedial veterinary care, or better nutrition, is currently unknown.

What's the bottom line on raw food? The benefits are theoretical and unproven. The risk to animal health is proven. And even more worrying, there is a significant risk to human health of feeding raw food to household pets.

Owners who choose to feed their pets raw should be aware of the risks to their pets and themselves and take proper hygienic precautions in food preparation. Vets who recommend raw food diets should make sure that owners are fully aware of the risks to pet and human health of these diets, and the lack of strong evidence at this stage for benefit.

Raw feeding is somewhat unusual among alternative practices, in that it has a scientifically plausible rationale. However, it belongs firmly in the realm of complementary or alternative veterinary medicine because of its lack of evidence for efficacy. Maybe one day studies will prove that raw is the optimal way to feed our pets. Until such evidence emerges however, the known risks to humans and animals from the practice, and the lack of known benefit, precludes recommending raw food diets for our pets.

# CHAPTER EIGHT

# *Acupuncture*

'*Even in China, where strenuous efforts have been made, there is still no agreement on whether acupuncture meridians or Oriental viscera such as "kidney" correspond to any known anatomic structures.*'[1]

## The myth of acupuncture

'Acupuncture: an ancient medical art that promotes natural healing by using fine needles to adjust the body's natural energy, or Qi, as it flows between fixed points on and within the body along channels known as meridians. Harmonious, balanced and gentle, it has been practised for thousands of years, its origins dating back to the roots of the oldest nation on Earth. An integral part of Traditional Chinese Medicine, acupuncture is uniquely Chinese, a unified system operating on principles previously unknown in the West which is nevertheless now being substantiated by science and embraced by the medical profession.'

The paragraph above wouldn't seem out of place in an acupuncture textbook or the glossy brochure or website of a high street acupuncture salon. Most of us, being trusting in nature, would probably accept such a statement at face value. But how much of it is truth and how much is feel-good spin? It turns out there is very little of the former and rather a lot of the latter, as we will see.

With the increasing consumerisation of the New Age has come a subtle and pervasive propaganda that has been influencing hearts and minds throughout the latter half of the twentieth century and beyond, almost without us realising. The fact this description of modern, Western acupuncture seems to ring so true is a testament to this promotional effort and the lure of counter-culturalism and idealised, romantic notions of a 'mysterious orient' (so-called Orientalism).[2] Sentiments of this sort however, no matter how loosely based in fact, are central to the continuing commercial success of acupuncture today.

Little is as it seems, or as we have been led to believe about acupuncture. In the same way that the legendary ancient kingdom of the *Xia* dynasty of 4,500 years ago would be unrecognisable, after so many upheavals and reinventions, as the present day China it has become,[3] so it is with Traditional Chinese Medicine (TCM), which bears very little resemblance to true historical Chinese medical practices, and with acupuncture in particular, the modern incarnation of which is actually quite the new kid on the block.

In this chapter we will cast light on the claims of present day advocates of acupuncture, discover what really lies behind the legends and misinformation, and consider the implications for the use of acupuncture in animals.

## Acupuncture – A questionable history

The idea that modern acupuncture, with its filiform needles, meridians and written texts, extends back in an unbroken line back to the origins of Chinese civilisation is no more true than the idea that European medicine, with its anaesthetics, pharmaceuticals and ingenious diagnostics, could be said to date back directly to the practices of the ancient greats such as Galen, Hippocrates or, to even earlier times, those priest–physicians who worshipped at the shrines of Asclepius. While there are certain fundamental similarities (holism and naturalism in particular) between modern Western medicine and the practices of the Mediterranean civilisations of the Hippocratic age nearly 2,500 years ago,[4] few would claim it has descended to us unchanged from the Classical World.

Yet contemporary proponents maintain this supposedly enduring nature is one of acupuncture's major claims to credibility, with the strong suggestion it has come down through the millennia more or less in its original form. 'Veterinary acupuncture has been used in practice for thousands of years in China', we are told in the opening sentence of one text book of veterinary acupuncture.[5] The Association of British Veterinary Acupuncturists too, claims acupuncture '... has been practiced by the Chinese and other Eastern cultures for thousands of years.'[6] One author goes for the record by claiming a provenance of 10,000 years for TCM and acupuncture,[7] taking it right back to the Stone Age. Even mainstream veterinary works now perpetuate the same story with one respected text informing us, 'The commonly accepted explanation for the methods of acupuncture can be traced back over 3,000 years ...,'[8] while another claims, 'Acupuncture is a science of energy medicine, having its origins in ancient China anything up to 4,000 years ago.'[9]

The reality is that acupuncturists today would be hard-pressed to recognise any vestige of their trade in the practices of Chinese healers much before the middle of the twentieth century. Acupuncture, as it is currently recognised, is a modern construct, and the idea that 'Chinese Medicine' can be characterised as an identifiable and coherent system is described as 'both ahistorical and selective'.[10]

## Creation myths – A questionable heritage

Studying the origins and development of Chinese medicine – its attitudes to health and sickness, to people and animals and their place in the great scheme of things – is a rewarding occupation that gives great insight into one of the most ancient and populous nations on earth. But when works are consulted, not written by practitioner–advocates seeking to garner only supporting evidence, but by authors who have analysed primary sources and have an understanding of Chinese language and culture, it quickly becomes apparent that the creation myths of contemporary human and veterinary acupuncture that are repeated with such conviction in modern texts are just that – myths.

An excellent 2001 article in the equine section of the *Compendium on Continuing Education* by veterinary surgeons David Ramey and Robert Imrie, and Sinologist and historian of Chinese medicine, Paul Buell, has selected a few of the more beguiling of these myths for us and subjected them to the type of scrutiny rarely seen from acupuncturists themselves.[11]

Take the story of so-called 'elephant acupuncture'. One popular acupuncture text informs the reader '[a]cupuncture was used on animals as long as 3,500 years ago, when, legend has it, an elephant was treated for a stomach disorder ...',[12] others claim even earlier provenance. When the evidence for this story (which originates in Sri Lanka) was examined by Drs Ramey, Imrie and Buell however, the earliest texts from Sri Lanka and India were found to contain not a single reference to acupuncture of any kind. Instead the story seems to originate, not from a verifiable, physical document, but from a single conversation that took place on 30 September 1975, mentioned in a paper written in 1979, which claimed the existence of a 3,000 year old written treatise on elephant acupuncture in Sri Lanka.[13] This claim is surprising, not least because the use of writing in Sri Lanka is considerably less than 3,000 years old.[14] Neither the original document or a transcript of the conversation has ever been produced to allow the claim to be properly studied.

Then there is 'equine arrowhead acupuncture'. The typical claim for this alleged ancient medical practice runs along the (somewhat implausible) lines that certain lame horses became sound after being hit by arrows at specific points on their bodies during battle, these observations then being developed into a therapeutic system.[15]

Supporting evidence seems to hinge on one particular bas relief, dating from 649 AD, during the Tang Dynasty. It is beautifully carved in limestone and purportedly shows a Chinese warrior performing 'arrowhead acupuncture' on a horse. This is said to be the first illustrated use of acupuncture in horses.[16] According to the University of Pennsylvania Museum of Archaeology and Anthropology, where the carving is currently on public display, the warrior in question is General Qiu Xinggong; but the museum's website has a completely different explanation for the carving than that given by acupuncture proponents.

In a tale worthy of Shakespeare, we are informed that when the Emperor's horse, *Autumn Dew*, was struck by an arrow during battle, General Qiu gave up his own unwounded charger to the Emperor, allowing him to fight on and win the day. The carving depicts this most loyal of officers, not performing battlefield acupuncture, but in the process of removing the arrow from the injured *Autumn Dew*.[17] The carving has nothing to do with acupuncture, modern or ancient, and common sense alone would dictate that even if a weapon such as an arrow was to be used in an ancient approximation of acupuncture the effect on the horse would be considerably more bloody and more painful than would be expected from the use of the delicate, filiform needles employed today.

Even the alleged 'father of Traditional Chinese Veterinary Medicine', Bai Le (also known as Sun-Yang), supposedly a 'skilled veterinary acupuncturist',[18] when examined closely turns out to be a most elusive figure. No actual text from Bai Le is known to exist and the earliest his name appears is in documents written about (not by) him 1,000 years or more after his death, these documents containing information so scant it is impossible to say what his connection with acupuncture (if any) was. In later texts, around 1125 to 1278 AD, the name Bai Le begins to be associated with 'needling' but even then no mention is made of the manipulation of *Qi* by this means, needling at that time being more associated with bleeding and cautery.[19]

The earliest surviving Chinese veterinary text, the *Simu anji ji*, dates from no earlier than 1384 and in it acupuncture is conspicuous only by its absence. While pre-modern Chinese veterinary texts make reference to the word *zhen*, this term has been consistently mistranslated as 'acupuncture' when it actually refers to 'incision' or 'penetration' (the ancient text *Baile Zhen Jing* for instance has been mistranslated as *Baile's Canon of Veterinary Acupuncture*[20] rather than the more correct *Baile's Canon of Veterinary Medicine*.[21] This is to say pre-modern Chinese veterinary medicine employed, not acupuncture as we would know it, but lancing, bleeding and firing (so-called 'fire-needling'), which, of course, were all practised by European physicians, veterinary and human, during the same period.[22]

In fact, there is very little of modern veterinary acupuncture's so-called ancient heritage that stands up to scrutiny. A diagram from one of the earliest manuals of horse medicine, the *Yuan Heng liaoma ji* (*Yuan and Heng's Collection for Treating Horses*) is claimed by modern acupuncturists to represent acupuncture points in the horse[23] but on closer inspection proves to be nothing more than diagrams of the bowel indicating likely points of faecal impaction that cause colic (see Figure Two) – there is even a later illustration in the same text showing an arm inserted into the horse's rectum illustrating how these impactions may be cleared.

It transpires there is not a single mention of acupuncture in the original text, although again cautery and bleeding are described.[24]

Acupuncture charts – supposedly crucial to the correct placement of acupuncture needles – are discussed in excruciating detail in every available contemporary text on veterinary acupuncture. Yet veterinary charts prior to the fourteenth century showed only small numbers of unconnected points (just as likely to be used for bleeding or cautery as acupuncture) with no connecting channels (meridians). While human charts had acquired connections by the fourteenth century (although their number, positions and routes were prone to change with time,[25] veterinarians had to wait until the 1970s before veterinary acupuncture charts finally acquired them, when they were simply drawn in at the insistence of the equine practitioners of the day. They are still considered only hypothetical[26] and there are concerns that since in the East animals are regarded as not possessing souls and cannot therefore have circulating *Qi*, this means meridians are an irrelevance in veterinary acupuncture.[27]

Many veterinary acupuncture points and meridians were simply transposed from human charts, a process that is questionable at best given the great differences in physical appearance, size and posture between humans and animals.[28] This illogical process of transposition almost certainly explains

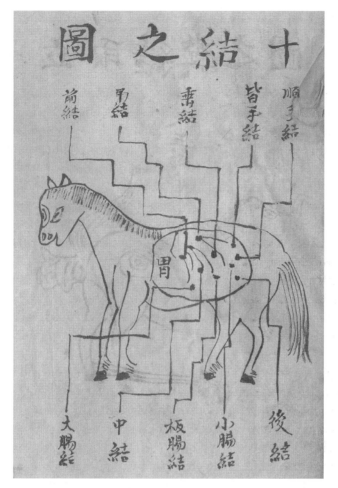

*Figure 2*    Page from Yuan Heng liaoma ji. With thanks to David Ramey

why horses have a gall bladder meridian while not actually being possessed of a physical gall bladder, and why even a casual glance at a few different veterinary texts is sufficient to demonstrate there is little or no agreement between the number or location of acupuncture points and meridians in the same species from author to author.

Even the term meridian (previously confined to geography texts) was not used by acupuncturists until it was coined in 1939 by George Soulié de Morant, a French diplomat with an enthusiasm for Chinese Medicine. In traditional Chinese practice, these vessels were properly referred to as *mai*, *jing*, or *lo* (it was also Morant who first equated the Chinese concept of *Qi* with 'energy'.[29, 30] Ear (or auricular) acupuncture, with its own set of points and lines, far from being an ancient practice, was the invention of a French physician and has a provenance dating back no further than 1950.[31]

Despite the assertions of its proponents, the only way by which acupuncture can be truly said to date back to ancient times is by redefining the term so widely as to include the act of penetrating the skin with any instrument, from Stone Age *bian-stones* to arrows and lancets. But if this is done, what is being described is no longer what modern practitioners would regard as acupuncture at all, but simply bleeding (phlebotomising) at specific points on the body, which was practised widely throughout the ancient world, having no special affinity with the East or with China.[32]

The lack of a specifically Chinese provenance is further apparent in the form of the clear influences on Chinese medicine, dating back to its earliest periods, from Egypt, Persia, Mesopotamia and the mystery cults of the Eastern Mediterranean, as medical practices and schools of thought were exchanged freely along the trading routes of the Silk Road in both directions within the continent of Eurasia. Medical informatician Ben Kavoussi highlights the unmistakable evidence of a rich and productive cross-pollination of ideas between East and West over the centuries, '… acupuncture's underlying belief system is significantly similar to concepts of health and disease that underlined European and Islamic astrological medicine and bloodletting throughout the middle ages …' Kavoussi also points out that, '… a postulated relationship between specific points on the skin and internal organs or between points and various effects on the body is not uniquely Chinese, nor is it unique to acupuncture …'[33]

He illustrates this link using charts comparing medieval European leech and phlebotomy points and Chinese acupuncture points from the same era showing a considerable degree of overlap. The notion that ancient European medicine employed concepts such as non-physical channels connecting points in the body almost identical to Chinese meridians is further demonstrated by British Library tutor, Julian Walker, as he reports 'Early theories of [European] anatomy proposed a system of veins running the length of the body, with two connecting the navel and the genitals.'[34]

Connections with Ancient Greece are also to be found, for instance in the names of diseases such as the Chinese *fèi xiāo* meaning consumption or pulmonary wasting, a literal equivalent of the Greek term for the same condition, *phthisis*; while the Chinese term for Cholera (*huò luàn*) may be a direct transliteration from the Greek. Even the central concept of *Qi* is virtually identical in its original meaning to Hippocratic *pneuma*, both terms translate as 'food from vapour', both later developed to embrace more complex ideas, ultimately being perceived as substances 'of the finest matter' that pervaded the whole world and linked the body to the wider cosmos as well as being contained in food and drugs. It can even be argued that *Qí Bó*, the most important interlocutor of one of the most fundamental texts in Chinese Medicine, the *Inner Canon of the Yellow Thearch*, supposedly a minister to legendary ruler, the eponymous *Yellow Emperor*,[35] yet a character who has no historical background in China, may be none other than Hippocrates himself, his teachings having reached China two centuries after his death.[36]

Whatever its origins, in China itself the practice of needling, mainly carried out by itinerant healers with their traditional 'nine needles' of various shapes and sizes (only three of which resembled coarse needles and pins, the rest being more akin to the instruments of bloodletting and surgery), had fallen into disrepute by the sixteenth century and in the nineteenth century steps were taken to ban it completely.[37, 38]

It might seem surprising that acupuncture should be suppressed in its purported country of origin but there were good reasons for it. One particular text gives a disturbing insight into a little-known aspect of acupuncture's history, suggesting it was far from the kindly folk medicine portrayed in recent decades.

Dugald Christie was a Scottish doctor who lived and worked in Manchuria, China, for thirty years from 1883 to 1913. The account of his time there makes fascinating reading but it is this passage, describing indigenous Chinese medical practices, which has particular relevance here:

'*The only mode of treatment in vogue which might be called surgical is acupuncture, practised for all kinds of ailments. The needles are of nine forms, and are frequently used red-hot, and occasionally left in the body for days. Having no practical knowledge of anatomy, the practitioners often pass needles into large blood-vessels and important organs, and immediate death has sometimes resulted. A little child was carried to the dispensary presenting a pitiable spectacle. The doctor had told the parents that there was an excess of fire in its body, to let out which he must use cold needles, so he had pierced the abdomen deeply in several places.*

'*The poor little sufferer died shortly afterwards. For cholera the needling is in the arms. For some children's diseases, especially convulsions, the needles are inserted under the nails. For eye diseases they are often driven into the back between the shoulders to a depth of several inches. Patients have come to us with large surfaces on their backs sloughing by reason of excessive treatment of this kind with instruments none too clean.*'[39]

It took seventy years and a brutal revolution before accounts such as those of Dugald Christie were forgotten and acupuncture received the serious make-over and positive publicity it needed in order to become acceptable to contemporary tastes in the West. In contrast, its acceptability in China remains less enthusiastic, as we will discover.

## Brand acupuncture – the relaunch

A few attempts were made to introduce acupuncture to Europe early on. In 1683, Dutch trader and adventurer Ten Rhyne's treatise, *De Acupunctura*, exhorted patients and physicians to experiment with and assess acupuncture, following his experiences of the practice in Japan. This got little reaction at the time, partly since the operation employed a finely ground needle of silver or gold and these instruments were far from commonplace, but also because of the perceived risks associated with the 'highly dangerous' act of penetrating the body's surface in an age before the discovery of antiseptics and antibiotics. Later, in the early decades of the nineteenth century, acupuncture had a brief 'flush of glory' that was all but extinguished by the 1840s.[40]

It wasn't until more than a century later, in 1971, that acupuncture as we know it today hit the mainstream. It began with a newspaper report by journalist James Reston, who had travelled to the People's Republic of China in order to cover the visit of the US table tennis team.[41]

During a visit to Beijing (then known as Peking) Mr Reston developed appendicitis, which required surgery. He gave an account of his experiences during and after the procedure, including the use of acupuncture and moxibustion (the practice of burning fragrant herbs at acupuncture points), in an article in the *New York Times*. It is important to note that his operation was carried out under an entirely conventional anaesthetic regime, not (as has often been reported) using 'acupuncture anaesthesia'. His immediate post-operative pain was again controlled using conventional medicine but it was during the second night after his operation that acupuncture (which he described as sending 'ripples of pain through my limbs') was employed to provide relief – not least, according to Reston himself, by means of distraction – from the bowel distension that was causing him discomfort.[42]

In February of the following year, US President Richard Nixon made his historic visit to China at a time when relations between Communist China and the USA were just beginning to thaw. During the trip the visiting delegates and members of the press corps were treated to demonstrations of surgical procedures supposedly performed under acupuncture anaesthesia. These demonstrations were accepted at face value and from that time acupuncture and TCM took hold in the popular imagination, undergoing an unprecedented flowering in the West. Numerous practitioners set up in business and countless texts of variable quality were published in an effort to enlighten and entice a curious public into discovering acupuncture for themselves. Today it is almost impossible to walk down any city high street in the world without passing at least one establishment providing acupuncture to all comers.

But what is it exactly that is being offered by these eager practitioner–advocates if it's not an ancient Chinese practice dating back more than thousands of years? In fact, modern-day acupuncture as we know it originates no earlier than the early 1930s when Cheng Dan'an, a Chinese paediatrician, resurrected and adapted the practice, believing its actions could be explained by neurology. Dr Cheng redesigned traditional acupuncture charts by moving points previously used for bloodletting away from blood vessels and relocating them where they would be more in keeping with modern ideas of the nervous system. He also exploited modern technology to introduce filiform needles for the first time, replacing the coarse instruments used previously.[43]

Crucially, shortly afterwards this revival perfectly suited the agenda of the central authorities following the 1949 communist revolution. Dr Cheng's variations were adopted wholeheartedly at a time when indigenous medicine was a matter of national pride and, more practically, when modern medical health care was both prohibitively costly and extremely thin on the ground. The network of traditional folk healers (the so-called barefoot doctors) that grew up by decree did so, not in accordance with medical knowledge but with Communist Party ideology.[44]

Thus the TCM and acupuncture, adopted by the Western world with such gusto in the latter decades of the twentieth century was, unbeknown to Richard Nixon and James Reston, largely a modern construct; the result of political and economic expediency. As Dr Paul Unschuld, one of the world's leading authorities on Chinese Medicine states, '... few people are aware that TCM is a misnomer for an artificial system of health care ideas and practices generated between 1950 and 1975 by committees in the People's Republic of China ...'.[45] Kavoussi calls TCM simply, 'a conceptual chimera ... which reflected more post-Counterculture and New Age ideas and ideals than the historical reality of the history of medicine in China ...'.[46]

But even this isn't the full story, and while texts such as *Chinese Acupuncture and Moxibustion*, compiled by the state-sponsored Acupuncture Institute of

China, extol the virtues of acupuncture in order to satisfy a 'global interest ... and special enthusiasm', and describe how the Communist Party revived acupuncture during the 1940s and '50s,[47] they fail to mention there was a dark side to the widespread imposition of this national system of medicine. It transpires the so-called acupuncture anaesthesia demonstrated to credulous visitors in the early 1970s was nothing more than a cynical sham.

It wasn't until the opening of China in 1978, as state repression gradually eased and the climate of fear that had prevailed during the Cultural Revolution began to lift, that witnesses began to feel safe enough to speak out about the reality of the Chinese National Health System.[48] What they revealed was a situation almost as brutal as that noted by Dugald Christie nearly a century before. This time though, the horrors were reported not by outsiders, but by Chinese practitioners themselves.

In a 1980 article in the newspaper *Wen-hui pao*, two experienced Chinese surgeons, who between them had conducted more than 30,000 surgical procedures under acupuncture anaesthesia, were finally able to lift the lid on the truth behind the propaganda, coercion and cruelty that went on under the guise of Traditional Chinese Medicine. The authors recorded tales of great suffering in the name of political dogma: doctors under orders to use acupuncture anaesthesia and patients going to great lengths to 'go through the back door' and use any influence they had to avoid it; the frequent need for the use of conventional drugs in addition to (or instead of) acupuncture; and the ever-present fear of the consequences of speaking out. Of so-called acupuncture anaesthesia they said its effects were weak, and it was used, '... at the expense of mental and physical suffering by the patient. The patient undergoes surgery in a state of full consciousness . . .'

Patients and doctors alike, '... had no choice but to have exceptional courage in order to carry out or undergo surgery, especially as the patients who felt pain could not cry out ... Only joy was reported but not sorrow; one did not dare to tell the facts.'[49]

The authors described patients having to resort to shouting political slogans in order to hide their pain during surgery and one leading ophthalmologist who, having tried acupuncture on himself and finding it ineffective, spoke out against it only to find himself severely reprimanded and at grave personal risk. They also reported that in many cases of so-called acupuncture anaesthesia, such as those witnessed by Nixon's entourage in 1972, patients were surreptitiously given conventional anaesthetic agents and painkillers prior to the surgery, with acupuncture applied during the procedure merely for show.

Despite all this, since the taking root of acupuncture in the West, it has continued to flourish. This is thanks in no small measure to a willingness on the part of practitioners and patients alike to turn a deaf ear to genuine accounts such as those above and instead believe in a version of TCM that owes more to Western desires and a fairy tale romanticism about the 'mysterious orient' than it does to actual Chinese history or philosophy.

According to Paul Unschuld '... more than 95 per cent of all literature published in Western languages on Chinese medicine reflect Western expectations rather than Chinese historical reality ... while they reflect Western yearnings, they fail to reflect the historical truth of Chinese medicine'.[50] Ben Kavoussi is of the same opinion, '... this mythical orient is a mere fiction that serves to represent the hidden desires of Western cultures, a mysterious 'other' onto which we project our fantasies.'[51]

Paradoxically, despite the enormous revenue it brings to present-day China (approaching $40 billion according to one account),[52] as a system of medicine, acupuncture is now regarded less highly in China than it is elsewhere in the world. 'Chinese medicine has been on the defensive in its homeland for a century ...'[53] A Chinese newspaper, the *People's Daily*, reports that even though the TCM industry makes up more than a quarter of China's total medical industry it is nevertheless falling out of favour when compared to Western medicine and there have been proposals to remove TCM practices from China's national health service.[54]

This attitude is reflected too in the veterinary literature. In 2014 UK Veterinary Surgeon Jason Kimm won a scholarship to travel to the city of Hangzhou in eastern China in order to study the use of acupuncture in animals. On a visit to Zhejiang University (where the university principal was an advocate of Chinese Medicine) Kimm described a distinct lack of enthusiasm for TCM and acupuncture among the veterinary students there, who maintained they only studied the subject in order to pass examinations and considered the practice 'outdated and of little relevance'. At one point Kimm's superviser told him most emphatically that acupuncture in animals was rarely employed in China now, its main use being to teach to foreign veterinary surgeons, who would then use it in their home countries.[55]

The inescapable conclusion for any impartial observer with a genuine interest in the truth of Chinese Medicine and its history is that modern acupuncture has very little to do with ancient practices. At best it is a modern caricature, dating back no further than a few decades, a sanitised version of sometimes quite brutal traditional practices including bleeding and cautery that themselves date back with certainty no more than 2,000 years or so and, rather than being uniquely Chinese, have much in common with almost identical modes of treatment of the same era elsewhere in the Eurasian continent and North Africa.

We are in danger of becoming unable to distinguish between truth and spin in the race to capitalise on the alleged benefits of acupuncture. It is a matter of regret to many commentators that the history and heritage behind Traditional Chinese Medicine is being obscured and rewritten to suit contemporary Western palates – what Paul Unschuld describes as the 'simplistic and often naive historical accounts found in modern Western secondary literature on acupuncture and Oriental medicine'.[56]

This matter is so troublesome that Dr Unschuld has even proposed a subtly different term – Chinese Traditional Medicine – for the study of the true historical entity, in order to set it apart it from the commercialised Western version, Traditional Chinese Medicine.

§

## Acupuncture and science

What then remains when acupuncture is examined for what it is, without its metaphysical trappings and questionable provenance? Is acupuncture a technique with scientific credentials?

## The theory – Acupuncture's mechanisms

Attempts to discover acupuncture points and meridians by means of dissection, histological and electrical analyses and the injection of dyes and radioactive agents have been inconclusive at best, being plagued with errors and methodological shortcomings, giving results that are inconsistent, fail attempts at replication or are easily explainable by other means.

Injectible tracers obstinately insist on draining away along unremarkable lymphatic and blood vessels, not 'meridians';[57, 58] variations in cutaneous electrical resistance turn out to correlate more with pressure between skin and probe rather than locations on anatomical charts from the Ming dynasty;[59] and descriptions of so-called primo-vessels proposed as physica–anatomical manifestations of meridians, instead bear an uncanny resemblance to the more mundane channels of the lymphatic system.[60]

Advanced techniques such as functional magnetic resonance imaging (fMRI) scans of the brain do indeed show changes during acupuncture nee-dling but such changes are not specific to any particular acupuncture point and it has not been determined whether they are any different to those seen with other types of stimulation such as non-specific needling or even a simple skin pinch.[61]

Small wonder acupuncture points are so hard to pin down when one reads 'there are about 1,600 Extra-Jing (Extra-Meridian) Old Acupoints and New Acupoints scattered all over the body'.[62] When this statement is considered alongside another study that reveals wide variation in the size (or 'fuzziness') of acupuncture points used by practitioners, being on average 19.4 cm$^2$ and occasionally more than 41cm$^2$,[63] it quickly becomes apparent there is hardly a square inch of the body surface that is not an acupuncture point of some kind.

Recognising this lack of success in discovering evidence-based explana-tions for the underpinnings of acupuncture, many modern practitioners are distancing themselves from its philosophisings and making efforts to estab-lish a scientific basis for so-called 'Western Acupuncture'. Many proponents now recognise classical acupuncture points are of limited importance '... needles put anywhere in the body are likely to have some effect.'[64] This is not an easy path however, and in doing so some have been subject to attacks from more 'traditional' colleagues. One leading veterinary acupuncturist, by taking an evidence-based approach to the subject, has been accused of insult-ing her fellow veterinarians and even of racism, while others have called for her regular news column to be replaced with something more 'positive' about acupuncture.[65]

## The practice – Clinical evidence

Clinical acupuncture research has a particular set of challenges, particularly the development of an acupuncture equivalent of the placebo, so essential in medical research when conducting controlled studies, in order to measure the true effect of acupuncture over and above any incidental effects from non-specific needling or the prolonged patent–practitioner interaction.

In the main two approaches are used. The first are sham needle systems where cleverly designed telescopic needles are employed that initially contact the skin, giving the sensation of acupuncture, but when further pressure is applied, instead of penetrating the skin they disappear into the handles rather like a stage dagger. The second approach uses sham acupuncture points, where acupuncture needles are used to penetrate the skin in the usual way, but the points chosen are either some distance from classical acupuncture points (non-points) or deliberately chosen to be incorrect for the condition being treated (wrong-points). There is good evidence to show, by interviewing trial participants afterwards, that both types of placebo are largely indistinguishable from true acupuncture.[66]

Clinical research in acupuncture is limited and often flawed.[67, 68, 69] Such good quality trials as have been performed (including double blind placebo controlled ones) consistently suggest there is little or no effect from acupuncture, and any effect that is found is independent of so-called meridians and of questionable clinical relevance.[70, 71, 72, 73, 74] Perhaps the most comprehensive study of veterinary acupuncture in recent years was published in the *Journal of Veterinary Internal Medicine* in 2006.[75] This was a systematic review looking at thirty-one of the best trials; which even so the authors described as generally of low quality. While there were some results that, in the authors' view, warranted further interest, they also reported evidence for the effectiveness of acupuncture in domestic animals was weak and concluded, 'There is little strong evidence to support the use of acupuncture as a clinical treatment in veterinary species', a phrase quoted verbatim by veterinary acupuncturist, researcher and lecturer, Samantha Lindley, in her 2006 article, *Veterinary acupuncture: a Western, scientific approach*.[76]

There is a lack of consistency, however, even among acupuncturists who claim a more science-based rationale for the practice. The systematic review above, which gave such poor results for acupuncture, was criticised for including common variations on traditional needle acupuncture such as gold bead implantation, laser acupuncture and injection techniques (so-called aquapuncture). These techniques we are told, in no uncertain terms, are 'not acupuncture' so should not be included in assessments of this kind.[77] Perplexingly though, another UK veterinary acupuncturist, after giving the generally accepted definition of acupuncture as 'insertion of a very small needle into the body in order to cure or prevent disease' has further defined it to include gold bead implantation as well as electro-acupuncture, aquapuncture (using injections of B-vitamins or bee venom), acupressure, and 'thermal' techniques such as moxibustion and laser acupuncture.[78]

Despite Dr Lindley's reservations, gold bead implantation has been an area of particular interest in veterinary acupuncture research although trials have shown inconsistent results, some showing results in dogs which are indistinguishable from placebo.[79, 80, 81] One group of authors proposes if there is any effect from this technique it may be due to sustained local inflammation and release of soluble mediators caused by the implants, suggesting a more pharmacological explanation rather than anything peculiar to acupuncture.[82] Others go further and point out, given the lack of evidence for its effectiveness, the implantation of gold beads has been condemned as malpractice.[83]

There is little question that acupuncture does something – it shouldn't come as a surprise to anyone that sticking a needle into an animal will get a response of some kind, whether in endorphin levels in the bloodstream or the central nervous system, or changes in brain activity seen on fMRI. The challenge is to decide whether acupuncture has any unique properties distinguishing it from non-specific factors such as random needling, or other forms of stimulus. There have been a number of trials carried out in human medicine that have used sham acupuncture to control for these incidental effects. They have consistently shown the effects of sham and true acupuncture are indistinguishable, both giving almost identical results in the final analysis.[84, 85, 86]

Yet presentation is everything, and it is common to see the conclusions of such trials presented in an undeservedly positive light by some authors, suggesting in their discussions first that there is an effect due to acupuncture before later mentioning, almost as an afterthought, the placebo arm also produced a similar effect. This negates the whole point of including a placebo control group in the first place and would be the equivalent of a pharmaceutical company launching a new drug on the basis it performed as well as a sugar tablet.

The importance of these non-specific factors is demonstrated most convincingly by two studies in particular. In 2008 a research team led by Ted Kaptchuck, associate professor of medicine at Harvard Medical School, studied 262 patients, all with Irritable Bowel Syndrome (IBS). The participants were divided into three study arms. For six weeks one group (the 'waiting' group) received no treatment while the other two *both* received sham acupuncture – one (the 'limited' group) having needling with minimal interaction with the physician, the other receiving an 'augmented' treatment of needling plus 'a warm, empathetic, and confident patient–practitioner relationship'.[87]

When the final results were analysed the limited interaction sham group was seen to have responded better than the waiting group but the 'enhanced' group performed better still, to a degree that was both statistically and clinically significant in scores including quality of life and symptom severity. The authors concluded '[n]on-specific effects can produce statistically and clinically significant outcomes and the patient–practitioner relationship is the most robust component'. In other words it's bedside manner, not needle placement, which makes the difference.

Another study took this concept one step further by persuading seventeen participants to temporarily accept a dummy hand as their own by allowing them to observe it being stroked for a period of three minutes at the same time as their own (a phenomenon known as the *rubber hand illusion*). Once this 'incorporation' process was completed, the participants then watched while the dummy hand was needled – their own hand remaining unobserved and untouched throughout.[88]

Incredibly, it was discovered the participants experienced identical neurological (according to fMRI scans) and physical (the *DeQi* sensation) responses to those seen during acupuncture – it was as if the needling was being performed on their own hand. This has been referred to as *phantom acupuncture* and demonstrates beyond doubt the enormous power of suggestion in the patient–practitioner relationship as the ritual surrounding the act of acupuncture and the visual input from observing the process completely override the knowledge that no physical needling is taking place. This is precisely the effect placebo-controlled trials are designed to allow for.

Because of findings such as these – highlighting the importance of acupuncture's elaborate rituals, with needles reduced to mere props – some commentators have described acupuncture as a 'theatrical placebo'.[89] This raises valid questions in human medicine and if patients benefit from prolonged and empathic practitioner interaction there may be lessons to be learned for conventional health providers in overstretched clinics, and implications for funding and staffing levels. But such debates, important as they are, have little to do with the claimed effectiveness of acupuncture as such, with its emphasis on needling as the lynchpin.

Furthermore, in the veterinary world, our patients derive no benefit from extended interaction with the clinician, no matter how elaborate (indeed many would probably be grateful for rather less interaction!). There is no placebo effect in animals in the sense it exists in humans, but it is recognised we, as caregivers, can be misled into believing we are witnessing an improvement even when, objectively, there has been none.[90, 91, 92]

There is partial support from basic research for a number of theories that might explain the effects of needling, albeit without the need for 'theatrics', specific acupoints, meridians or *Qi*. These include the release of pain modulating compounds and neurotransmitters in the brain and spinal column, and activation of other pain-control mechanisms including the hypothalamus and limbic system.[93] Veterinary advocates for acupuncture refer to its possible effect on inhibitory nerves, C–fibres and A–delta fibres (both of which transmit pain signals) and N–methyl–D–aspartate (NMDA) receptors. The release of hormones such as adrenocorticotropic hormone (ACTH) and oxytocin is also suggested as a mechanism, as well as possible beneficial competition between the fast, acute pain signals from an acupuncture needle and the slow, chronic pain signals from long-term conditions such as arthritis; and the 'gate theory' of Melzack and Wall.[94] But the precise clinical significance of all this is still uncertain,[95, 96] and the effects are independent of what techniques or needle points are used. At the same time we also know acupuncture 'works' whether or not the needles penetrate the skin and even whether or not it is performed on the patient or a dummy hand. We also know the effects of needling are entirely attributable to well understood neurological mechanisms and the effects on sensory receptors and pain pathways are easily replicated by other means including finger pressure or even toothpicks.[97] Some researchers go so far as to regard 'sham' acupuncture as simply another form of acupuncture.[98]

But are these physical effects useful in the clinical setting or are they merely 'surrogate outcomes' – interesting, but of little real relevance?

Practitioners of Western veterinary acupuncture, of course, argue there is a useful clinical effect despite the obvious contradictions noted above. For instance, even though one article reports '[t]here is little strong evidence to support the use of acupuncture as a clinical treatment in veterinary species', later in the same paper the author also claims '[p]ain is the most common indication for veterinary acupuncture' and 'acupuncture is used to great effect in the treatment of acral lick granuloma'.[99]

US acupuncturist Narda Robinson acknowledges, 'Acupuncture is simply neuromodulation, as is placebo', yet still maintains there is something 'extra' about acupuncture, '[w]hile the brain pathways leading to effects related to placebos overlap with acupuncture, the peripheral and spinal nerve stimulation engendered by ... acupuncture is discrete, measurable and purposeful.'[100] Other, less partisan commentators point to a continued lack of evidence, even after a total of roughly 3,000 clinical trials in humans.[101]

### The future – The need for the needle

*'If needles are unnecessary, then let us dispense with them'*
(Moffet, 2009, 'Acupuncture: Will Ugly Facts Kill the Beautiful Theories')[102]

Of all the complementary and alternative practices used in veterinary medicine, acupuncture is one of the most popular with owners and practitioners alike and, judging by the flavour of articles that appear in the veterinary press, possibly one of the most pragmatic. Modern day practitioners seem increasingly to acknowledge the science behind much of what underlies acupuncture; the demand for *acupuncture lite* – without the historical and metaphysical accoutrements – is growing. There has previously been dissatisfaction with the high proportion of TCM taught and required to pass examinations in veterinary acupuncture in the course run by the Association of British Veterinary Acupuncturists (ABVA), so much so that a course in Western Acupuncture was launched in 2001.[103] The foundation of the Western Veterinary Acupuncture Group (WVAG) by Samantha Lindley and Mike Cummings took the process a step further. This is a clear signal of the movement towards a more grounded approach to the subject from a few practitioners with an honest and forthright view of acupuncture's scope and applications. Acupuncture seems to be doing its best to become plausibly mainstream and it is common to find an interest in the subject in veterinary surgeons running pain clinics and with specialisms in anaesthesia.

There is, however, an elephant in the room. A crucial issue, pointed out in 1999 by acupuncturist and researcher Howard Moffet, is not being addressed. What about the needling?

Knowing the effects of acupuncture on nerves and neurotransmitters, we also know these effects can be achieved in other ways, without the need for relatively invasive needling and besides, there is limited certainty as to their clinical relevance. We know now there is little that is ancient, traditional or mystical about contemporary acupuncture but through scientific investigation we are also coming to realise it isn't rocket science either. As more research is carried out, it becomes increasingly apparent there is less that is special about acupuncture in general, and needling in particular. It remains to be seen how or even if these developments will be embraced by the more progressive elements among acupuncture's practitioner–advocates and whether needles will ever be 'dispensed with' as Moffet proposes.

§

At the 2008 British Association Festival of Science Professor Francis McGlone of Liverpool University gave an address on the subject of touch and grooming behaviours in humans, particularly the effects of stroking. He and his team discovered (using a special machine he invented for the purpose, the Rotary Tactile Stimulator), that stroking excited specific nerve fibres in the skin. When stimulated, these 'mechano-sensitive C-tactile afferents', which project into the brain in areas involved with emotion and well-being, make us feel good. He also outlined the work of another team carrying out related work on the mechanisms involved in scratching to relieve an itch (also mediated by C-fibres) and asked the question why these types of stimuli are so pleasurable and rewarding.[104]

The answer, he feels, lies in the 'interplay of traffic in the C-fibres … one balancing the other'. In other words, one type of sensation (the scratch) masks another (the itch). The similarity with some of the suggested mechanisms of acupuncture and its supposed effect on inhibitory neural pathways and on the interaction of signals from slow and fast nerve fibres is striking.

Could it be, in the final analysis, that acupuncture will turn out to be little more than good, old-fashioned 'rubbing it better' with a New Age twist?

# CHAPTER NINE

# The Anti-Vaccination Movement

W HY are we discussing vaccinations in a book about complementary and alternative medicine? Vaccinations are surely a science- and evidence-based intervention? But in both human and veterinary medicine there is a vocal movement opposing the use of vaccinations, and in many cases the voices raised in opposition to vaccinations are closely related to the practice of alternative medicine, particularly homeopathy.

In this chapter, I explore the history of vaccinations, the history and arguments of the anti-vaccination movement, the attitudes of the alternative medicine community to vaccination and the evidence regarding the safety and efficacy of veterinary vaccines.

§

## History of vaccinations

The Centre for Disease Control (CDC), the leading national public health institute of the United States, reports that during the twentieth century the average life expectancy of a person living in the US increased by more than thirty years. It attributes twenty-five of these gained years to improvements in public health, such as control of safer and healthier foods, recognition of tobacco as a health hazard, and healthier mothers and babies. However, the first item on its list of *Ten Great Public Health Achievements* is vaccination.[1]

Vaccination is the administration of a material (the vaccine) with the intention of stimulating an immune response in order to develop a resistance (or immunity) to an infectious disease. If immunity is successfully induced either naturally or by vaccination, when an individual is exposed to an infectious organism to which they have immunity, they will either not develop the disease that that organism causes, or will develop a milder form of the disease.

The ability to develop immunity has been known since the classical era, when Thucydides observed that Ancient Greeks infected with smallpox who survived did not contract the disease in future. A primitive form of vaccination called variolation, which involved exposing healthy people to the scabs of others infected with smallpox, was used in India from the tenth century, and spread to Europe via Turkey in the eighteenth century. At this time, smallpox was the most serious infectious disease of all, with numerous epidemics killing up to 20 per cent of everyone infected.

Towards the end of the eighteenth century, it was observed that milkmaids, who commonly suffered from a disease that was similar to smallpox, but with milder symptoms, namely cowpox, rarely developed smallpox. Edward Jenner, in an experiment that would have not gained ethical approval in modern times, took samples from the pustules of a milkmaid with cowpox, and rubbed them into scratches he had made on the arm of the 8 year old son of his gardener. Not content with this minor assault on the young boy, Jenner went on to expose the boy to smallpox, with the fortunate result that the boy did not develop the deadly disease. Many would forgive Jenner in hindsight, given the way he went on to promote vaccination, and begin a practice that would go on to save millions of lives over subsequent centuries.

Pasteur took Jenner's work further, developing vaccines for anthrax and rabies using inactivated disease agents that had lost their ability to cause the disease. Since then, vaccines have been developed against numerous, formerly rife and fatal diseases, such as polio, measles, hepatitis A and tetanus.

While vaccinations are highly effective at preventing or reducing the impact of disease to an individual, no vaccine is 100 per cent effective. Furthermore, some individuals cannot receive certain vaccines, for example those that are too young, or suffer from a reduced ability to mount an effective immune response (e.g. HIV sufferers or patients being treated with chemotherapy). However, individuals not directly protected can still benefit from vaccination within the population due to the concept of 'herd immunity'.

The term herd immunity is defined in various ways, for example as the proportion of immune individuals in a population, or the threshold of immune individuals, beyond which the ability of a disease to spread within a population will reduce. Generally though, herd immunity refers to the concept that if enough members of a population are immune, protection will be afforded to the susceptible members of that population. The term herd immunity was first used in the 1920s, when it was recognised that after a measles epidemic, the number of new infections temporarily decreased, even among those that were not immune. In the 1970s, simple mathematical formulae were produced to describe the proportion of a population that should be vaccinated to provide herd immunity.[2] Although this simple threshold model has been challenged because of the variations in different populations, it is still widely used, and is likely to be a valid approximation of the real situation.

Herd immunity occurs because a disease requires the presence of susceptible individuals to spread throughout a population. Chains of infection are interrupted as the pathogen encounters individuals in which it cannot reproduce, or be spread from. The higher the proportion of individuals within a population that are immune, the less chance a disease has of interacting with susceptible individuals.

Naturally occurring examples of herd immunity after epidemics have been noted following outbreaks of measles, as noted above, and other diseases such as mumps, rubella, chickenpox and polio. It has also been noted that after the introduction of certain vaccines such as pneumococcal and *Haemophilus* infections, there has been a reduction in the disease, even in groups that were too old to have been included in the vaccination campaign. In these particular cases, herd immunity has been improved by the ability of these vaccinations not only to protect against disease, but also to reduce nasal carriage of the pathogen. A reduction in influenza was noted in the elderly in Japan after the introduction of flu vaccination in children.[3]

Vaccination of individuals, with the additional benefit of herd immunity, can be so successful that it is possible to consider the complete elimination of certain diseases, which has led to the worldwide eradication of both smallpox and rinderpest, the dreaded cattle plague.

Sadly, diseases that appeared to have been on their way to eradication, at least in certain countries, have started to make a comeback because of declining levels of vaccination allowing the proportion of immune individuals to fall below the threshold needed to prevent the spread of the disease.

In the year 2000, the CDC in the US considered measles to no longer be endemic in that country. Between 2004 and 2011, most cases of measles in the US were in individuals who had caught the disease in another country and brought it back. More recently though, in both the UK and the US, measles outbreaks have occurred because of declining vaccination rates, the reasons for which are explored below.

Vaccination in the veterinary field has developed alongside human vaccination, with certain diseases being important in both human and animal medicine, such as rabies and anthrax. In some diseases, the animal vaccination was developed before the human version, while in other cases the reverse was true.[4] Interestingly, the focus of early vaccinations in the veterinary field was on herd immunity, reflecting the predominantly large animal nature of veterinary work prior to the Second World War, which generally aims to maximise revenue from the herd rather than protecting an individual. Early human vaccinations focussed on individual protection. With the rise of small animal work dominating the veterinary profession in the UK and US, the focus in veterinary medicine has shifted to the protection of individual pets to which there is an emotional rather than a financial investment, while in human medicine the concepts of public health has increased the push towards protection of whole populations. It has even been suggested that vaccinations that block the transmission of malaria should be used, which leads to difficult ethical questions, since those vaccinations do not directly benefit the protected individual.[5]

Prevention and control of epizootics (the animal equivalent of an epidemic), are major issues for the veterinary profession and government organisations with responsibility for animal health such as the Department for Environment, Food and Rural Affairs (DEFRA) in the UK. I was a young farm animal vet when the foot and mouth outbreak hit the UK, and though I was fortunate that my area remained disease free, many of my colleagues were traumatised by the mass slaughter that was carried out to control the disease.

A little further back, a colleague who still works with me in my practice, Andrew 'Chiv' Chivers, recalls when canine parvovirus hit the UK, with its devastating impact on dogs of all ages. Chiv graduated from Liverpool University in 1969, a time before veterinary vaccinations were available. I asked him about the onset of the parvovirus epidemic. He told me about breeders losing whole litters of puppies, and being unable to help. However, within a year or two, an effective vaccination had been developed, and the incidence of the disease dropped dramatically. Chiv also remembers when canine distemper was rife, and saw many cases of canine viral infectious hepatitis or 'blue eye', a disease I have been lucky enough to have never seen in twenty years in primary and referral practice. Nowadays, when Chiv is asked by clients whether it is really necessary to vaccinate dogs and cats, he says that he is old enough to remember the days before many of these vaccines existed, and as a consequence he is a firm advocate of vaccination.

Although vets now see far fewer cases of these distressing and fatal diseases, outbreaks are still common among unvaccinated individuals, partly because of the ability of the virus to survive for long periods of time in the environment. Vaccine technology continues to move forward, and new vaccines are often being developed to combat new strains of diseases, or diseases for which vaccines were previously unavailable. An interesting very recent example in my own region involved an outbreak of leptospirosis. My practice had recently adopted an improved version of the *Leptospira* vaccine that covered more strains (or serovars). Consequently (or possibly fortunately, bearing in mind this is anecdote!) we saw no cases of leptospirosis during this outbreak, whereas other practices that had been slower to adopt the new vaccine saw high numbers of cases, including a number of fatalities. The outbreak was reported to be the *bratislava* serovar, which the older vaccination did not protect against, but the newer one did, and since local practices have adopted the new vaccine, the outbreak seems to have abated. Interestingly, anti-vaccine campaigners were quoted in the press as warning against vaccinating, even in the face of an outbreak that was killing dogs.

The introduction of vaccinations in both human and animal medicine has hugely decreased the impact of diseases for which vaccines are available, both through protection of the individual and by herd immunity. However, vaccine levels are often not as high as they need to be within a population to protect individuals and to provide herd immunity. There are a number of reasons as to why this is the case, including lack of education and financial issues. Particularly in the developed world, however, a large cause of failure to vaccinate is the anti-vaccination movement.

§

## The Anti-Vaccination Movement

Although opposition to vaccination appears to have grown in the social media age, it is not a new phenomenon. Opposition to vaccination has been around for almost as long as vaccination itself. In the UK, various Acts of Parliament were made between 1840 and 1898 to make vaccination compulsory for children.[6] The introduction of an Act in 1853 making vaccination compulsory in infants in their first three months of life led to riots in several English towns and the formation of the Anti-Vaccination League in London. In 1866 the Anti-Compulsory Vaccination League was formed, and 1896 the National Anti-Vaccination League was formed with the aims of repealing the anti-vaccination Acts and the disavowal of the practice of vaccination. A Royal Commission in 1896 concluded that vaccination against smallpox was effective, but after continued pressure an Act was passed in 1898 that allowed parents who did not believe vaccines were safe or effective to obtain a conscientious objector exemption.

In the US, successful use of the smallpox vaccine in the early nineteenth century led to a decline in the disease and a subsequent decline in vaccination. Epidemics occurred among the susceptible in the late nineteenth century, and when states tried to impose or enforce new or existing compulsory vaccination laws various anti-vaccination societies sprang up, and succeeded in repealing vaccination laws in many states.

The arguments of the early anti-vaccination movement mirror many of the arguments of the modern movement, and Wolfe and Sharp argue that the modern movement is directly descended from the nineteenth century one. Similar arguments advanced against vaccination in both the nineteenth and twenty-first centuries include a belief that vaccinations cause disease, that vaccinations are recommended out of a desire for profit, that vaccines contain poisonous chemicals, that vaccine side effects are covered up, that vaccines are ineffective, and that a healthy lifestyle is just as effective or more effective than vaccination.

Other early opponents of vaccination included chiropractors and homeopaths.

Chiropractic is based on the belief that all diseases are caused by subluxations (misalignments) of the spine, which interfere with the body's function. More detail about the theory and evidence for chiropractic can be found in Chapter Eleven. What is important for this discussion though is that early chiropractors, and many modern ones, do not believe in 'germ theory', the well-proven fact that some diseases are caused by micro-organisms. Since vaccination is aimed at stimulating the immune system to defend the body against these micro-organisms, it runs in direct contradiction of the fundamental tenet of chiropractic. Daniel David Palmer, the founder of chiropractic, stated, 'It is the very height of absurdity to strive to "protect" any person from smallpox or any other malady by inoculating them with a filthy animal poison.'[7]

A minority of modern chiropractors reject germ theory, with one-third of chiropractors in a 1994 study agreeing that there is no evidence that vaccines prevent disease, that vaccines cause more disease than they prevent, and that it is safer to contract a disease than be immunised.[8] Although most modern chiropractors seem to accept that germ theory is true, a simple web search will reveal plenty of them who deny this. One consequence may be reduced levels of hygiene in chiropractors' offices, with a 2007 study culturing various pathogens from chiropractors' tables, including MRSA.[9]

In order to hold on to their beliefs and avoid uncomfortable cognitive dissonance (discomfort caused by having beliefs challenged with conflicting information), germ theory deniers, as with many other alternative practitioners and pseudoscientists, can go to extraordinary lengths to justify their beliefs, including just making things up. One common myth is that Pasteur recanted germ theory on his deathbed, for which there is no recorded evidence, and seems to have been made up by germ theory deniers. Harriet Hall discusses a fascinating conversation with a germ theory denier on the *Science Based Medicine* blog.[10] Dr Hall's correspondent did not believe smallpox existed, believed that viruses visible under electron microscopes were just cellular debris, and that the Black Death was caused by inadequate diet.

Samuel Hahnemann, the founder of homeopathy, in contrast to the views of early chiropractors and to many modern day homeopaths, supported Jenner's use of vaccination, citing it as support of his belief that 'like cures like' (see Chapter Ten). However, homeopaths soon became concerned about side effects of vaccination, and the homeopath J. Compton Burnett coined the term 'vaccinosis' in his work *Vaccinosis and its Cure by Thuja*. Vaccinosis is not a medically recognised term, but is still used by homeopaths to describe a plethora of supposed side effects from vaccinations that are often either exaggerated, disproven, or for which no evidence exists.

Homeopaths often recommend a nosode instead of a vaccine. Although the official positions of homeopathic groups is usually measured, the reality can be very different. The British Homeopathic Association (BHA) states in the FAQs section of its website that there is no evidence that homeopathic medicines can be used instead of vaccines and that immunisation should be carried out in the normal way.[11] Yet when Schmidt and Ernst performed a survey of 168 homeopaths, who were asked advice about vaccination with the MMR vaccine for a 1 year old child, 77 per cent advised against the vaccination, although some of these withdrew their answers when they were subsequently advised that this was part of a research project.[12] The response rate from homeopaths to the letter was 72 per cent, while frustratingly, not a single general practitioner out of 111 contacted responded. This study is an excellent example of how alternative practitioners may state one thing publicly while advising patients differently, but also shows how easy it is for alternative practitioners to take control of the message given to the general public, when conventional practitioners do not engage in discussion.

Similarly, the British Association of Homeopathic Veterinary Surgeons (BAHVS) states on its website that where there is no medical contraindication, immunisation should be carried out in the normal way with conventionally tested and approved vaccines. However, it does go on to raise concerns about the safety of vaccines, and also states that if an animal cannot be vaccinated, it may be appropriate to consider the use of a homeopathic alternative.

A letter concerning the safety and practice of annual vaccination was written to the *Veterinary Times* in 2004. While this was quite a measured piece, and questioned the need for annual vaccination, which is a sensible issue to raise, it did also raise concerns about vaccine safety. It later emerged that out of the thirty-one signatories of this letter, twenty-four were on the RCVS register of homeopathic veterinary surgeons, although they all omitted their homeopathic qualifications from the letter. While the fact that they are homeopaths does not automatically invalidate their arguments (see the ad hominem fallacy in Chapter Four), it does help to demonstrate the attitude of suspicion or outright condemnation many homeopaths harbour towards the practice of vaccination.

Controversies surrounding vaccination in humans came to the fore again in 1998 with the publication of a paper by British doctor Andrew Wakefield that purported to show a link between the measles, mumps and rubella (MMR) vaccination, and autism. Despite the fact that the initial study, published in the *Lancet*, included only a very small number of patients, Wakefield announced, prior even to publication, that there was a link between MMR and autism, and argued for use of the vaccine to be suspended until further testing had been performed. The British national press over the next few years widely reported the suspected link, scaring parents away from the vaccination and leading to a fall in vaccination rates and a rise in these preventable diseases.

After an investigation by *Sunday Times* journalist Brian Deer, it was discovered that Andrew Wakefield had undisclosed financial links, in which two years prior to his 1998 paper, he was paid more than £400,000 to build a case against the MMR vaccine. He also performed invasive and potentially dangerous tests on the children in the study without ethical approval, such as colonoscopy and lumbar puncture. Eventually it emerged that even the weak findings that were present in the initial paper had been falsified, particularly that the histopathological diagnoses were changed from the original findings. It was also discovered that some of the children had behavioural changes before the MMR vaccine had been administered, that the timings of the report between the vaccine and the onset of autism signs had been tampered with and that three of the children in the study did not have autism at all.

The *Lancet* fully retracted the paper, and Wakefield was struck off by the

General Medical Council for acting against the interests of his patients and acting dishonestly and irresponsibly in his research.

Interestingly, medical doctor and journalist Ben Goldacre, in his book *Bad Science*, blames the press more than Wakefield for the MMR scare, because of its willingness to publicise the controversial study despite the clear flaws.

Since the 1998 Wakefield paper, numerous studies have been performed to investigate a possible link between autism and vaccination, and two reviews of these studies, one involving a million patients, and another involving more than 14 million patients, have proven there is no link between MMR and autism.

Despite all this it is still widely believed, in anti-vaccination circles, that MMR causes autism, and high profile celebrity anti-vaccination campaigners have helped to perpetuate what has been described as perhaps the most damaging medical hoax of the last 100 years.[13]

Concurrent to the rise of the human anti-vaccination movement, a similar movement has arisen in animals. In 1994, Canine Health Concern (CHC) was founded by Catherine O' Driscoll after the loss at a young age of two of her dogs. O' Driscoll and CHC has been vocal over subsequent years in the veterinary and national press. The CHC website calls pet vaccination 'an institutionalised crime' and states that 'pet owners should be aware that vaccines compromise the health of their cherished pets causing serious side effects including allergies, arthritis, behavioural problems, cancer, paralysis and, at worst, death.'[14]

CHC also states that it 'advocates the use of alternative health care for pets, including the homoeopathic vaccine alternative, natural flea and worm prevention, and a range of complementary therapies such as Bach flower remedies, chiropractic, emotional freedom technique, Reiki, nutritional therapy, acupuncture, and more.' This highlights again the link between the anti-vaccination movement and alternative medicine.

§

So what is it that modern pet anti-vaccination campaigners are concerned about? I performed a web search for 'dog vaccine side effects' and 'cat vaccine side effects' on 24 January 2016 and scrutinised the anti-vaccination sites that were listed to assess their main arguments. (Interestingly there appeared subjectively to be far fewer anti-vaccination sites in the top results when searching for cat side effects than dogs, despite the fact that as we will see below, there is more evidence for serious long-term side effects in cats than dogs as a consequence of vaccination, even though this is still very rare.)

The main argument against vaccination appears to be a concern that vaccination may be contributing to or causing chronic disease in pets. As we have seen, vaccinosis was a term coined by a homeopath to describe the perceived long-term adverse effects of vaccination, and is used almost exclusively in the alternative medicine and anti-vaccination field.

In an article on the Canine Health Concern website, vaccinosis is stated to be 'understood as the disturbance of the life force or *Qi* of the patient that results in mental, emotional and physical changes induced by laboratory modification of a viral disease to make a vaccination.' (For discussion of the mythical life force and *Qi*, see Chapter Eight). A long list of clinical signs and diseases are attributed from various sources to vaccinosis, including polyarthritis, infertility, embryonic death, thyroiditis, myocarditis, glomerulonephritis, respiratory disease, immunosuppression, lymphoma, seizures and behavioural changes. It is asserted that these problems can occur months or even years later. If you haven't read Chapter Four on logical fallacies yet it would be worth referencing the post hoc fallacy at this point, but suffice it to say at this point that just because one event occurs after another it doesn't mean the first event caused the second.

Anti-vaccination campaigners also believe that many or all vaccines are unnecessary. More moderate anti-vaccinationists believe that vaccines should be used less frequently, but still recommend some vaccination, while the more extreme voices recommend avoiding all vaccination.

Other arguments against vaccination include the assertion that vaccines are often ineffective, that the risks outweigh the benefits, and that the diseases that are being vaccinated against are rare.

If it is so obvious to some pet health advocates and vets that vaccines are dangerous and unnecessary, why do most veterinary surgeons and veterinary professional and scientific bodies recommend their use?

Two answers frequently come through on anti-vaccination and CAVM websites, and they are similar to the arguments used against vaccination in humans.

The most benign explanation is that vets are simply uneducated, and are not up to date with the latest research, or were inadequately taught on the subject at college. More antagonistically, some assert that vets are preying on vulnerable pet owners to make money, with 'Big Pharma', being the worst offender. A *Daily Mail* article in 2010 on pet vaccination ran under the headline, 'Vaccines "are making our dogs sick as vets cash in."'[15]

Both arguments are incredibly offensive to vets. They assume that the vast majority of vets are scientifically illiterate and/or profit driven to the point of being prepared to harm pets to make more money.

My experience of the veterinary profession spans from being an employee, to owner of a small veterinary practice, to partner in a large veterinary practice, to a clinical director of a practice that is part of a large national veterinary group. In my current role, I am a member of the clinical board that advises the company on clinical matters. We have discussed vaccine safety and efficacy extensively, and have recommended rejecting the use of a new vaccine that we considered to have too many side effects compared to the rarity of the disease being protected against. This was agreed to by the management without argument, despite the fact that recommending this vaccine routinely across the group would have generated a lot of extra income. We also recommended moving to the L4 Leptospira vaccine, which as described above, likely saved lives in my own practice. This move actually cost us significant amounts of money, since the new L4 vaccine required all animals, including adults, to have a booster one month later, which we performed free of charge during the twelve-month changeover period.

It is hard to understand the argument that the vast majority of a profession that has some of the brightest and most highly educated members in the world, with high ethical standards, regulated by independent professional bodies, would willfully carry on a practice that was known to be harmful, not beneficial, and only performed for profit.

What is the truth of the matter? What evidence is there that vaccines are safe and effective, or is there evidence to the contrary? Like most things in medicine, the answer is not black and white, so let's look at the research.

§

Three studies in particular are often quoted as showing evidence for long-term side effects of vaccines. One was a survey performed by Canine Health Concern, which is available in summary form on its website.[16] This survey of 3,800 dogs found that 66 per cent of all sick dogs started being sick within three months of vaccination, and 49 per cent within one month. It found high proportions of specific conditions such as colitis, dry eye, cancer, kidney disease and behavioural problems occurred within three months of vaccination. The summary states that these findings were highly statistically significant.

On the face of it, this seems pretty damning evidence. But this study has some problems. Most importantly, it has not been peer-reviewed. Peer review, although not perfect, is an important process to attempt to ensure scientific research is accurate. Without publication of the full data, the methods and results, a number of questions stand out about this research. How were the 3,800 dogs selected? Was it a truly randomised survey? If there was any degree of self-reporting involved, then we are likely to have seen reports from owners who were already concerned that vaccines had caused their dog's illness, similar to one of the problems of the Wakefield autism study. What statistics were used – were they appropriate? How were the diagnoses of illness made? Were they based on veterinary opinion or owner suspicion, and if they were made by vets, were they based on a clinical examination or clinicopathological data such as blood tests and biopsies?

The findings of this study don't correlate with my personal experience (during my history taking in a medicine referral consultation, I always ask if vaccinations are up to date, and it's amazing how often owners look shifty and say, well they are maybe a little overdue), but this is anecdote and I haven't done the statistics.

One group that did do the study and the statistics however, was the Animal Health Trust (AHT). This independent charity based in Newmarket, Suffolk, is internationally renowned for the quality of its research, and when pet vaccine safety fears were raised in the late 1990s, the AHT performed what was known as the POOCH study (Practice Overview of Canine Health). This epidemiological study was subsequently published in the journal *Vaccine*.[17] Some 9,055 postal questionnaires were sent out at random and 4,040 of these were returned. After statistical analysis to ascertain whether the findings were likely to be real or related to chance, the authors concluded that vaccination within the previous three months did not increase ill health by more than 0.5 per cent, and might in fact decrease ill health by up to five per cent.

Of course, no one is saying that vaccines are 100 per cent safe. The data sheets of vaccines, produced by the manufacturers often list anaphylaxis, a dangerous allergic reaction, as a possible adverse effect. This reaction though, is extremely rare. Other adverse effects include the possibility that autoimmune diseases could be provoked by vaccination. One study looked at the immediate adverse effects of vaccines, reported within three days of the injection.[18] More than 1.2 million dogs at 360 veterinary hospitals were included in this study, a massive amount of data in order to produce believable results. A total of 4,678 adverse events were found, about 38 per 10,000 dogs vaccinated. These were mainly allergic reactions and anaphylaxis. Another study, from Japan, surveyed 573 animal hospitals by questionnaire to assess the number of non-rabies vaccine-associated adverse reactions in the last 100 dogs to be vaccinated in each hospital. Of these 53,700 dogs, 359 showed signs of adverse reactions, 244 with dermatological signs, 160 with gastrointestinal signs, forty-one with anaphylaxis, and one death. Vaccine reactions usually occurred within twelve hours and anaphylaxis within sixty minutes, with half the cases of anaphylaxis occurring within five minutes. The authors note that even these relatively low numbers of significant side effects is higher in Japan than is noted in other countries.[19]

One paper from 1996 seemed to show a temporal (i.e. time-related) link between vaccination and the blood disease autoimmune haemolytic anaemia or IMHA.[20] In this study, the vaccination dates of fifty-eight dogs with IMHA were ascertained, and compared to seventy control dogs with diseases other than IMHA. It was found that 26 per cent of dogs with IMHA had been vaccinated in the month prior to developing the disease, while in the control group no marked increase in the likelihood of being vaccinated was seen in the month prior to presentation at the vets. Further studies however, have failed to confirm this finding. In a retrospective study of seventy-two dogs with IMHA, no difference was found in vaccination timing between the IMHA group and the control group.[21] Another review of sixty cases of dogs with IMHA also failed to find a statistical correlation between recent vaccination and IMHA.[22]

There is also conflicting data as to whether IMHA is more common in warmer months.[23] However, data from my own practice of nearly 10,000 canine vaccinations over a twelve-month period (January to December 2015) showed a clear increase in the number of vaccinations in the summer months (more than 1,000 in each of June and July compared to under 600 for December and January). If IMHA is associated with warmer weather or something that occurs more frequently in the summer months (e.g. allergies or flea infestations), and vaccines are also more commonly given in summer months, then any apparent temporal link between vaccines and IMHA may be pure coincidence.

In conclusion, the jury is still out on IMHA and its association with vaccination. The World Small Animal Veterinary Association (WSAVA) guidelines on vaccination currently state that 'vaccines themselves do not cause autoimmune disease, but in genetically predisposed animals they may trigger autoimmune responses followed by disease – as can any infection, drug, or a variety of other environmental factors.'[24]

Another known adverse reaction to vaccination is the formation of a vaccine-associated sarcoma (VAS), or injection-site sarcoma, seen mainly in cats. This is a malignant tumour that forms at the site of vaccination injections, though vaccines are not the only intervention that can provoke this – anything that stimulates an inflammatory reaction in cats has the potential to cause this cancer.

The incidence of this tumour in the UK has been estimated at a rate of 1/5,000 to 1/12,500 vaccination visits. This is a very low adverse reaction rate, but is still significant given the number of vaccinations that are performed on our pets. One recommendation regarding reducing the incidence of sarcomas is to use a non-adjuvanted vaccine, i.e. one without additional ingredients designed to improve an immune response. However, there is evidence in the case of the feline leukaemia virus (FeLV) vaccine that non-adjuvanted vaccines are less effective. In one challenge study (the gold standard way of assessing vaccine efficacy) ten out of eleven unvaccinated cats contracted clinical FeLV when exposed to the virus, as opposed to only five out of ten cats vaccinated with a non-adjuvanted vaccine, and zero out of eleven cats vaccinated with an adjuvanted vaccine.[25]

So if vaccines are very safe, but not 100 per cent safe, is there a good reason to be giving them?

To perform a medical intervention (such as vaccination), it is important that the benefits outweigh the risks. The risks of vaccination are very small, but if the benefits are also very small, this might suggest that vaccination isn't worthwhile.

Until recently, it has been difficult to assess the exact prevalence of the diseases that we vaccinate animals against. The Small Animal Veterinary Surveillance Network (SAVSNET) disease surveillance initiative is aiming to improve this. A recent report in the *Veterinary Record* looked at gastrointestinal disease, and found that 13 per cent of samples submitted to laboratories were positive for canine parvovirus (CPV-2).[26] Although this is not the same as a 13 per cent prevalence, it does indicate that the prevalence of parvovirus in the UK is high. A 1989 paper showed the feline leukaemia virus prevalence was 18 per cent in sick cats and 5 per cent in healthy cats.[27]

We can therefore see that at least some of the diseases we vaccinate against are common. But do the vaccines work?

In order for a vaccine or other prescription drug to be licensed for veterinary use, the manufacturer has to prove efficacy. John Helps, Veterinary Manager at MSD Animal Health, outlined the process of bringing a vaccine to market: 'The process for a pharmaceutical company to bring a new veterinary vaccine to the market is a major investment of time and resource. For all veterinary vaccines to receive a marketing authorisation within the EU the manufacturer is required to demonstrate, to the regulatory authorities'

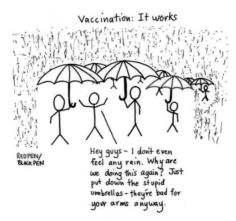

*Figure 3*   Vaccination, it works. With thanks for permission to John McDermott (http://jasonya.com/wp/category/comic)

satisfaction, its label claims for quality, safety and efficacy through a rigorous set of laboratory and field-based studies. Depending on the countries for which the product is licensed, the species it is authorised for and the intended indications, a dossier of between 5,000 and 500,000 pages is compiled for each product detailing the scientific evidence for the intended use. Registration itself may take up to three years on its own beyond the time required for research and development, so that bringing a new product on the market today may take between five and eleven years in all from initial inception and may cost up to 50 million Euros or more.'

There is also a vast amount of peer-reviewed data proving the effectiveness of vaccines, by both serology and the gold standard challenge method (i.e. exposing animals to the disease to prove protection of vaccinated compared to unvaccinated animals.) Examples include Darkauoi et al,[28] Spibey et al[29] and Abdelmagid et al.[30]

No vaccine is 100 per cent effective, but they are proven to work in the majority of cases, and if enough animals are vaccinated, then herd immunity will protect those that fail to produce a protective immune response to a vaccine. Unfortunately some individuals are happy to exploit the benefits of herd immunity while avoiding even the low risk of vaccination themselves (see Figure Three).

§

As we know that vaccines are not 100 per cent safe, and not 100 per cent effective, some people advocate titre testing instead of regular revaccination.

This involves taking a blood sample to check whether the antibody levels are sufficiently high to provide protection. The WSAVA vaccination guideline group state that titre testing for Canine Distemper Virus (CDV), Canine Parvovirus (CPV), Canine Adenovirus (CAV), Feline Panleukopenia Virus (FPV) and, for legal purposes, rabies virus, can be useful. However, titre testing does not measure cell-mediated immunity, the important 'other half' of the immune system that does not involve antibody production to fight disease. Since cell-mediated immunity is the mechanism by which, for example, leptospirosis is most effectively fought by the immune system, titre testing is useless for assessing immunity against this disease.

Titre testing is generally more expensive than vaccination, which can be a bar to some people ensuring that immunity is maintained in their pets.

Moreover, taking a blood test is an inherently invasive procedure, hence why it is considered an act of veterinary surgery, and would require a home office licence if performed for experimental purposes. Taking blood samples in cats can be particularly problematic, and can require sedation, a far riskier procedure than vaccination. Even restraining a fractious cat can entail some risk to the animal, and there has been one report of a freak accident in which a cat died after a blood sample when the carotid artery was hit instead of the jugular vein.

Titre testing may be a useful complement to vaccination in our fight against infectious diseases, but it is not without its own problems.

§

Vaccination is an extremely safe and effective procedure, which saves countless lives every year. There appear to be a variety of reasons that people don't vaccinate their pets according to recommendations, including neglect and financial issues, but also because of a vocal fringe movement, often strongly associated with the alternative medicine movement, that condemns vaccination as dangerous and unnecessary. The information in this chapter should enable professionals and pet owners to make a more informed choice about protecting their pets from these distressing and deadly diseases.

§

The authors of the WSAVA vaccination guidelines are internationally respected researchers in the field of immunology, and two of them kindly agreed to answer some questions from me (AG) regarding the guidelines.

§

193

Professor Michael Day (MD) is Professor of Veterinary Pathology at the University of Bristol School of Veterinary Science.

**AG:** Was there any pressure for a body such as the WSAVA to set up the vaccine guidelines, and if so did that come from the veterinary profession, pharmaceutical industry, the general public or anywhere else (e.g. special interest groups)?

**MD:** The WSAVA Vaccination Guidelines Group (VGG) was established in 2006 and produced the first WSAVA guidelines in 2007. The impetus to establish the VGG came from the WSAVA Scientific Advisory Committee (SAC) which keeps a broad oversight on contemporary scientific issues and oversees all WSAVA scientific projects. The SAC realised that vaccination guidelines had been produced for North America and Europe and some individual countries, but saw the need for global advice that could be used by all WSAVA member countries and veterinarians (currently some 158,000 veterinarians in eighty countries).

**AG:** Do you think there is sufficient published evidence to produce firm guidelines on vaccination frequency and adverse effects? What do you think the current evidence shows about the incidence of adverse effects from vaccination, and do you think the current reporting system means they may be either under or over-reported?

**MD:** The new 2015 WSAVA guidelines adopt an evidence-based approach to vaccinology and have proposed a novel classification scheme for the quality of evidence related to vaccinology. It is clear that the quality of scientific evidence related to vaccinology is not as great as we would wish. The types of studies required to provide such evidence are long-term and have cost and welfare implications. Increasingly, manufacturers are publishing such regulatory studies in the peer-reviewed literature, but this was not always the case.

Information about the prevalence of adverse events associated with companion animal vaccination comes from pharmacovigilance schemes (run by manufacturers and/or government regulatory authorities) or from academic studies involving questionnaire surveys or analysis of large practice management systems databases. The currently available evidence suggests that vaccination is a very safe procedure in dogs and cats, with a prevalence of adverse events (of any type, but mostly mild and self-limiting) within the range of 30 to 50 per 10,000 vaccinations administered.

Of course, voluntary (passive) pharmacovigilance schemes will not capture all adverse events and database mining will be a more robust means of gathering such data in the future. In the UK, the potential of projects such as SAVSNET and Vet Compass should impact in this area.

**AG:** Leptospirosis is listed as a non-core vaccine, and yet in the UK it is a common vaccine preventable disease. Do you feel the guidelines are clear enough when it comes to geographical variations of disease incidence?

**MD:** This question is frequently asked and reflects a lack of understanding of guidelines. Guidelines are not a globally applicable law of vaccination; they are simply a source of evidence-based scientific information that should be reviewed and adapted for regional, national or practice use. It is perfectly acceptable, and within the spirit of guidelines, for an individual country to classify a globally non-core vaccine as core; on the basis of scientific evidence that indicates that this process is justified. Leptospira vaccine can only ever be non-core globally, as there are geographical regions where this infection does not exist in the dog.

The 2015 guidelines try to make this concept very clear:

> 'These WSAVA vaccination guidelines do NOT serve as a set of globally applicable rules for the administration of vaccines to dogs and cats. It is simply not possible to produce a set of guidelines that applies equally to each of the eighty WSAVA member nations as there are vast differences between countries and geographical regions with respect to infectious disease presence / absence or prevalence, vaccine product availability, owned versus free-roaming dog and cat populations, practice and client economics and societal attitudes.
>
> 'Instead, these guidelines are intended to provide national small animal veterinary associations and WSAVA members with current scientific advice and best practice vaccination concepts. It is up to national associations or individual practices to read, discuss and adapt these guidelines for their own particular practice situations. These guidelines are not proscriptive; for example, it is entirely possible that what might be considered a non-core vaccine in many countries, or particular geographical regions, might be used as a core vaccine elsewhere.'

**AG:** How much weight do you put on the frequently quoted Purdue study showing autoimmunity following vaccine?[31] This is frequently quoted by anti-vaccination campaigners as evidence of harm and induction of autoimmune disease by vaccinations – do you feel this paper is robust enough to support this assertion?

**MD:** The association between vaccination and autoimmunity has been addressed by numerous studies (epidemiological, experimental and clinical) in both human and veterinary medicine. By virtue of the complexity of autoimmunity, no study has definitively demonstrated a mechanistic link (with high quality scientific evidence base), but there should be no doubt that in individual patients, vaccination can be a potential triggering or predisposing factor for autoimmunity … together with genetic background, immunological imbalance, gender, age, lifestyle, stress, diet, drug exposure, underlying neoplastic, infectious or chronic inflammatory disease and others.

**AG:** There is recent evidence that adjuvanted FeLV vaccines offer better protection that non-adjuvanted.[32] Was this taken into account in the guidelines and would it alter recommendations?

**MD:** This paper and the associated letters from the two companies involved were published after the VGG concluded its work on the 2015 vaccination guidelines … so no, the paper was not considered.

The VGG is careful to categorise vaccines generically and does not refer to product names or individual manufacturers. The VGG does not recommend specific vaccine brands over others. The only comment that is made with respect to feline vaccines is that we would recommend, where possible, the use of non-adjuvanted vaccines in order to lower the risk of feline injection site sarcoma.

**AG:** If pets are only given their primary puppy/kitten course and their first annual booster, do we know what percentage of pets will have lifelong immunity?

**MD:** The new 2015 guidelines redefine the core primary course as three vaccinations with the last given at sixteen weeks or older and now provide the option of either a twenty-six-week or fifty-two-week 'booster' (while redefining the purpose of that vaccination). Based on experimental and field studies, there is a belief that an appropriately vaccinated puppy or kitten will have long-lived immunity to CDV, CAV, CPV-2 and FPV. Experimental evidence for canine core vaccines shows seropositivity for up to fourteen years and field evidence for seropositivity up to nine years. Experimental challenge studies show protection with canine core vaccines for up to nine years and for feline core vaccines for up to seven and a half years. In the field, there will be individual animals for which long-lived immunity does not occur (or indeed any immunity in the case of genetic non-responders). The VGG believes that modified live virus (MLV) core vaccines will provide lifelong protection in 'the majority of animals', but we do not definitively quantify 'the majority'. The simple answer to the question is 'no, we do not know as the studies have not been done on sufficient scale'.

**AG:** Do you feel that the anti-vaccination movement is a threat to animal health and welfare?

**MD:** I think we need to be careful in use of the term 'anti-vaccination movement'. Most such lobby groups are not 'anti vaccination', but are against administration of unnecessary vaccines (i.e. with respect to individual components or frequency of revaccination). To that extent, over time, the acceptance of WSAVA (and other guidelines groups) recommendations have addressed the concerns of such groups. The concept of triennial titre testing for canine core vaccine antigen components (instead of automatic revaccination) is now also consistent with WSAVA advice and the wishes of the lobby groups. Provided the individual group accepts the fundamental principles of vaccination and minimum protective protocols, there should be no impact on animal health and welfare. It is for these reasons that the VGG produced a companion document to the veterinary guidelines that is for the information of pet owners and breeders.

§

Professor Ronald Schultz is Professor and Chair of the Department of Pathobiological Sciences at the University of Wisconsin–Madison. He kindly answered my questions regarding the vaccination guidelines with the following response:

*Dear Dr Gough,*

*Thank you for your email regarding 'vaccines and adverse events.'*

*Regarding your questions, the pressure to establish feline vaccine guidelines came from the American Association of Feline Practitioners (AAFP) when it was found that certain feline vaccines could cause feline vaccine associated sarcomas in healthy cats. Very few practitioners or owners ever thought about a vaccine causing a lethal sarcoma in cat. The prevailing attitude was 'vaccines protect from disease, not cause disease!'*

*The AAFP decided to develop vaccine guidelines when it was discovered that certain vaccines were associated with the development of VAS. Although there was no similar adverse event in the dog, it was decided to develop vaccine guidelines in part because I and my colleague Dr Fred Scott demonstrated long-term immunity (five to eight years) for certain feline vaccines. Similarly, I and my colleagues Dr Max Appel and Dr Skip Carmichael demonstrated long-term immunity (up to a lifetime) for certain canine vaccines (CDV, CAV).*

*At the time we did this work CPV-2 had not yet emerged. However, when it was found to be a mutated FPV virus, we knew that a CPV-2 vaccine would provide long-term immunity just like FPV provided long-term immunity! I knew there was sufficient evidence to produce firm guidelines on vaccination of the cat and the dog. We had published information very early (1960s and 1970s) showing that dogs that recovered from CDV or CAV-1 disease were immune for the rest of their life and cats recovering from FPV also were protected for life. We also knew that people who got measles, mumps, or rubella once in their lifetime had lifelong immunity. If immunity could persist for seventy-plus years in people, it surely could persist for seven-plus years in a cat or dog to certain viruses, especially when some of these viruses were closely related (e.g. CDV and measles virus.) In fact, as you know, measles virus is used to protect puppies with maternal antibody from CDV!*

*With regard to core vs non-core vaccines: If a disease is a significant threat in a certain country a vaccine to prevent it should be core, whereas if it is not a significant problem the vaccine should not be part of the core vaccines. I commonly get a question or comment, disease X is very common in our country or city or state – why isn't it core? It should be core if it is a significant disease problem.*

*Yes, I do think there is sufficient evidence (doesn't need to be published) from necropsy records, diagnostic microbiology laboratory testing, clinical studies, etc … to produce firm guidelines on vaccination. I think you, as a practicing veterinarian and your colleagues should be able to determine how important specific disease is in your country, state (geographic area) to determine the need for a given vaccine. It may be a core vaccine for one region and a noncore vaccine for another region of the country.*

*It is important to recognise that vaccines can cause disease (especially immune mediated diseases) in certain animals. However, the diseases or adverse reaction are rare, thus the vaccine should be given to all dogs and cats at risk. On the other hand, vaccines should not be given more often than is necessary. When vaccines like CDV, CAV, CPV-2 provide lifelong immunity, they don't need to be given more often than every three to five years or never again in the life of the animal.*

*I hope this helps,*

*RD Schultz*
*Professor and Founding Chair*
*Department of Pathobiological Sciences*
*University of Wisconsin–Madison, School of Veterinary Medicine*

I followed up Professor Schultz's email with the following question: 'One of the questions I asked was about whether you think vets are ignoring your work in order to prevent losing income, as you were quoted in saying in *Dogs Naturally* magazine.[33] Do you stand by this statement?'

His reply was as follows:

*Hello Alex,*

*The comment that I made to the person from Dogs Naturally was: 'There are some veterinarians that feel the only way some owners will bring their dog to the veterinarian is if it needs a vaccine'.*

*As you know any dog that needs a vaccine with a duration of immunity (DOI) of one year must be revaccinated yearly. However it would not need a vaccine yearly that provides five to seven or more years of immunity (CDV, CAV, CPV)!*

*I don't think veterinarians are ignoring my work, as the American and World Canine and Feline Guidelines are based in part on the research I and my colleagues at Cornell University (1970–1978), Auburn University (1978–1982), and the University of Wisconsin-Madison (1982 to present) have been doing for the last thirty-five-plus years! Furthermore, I have been a member of the Feline and Canine Vaccine Guidelines Committees, therefore I wouldn't allow them to ignore my work!*

*I hope this information is helpful.*
*Sincerely, Ron Schultz*

§

# CHAPTER TEN

# Homeopathy (Including Nosodes, Sarcodes, Isopathy, Bach Flower Remedies)

MISCONCEPTIONS abound regarding homeopathy. Such is the effectiveness of homeopathic 'spin', many users are convinced it is safe and effective and has firm scientific evidence behind it. Others may assume it is akin to herbal medicine, using small amounts of natural material to treat disease. In fact homeopathy is none of these; it is actually one of the most improbable and deeply strange manifestations of CAM in existence today. Its use has resulted in the deaths of humans and animals, yet in trials against blank placebo controls it is found to be utterly ineffective at treating disease.

Homeopathic texts claim it 'treats the individual', and that all disease is the result of a disturbance in a spirit-like 'vital force' as a consequence of a limited number of fundamental causes or 'miasms'. Originally it was said only three miasms – psora (scabies), sycosis (gonorrhoea) and syphilis – were sufficient to account for every known affliction,[1, 2] but modern authors consider there to be more including AIDS, tuberculosis and cancer.[3] It is also believed these malign influences can pass from generation to generation.[4]

When a homeopath is assessing a patient, the protracted case-taking will involve long lists of questions, not necessarily about the presenting condition, but about her personality, her likes and dislikes, family history, any fears or phobias and any particularly meaningful or shocking incidents during her life.

Only by doing this, homeopaths would have us believe, is it possible to determine the patient's *constitution* and come up with the all-important *similimum*, that painstakingly detailed list of symptoms that are unique to the individual and allow the practitioner to consult homeopathic texts, searching lists of remedies to find the one with the *signature* that most closely matches the signs and feelings described by the patient.[5, 6] Once this remedy is administered, we are told, the patient's symptoms will be 'cancelled out' and well-being restored.

That's the theory at least; the truth is somewhat different.

§

It was a lucky horse who, in the eighteenth and nineteenth centuries, was attended by a homeopathic rather than a conventional veterinary surgeon.

Compare these two accounts – one 'conventional', one homeopathic – of the treatment of a horse with inflammation of the lungs:

From the 1829 *Farrier and Naturalist:*[7]

'*... Bleeding was many times repeated, and in 14 days, no less a quantity than 48 quarts of blood by measure was drawn. A rowel was inserted on the sternum, and both sides of the chest were blistered. The blistering was afterwards several times repeated ...*

'*On the 27th [of May] the degree of dullness had increased, and so also had the pulse in frequency, though very low. Breathing was quickened, and the nostrils were expanded ... two plugs were inserted in the front of the chest, and two rowels on the sternum ...*

'*... on the 6th of June the mare dropped and died without a struggle.*'

From Dr Humphreys's book of 1860, *Manual of Veterinary Specific Homeopathy:*[8]

'*Give, the first twenty-four hours, the Specific for Inflammation, A.A., a dose of fifteen drops every two hours. After that, give the Specific for Cough and Inflamed Lungs, E.E., alternately with the A.A., at intervals of two or three hours between the doses.*

'*Continue this treatment steadily and uniformly by night, as well as by day ... After a day or two ... the medicines for Fever, A.A., may be omitted entirely, and only the E.E. given ... After the horse has commenced to improve, a dose of the E.E. every four hours during the day, will be sufficient to complete the cure.*'

Reading these contrasting excerpts, it is hard to disagree with Dr Humphreys as he wrote, concerning homeopathy, more than a century and a half ago, 'It is something to be emancipated from drugs, from lancets, leeches, blisters and poisons; but it is more, to be relieved from the fear of them ...'[9]

There can be no argument that the heroic medicine of past ages was as brutal as it was ineffective, and homeopathy, whether or not it was effective, must have been seen as a welcome contrast by owners, dismayed by the prospect of the bleeding, firing and purging that was virtually all mainstream veterinary surgeons had to offer at the time.

But things change and even by the 1880s, when Dr Humphreys published the third edition of his book, more enlightened authors such as Edward Mayhew were writing in disparaging tones about the excessive practices of the veterinary medicine of the day, advising practitioners to 'think twice before you bleed once, and shun the operation if it can possibly be avoided'.[10]

Since then, mainstream medicine has continued to move on, learning from its mistakes and adopting a progressive, science-based and self-critical approach to healing. It now bears no resemblance to the practices of days gone by. Yet homeopathy, founded some 220 years ago, seems to have failed to recognise this and still continues to tilt at the windmills of heroic medicine as if nothing had changed.

§

## Homeopathy – Origins

Homeopathy was invented in the eighteenth century by the German physician Christian Friedrich Samuel Hahnemann (1755–1843), the son of a painter in the Electoral porcelain factory at Meissen. Hahnemann initially studied medicine at Leipzig, later moving to Vienna, before finally qualifying at Erlangen in Bavaria, in 1779. Throughout his student years and during the start of his medical career Hahnemann supplemented his income by translating medical and other texts.[11]

As his career progressed he became an outspoken critic of the conventional medicine of his day, in particular the practice of blood-letting that he felt, probably with good reason, had contributed to the death of Kaiser Leopold II, King of Hungary and Bohemia, on 1 March 1792.[12] Gradually, as his disillusionment with his chosen profession grew, his income came to depend more on his work as a translator and less on medicine.[13]

One of the texts he worked on, the *Materia Medica* of Edinburgh professor of medicine, William Cullen, concerned the properties of the bark of the South American Cinchona plant that, when taken in powdered form, helped combat malaria, or marsh fever as it was then called. We know now this was due to the alkaloid, quinine, but in those days its curative properties were believed to be due to its bitter and astringent taste. Hahnemann disagreed and decided to test the treatment for himself. Having ingested four drachms of the powder twice daily for several days he found himself suffering a variety of symptoms that were described as '... "cold" fevers, similar to the fevers of the marshes'. Hahnemann, believing this couldn't be mere coincidence, 'sensed a law' that the curative powers of a substance are to be found in the effects of that substance on a healthy person.[14] In other words, if a healthy person takes a remedy that treats malaria then that person will experience the symptoms of malaria. This formed the basis, in 1796, of homeopathy's first and most fundamental principle – *Similia Similibus Curantur*; otherwise known as 'The Law of Similars', or simply, like cures like. This was the birth of homeopathy.[15]

After this initial, questionable leap of faith, Hahnemann began experimenting with other substances, now using his friends and family as subjects as well as himself. These so-called *provings* were used to determine what symptoms were produced by each remedy in healthy volunteers and consequently to discover what symptoms that remedy might be expected to address in a patient who was ill. Not surprisingly, after consuming quantities of deadly nightshade, aconite, leopard's bane and other toxic substances his testers and his patients started to become ill. This was such a feature of the early provings that the resulting text (*The Materia Medica Pura*) in which the various effects of poisonings and over-dosage were recorded, made a unique contribution to pharmacology in its own right.[16]

To reduce the risk Hahnemann started to dilute the substances under investigation and found, not surprisingly, the serious side effects diminished. More surprisingly, he also managed to convince himself that at the same time the positive effects also conveniently increased. This then became the second principle of homeopathy the *Law of Infinitesimals*, in other words, the more a substance is diluted, the stronger it gets.[17, 18] So convinced was Hahnemann of this 'less is more' principle that later in his career one of his most favoured means of administering his highly diluted remedies was to allow the patient merely to smell a single tablet.[19]

Hahnemann also decided better results could be obtained by *potentising* the remedies (making them stronger) by means of thumping (or *succussing*) them during preparation, as they were being diluted. The best medium for this he felt was 'an elastic body'; preferably a leather-bound book.[20] The more thumps, the more potent the remedy. The exact number of thumps required has been a matter of some debate, with Hahnemann advising, in his defining work, *The Organon of Medicine*, anything from two ('to avoid ill effects')[21] to one hundred.[22] These days a super-fast succussing machine is used by commercial homeopathic manufacturers and the number of blows can be as many or few as required. According to Hahnemann, the ability of succussion to increase the potency of homeopathic remedies was so great it could mean the difference between life and death. When he claimed a remedy made from sun-dew in a decillionth-fold dilution, 'cured whooping cough if shaken twice … whilst one drop in a teaspoon of the same dilution with twenty and more shakes would endanger a man's life' it engendered incredulity in even his most loyal biographer, Richard Haehl.[23]

And that, in a nutshell is it. The entirety of homeopathy is based on a single, initial experience of Hahnemann's, followed by a string of subjective impressions from various friends and family about the supposed effects of remedies on the individual. There is a difficulty though – unfortunately for Hahnemann and for homeopathy, that first experiment using the bark of the Cinchona plant was fatally flawed.

The reaction Hahnemann experienced after taking Cinchona powder is almost unheard of in anyone else who has taken the remedy – Cinchona bark simply does not produce the malaria-like symptoms Hahnemann recorded. Haehl, in his intimate and detailed life story of Hahnemann, tells us that a Dr Schwartz, of the local Board of Health, reported, '… Peruvian bark, even in the preparation advocated by Hahnemann, did not cause fever in either healthy people or animals', while Professor E. Behring, of Marburg, wrote in 1898 that, since Hahnemann's initial experiment on himself, '… Cinchona bark and quinine have been taken by people and have been administered to animals in the most varied forms without ever producing fever, let alone malaria …' Even Hahnemann's supporters were hard-pressed to rationalise away this weak-spot in the cornerstone of homeopathy, with Berlin pharmacologist and homeopath, Professor Lewin, claiming such a reaction could happened, but only in those with a 'special individuality'.[24]

In other words, what Hahnemann had experienced was anything but typical – it seems the basis for homeopathy was nothing more than an allergic reaction. Even if one is prepared to accept the quite arbitrary premise that like cures like, Hahnemann's conclusion that Cinchona bark cured malaria because it caused its symptoms in healthy people could not possibly be true.

§

## Homeopathy, there's nothing to it – The law of infinitesimals

Homeopathy today still depends on Hahnemann's two basic tenets – the law of similars (like cures like) and the law of infinitesimals (the more dilute a remedy is, the more potent it becomes). With the passing of time however, both these so-called laws have been taken to extremes.

Take the law of infinitesimals. One of the most astounding aspects of homeopathy is the extent of the dilutions employed in the preparation of remedies. Although the question of extreme dilution is only one of many reasons why homeopathy is so implausible to an impartial observer, it is worth considering the matter in detail just to get an idea of the true scale involved.

Many texts and websites will claim homeopathy uses tiny amounts of substances to achieve its results. They may suggest a similarity with say, hormone treatment, or vaccination, which do indeed use minute doses to obtain powerful therapeutic effects. These claims are wrong however, they massively under-estimate what is involved in homeopathic levels of dilution that, particularly with the most potent remedies, are quite literally astronomical, so much so that human minds have difficulty grasping them.

The level of dilution of any particular remedy can be seen on its label as a rather cryptic sequence of numbers and letters (although, since the letters are Roman Numerals, it is really a sequence of numbers and numbers). Consider a popular dilution for starters: *30X*. The '*X*' is the Roman Numeral ten and the '*30*' denotes the number of times a one in ten dilution has been made.

To carry out the 30X dilution the pharmacist will take a solution of the base substance to use as the *mother tincture* and dilute this one in ten. Then some of the resulting solution will itself be diluted one in ten. Then some of that solution will be diluted one in ten and so on until the process has been repeated 30 times.

Seeing this written down doesn't immediately suggest anything too startling. A quick glance at the figures might suggest the final level of dilution might be perhaps a one in 300 solution, possibly one in 3,000?

But it has to be remembered these dilutions are exponential, so the figures involved get extremely high extremely quickly. After a mere thirty dilutions of one in ten we arrive at a dilution of one in 1,000,000,000,000,000,000,000 ,000,000,000 (or one in $10^{30}$); a number that goes by the most appropriate of names, a *nonillion*.

If this is difficult to visualise, imagine walking to the seashore with a bottle of the mother tincture and taking from it a single drop that you then let fall into the ocean as it laps around your feet. Then imagine, as time passes, that one drop being carried by wind and current until it is spread out across all the oceans of the world. You would be correct in thinking that would be a phenomenal level of dilution. But is this literal drop in the ocean enough to get us to a 30X dilution? Well, no, not by a long shot – you would have to put one drop of mother tincture into the equivalent of 50,000 of the total world's oceans put together, to create a 30X solution!

Yet, in homeopathic terms a 30X remedy is really nothing to get excited about. By comparison with other remedies it's just getting off the starting blocks, and practising homeopaths routinely use far greater dilutions. Take the example of the 200C dilution used to prepare the homeopathic stalwart, *Oscillococcinum*, a remedy that starts with an infusion of the internal organs of a duck that have been allowed to putrefy. The letter C in 200C is the Roman numeral for 100, so in this case the mother tincture has been diluted at a ratio of one in a hundred, and this is repeated 200 times. Physicist Robert Park has done the maths on this one and tells us the dilution obtained at the end of the process is equivalent to one molecule of duck to $10^{400}$ molecules of water, which is to say the number one followed by 400 zeroes.[25]

Now we're way, way beyond the volumes of oceans, planets or even galaxies required in order to put things in perspective and give us an idea of the scale involved. For our unit of dilution only the entire universe itself will suffice. Professor Park tells us the known universe contains only $10^{80}$ atoms, so if we wanted to dilute a single molecule of duck with the further $10^{400}$ water molecules required, we would need several thousand universes-worth of water to do so. Even this unimaginable level isn't enough for some homeopaths – still higher dilutions include the M (1,000) potency; while the LM potencies are diluted at an incredible 1 in 50,000 ratio many times over.

Living in an age when molecules and atoms were unknown, Hahnemann wouldn't have realised dilution can only be taken so far before every last trace of the original substance has disappeared, although even he was uneasy with some of the extremes and expressed the opinion there 'must be a limit' to the matter of dilution.[26] It turns out he was correct, the *Avogadro limit* means once a molecule has been diluted in another $6.02 \times 10^{23}$ then the original molecule is effectively gone. The implication for homeopathy is that any remedy of 13C potency or greater will contain no trace of the base ingredient. After that any further dilutions make no difference – you are just diluting water. As Prof Park points out, there is simply no medicine in the medicine!

Homeopaths themselves are fully aware their remedies are nothing more than water, sugar (lactose) or alcohol but surprisingly say it makes no difference and continue to claim a remedy will get stronger the further it is diluted, despite a complete absence of any trace of the original ingredient.

## Enhanced potency and the memory of water

One of the main reasons for the imperturbability of the homeopath when it is pointed out remedies contain no active ingredient is they have come to believe water has a 'memory' and can recollect what was dissolved in it, even after no physical trace remains.

But this in turn gives rise to a further set of problems and homeopaths have had to come up with a variety of theories about the mechanism by which simple H2O is imbued with a sense of history and can retain information, a phenomenon no one else apart from homeopaths (and possibly a few ice sculptors) has ever claimed.

In his *Organon of Medicine*, Hahnemann writes that medicinal powers are 'lying hidden in the soul of natural substances' and he believed when succussed, the base material became 'spiritualised'. It was this succussion – the banging of remedies on a leather pad during preparation – he maintained, which set homeopathic dilutions apart from 'simple dilutions' where the solution was merely stirred gently, and allowed his remedies to retain their healing properties even after extreme dilution.[27]

Such overt spirituality though, doesn't sit comfortably with the scientific credibility to which homeopathy now aspires. These days homeopaths have been obliged to devise other explanations to fit the bill.

Veterinary homeopaths tell us succussion (which apparently has to be in the vertical plane, suggesting water not only has a memory but also a sense of direction) 'encourages a spiralling movement and the formation of vortices, which is necessary for ... molecular clusters to form'.[28] What these molecular clusters do to impart memory exactly, how long they last in solution or why their effect has never been demonstrated to the satisfaction of the scientific community isn't made clear.

But anyone unhappy with the limitations of molecular clusters needn't worry, a wide assortment of other theories can be found to suit every taste in virtually every homeopathic website and textbook one cares to read.

Nanotechnology is an astounding, cutting-edge field of research involving the manipulation of matter at the atomic or sub-atomic level by machines the size of molecules. The subject is incomprehensible and baffling to many but a simplistic argument by some homeopaths would have us believe since nanotechnology involves things that are really tiny, and homeopathic remedies involve really tiny amounts of base ingredient, the two must be connected.

One study, which has been embraced by many in the homeopathic community, announced the discovery of so-called nanoparticles in homeopathic remedies that the authors had purchased from the local market. Electron micrographs included in their paper reveal these particles to be amorphous blobs of varying shapes and sizes. Their chemical constituents were determined and measurable quantities of mercury, iron, zinc, gold and copper detected. Yet, in keeping with the inverse logic of homeopathic research, these results were interpreted as indicating, not worrying levels of heavy metal contamination, but evidence in favour of nanoparticles being the mechanism by which homeopathy has its effect.[29] However, the authors fail to address some obvious questions that arise if their conclusions are true. For instance, if metal-based remedies are claimed to retain starting materials in the form of nanoparticles, what about those made from say lymph from smallpox sores, Ebola, Human Immunodeficiency Virus (HIV) or other, smaller viruses – do they contain actual viral material? And what about remedies made from those altogether more insubstantial base materials that we will discuss later in this chapter; how is it possible to have nanoparticles of storms (*Tempesta*), shipwrecks (*Naufragium Helvetia*), light from the planet Venus (*Venus Stella Errans*) or anti-matter (*Positronium*)?

Ironically, and in somewhat of an own goal, the chief advocacy group for organic farming, the Soil Association, while on the one hand suggesting homeopathy must be used in preference to science-based medicines in the treatment of diseased animals, on the other hand has also banned the use of nanoparticles.[30] It seems organic producers will have to find another theory about how homeopathy works to believe in if they are not to fall foul of either their regulating body or of the Veterinary Medicines Directorate (VMD), which regulates the use of medicines in animals and requires homeopathic remedies to be 'sufficiently dilute to guarantee safety'.[31]

The incomprehensibility of quantum physics may help resolve the dilemma. This branch of science is almost irresistible as a means to explain the equally incomprehensible principles of homeopathy, although curiously it is only homeopaths who claim this, never nuclear physicists. One pioneering practitioner believed succussion generates enough energy to split the atoms of the solute and release nuclear energy in a process known as spallation.[32] Fortunately for both practitioners and patients this homeopathic form of atomic radiation doesn't seem to have the same deleterious effects as the identical process customarily viewed from behind thick sheets of lead glass in nuclear reactors.

Others propose a relationship between homeopathy and '... quantum physics and vibrational qualities of matter' by way of explanation. This process is so powerful we are warned of the sobering case of a US homeopath who described how the rapid flow of water around pipes in New York led to an inadvertent potentising of fluoride (added by the authorities to reduce the incidence of dental disease), leading to all sorts of problems such as unsociable behaviour, sexual over-excitement and mental exhaustion. Fortunately for the good citizens of the Big Apple the same enterprising practitioner was able to reverse the damage by marketing a homeopathic antidote to this unexpected form of pollution.[33]

A homeopathic diploma holder tells us (at considerable length) '... the process of succussion acts to add more electrons to the solution through the addition of oxygen to it ...' claiming each succussion crams more and more electrons into oxygen atoms, while the increasing dilution provides the extra space required. The author doesn't explain why this accumulation of negative charge has never been detected by any experimental process, or why it doesn't simply dissipate into the surroundings in the same way any other form of static electricity might.[34]

In a melange of New Age thinking and quantum- and meta-physics, one website attempts to explain things in a way that is as poetic as it is cryptic, 'While the potentising process "de-spaces" substances and carries them from space over into time, into a state of pure life, the radioactive decay of matter implies a "de-timing" of substance, a death process of matter that instead completely carries it out of time over into space, thereby necessarily leading to an "atomizing" of the substance.'[35]

Inventive as these explanations are, they are free of content and devoid of meaning; amounting to nothing more than metaphor or wishful thinking. None have any firm evidence behind them. They coin scientific-sounding language and exploit a few genuine scientific phenomena – clusters of water molecules can form in liquid water, for example but carry no information and have a duration of fractions of a second – but are themselves profoundly unscientific, and many are mutually exclusive. For this we should be deeply grateful, it means so far no one has been able to split an atom by banging it on a leather-bound book, but it does mean we're still none the wiser about the memory of water.

Research into the subject is limited and characterised by a disproportionate optimism, considering its meagre quantity and quality. In the first and best-known 'memory of water' experiment, charismatic French homeopath Jacques Benveniste and his team, took a solution of antibodies known to 'degranulate' suitably primed cells (known as basophils) and diluted it to a point where no antibody was present. They reported that this highly dilute preparation continued to exhibit the same property of causing degranulation when exposed to target cells.[36]

Basophils are delicate creatures, notoriously sensitive and they will degranulate (effectively burst) with very little prompting, even without the presence of the antibodies used in this experiment. But, after getting his results, rather than doing what anyone else might have done – checking for contaminants and having a stern word with the people responsible for cleaning the glassware – Benveniste turned a blind eye to the possibility of error and chose instead to believe the solute had developed a 'memory' and published a paper to that effect.

This result and the conclusions of Benveniste and his colleagues seemed so implausible the experiment was repeated a short while later in the presence of a team from *Nature*, the journal in which the original article had been published (Benveniste had agreed to this in advance of publication). Once the statistics were properly controlled, the risk of bias removed and the results from all the experiments looked at – not just the ones that gave the expected answers – the final data were found to be entirely in keeping with real-world expectations. The concept of the memory of water was deemed 'as unnecessary as it is fanciful'.[37]

Subsequently many other attempts have been made to replicate Benveniste's original results, none have succeeded in any credible or repeatable way and the conclusions arrived at are now regarded as an example of the *observer expectancy effect* we discussed in Chapter Four. This however didn't stop Dr Benveniste from going further still and, using dissected guinea pig hearts to measure the effect, claiming he had managed to isolate the 'bio-electric signals' unique to homeopathic remedies in a way that allowed them to be sent (and sold) along telephone lines, across the internet and captured on compact disc.[38]

Another paper frequently quoted as evidence for the memory of water was published in a special 'memory of water' edition of the journal *Homeopathy*, mentions the word 'water' twice in the abstract and has the phrase 'structure of water' in the keywords section, yet bizarrely has nothing at all to do with water. Instead the paper concerns itself with the properties of alcohol.[39] In the final outcome, however, the only thing demonstrated was that alcohol samples from different sources have different appearances when analysed.

The researchers had spent time, hard work and money only to discover they could distinguish between different types of impurity, not homeopathic remedies.[40]

But the problems aren't limited to the questions of whether or not water has a memory. It remains a mystery why, if it exists, this memory is selective and obligingly fails to recall any details of the contaminants, unavoidably present in the purest of distilled water. Remember, in comparison with the dilutions employed in homeopathic remedies, the smallest impurity – just one stray molecule in billions of gallons – is still a massive level of contamination. Why is it that during the process of serial dilution and succussion the water retains only the imprint of the mother tincture – the bee, but not the glass; the daisy, but not the metal; the sunbeam, but not the plastic?

Neither are any of the above theories able to account for the crucial claim that homeopathic remedies get stronger as they are diluted. Why the concentration of any of these elusive phenomena – micro-clusters, nanoparticles, electrically charged oxygen atoms, energy signatures and the rest – should increase with dilution eludes even the most creative of homeopathic minds.

Nor do the most ingenious proposals for the memory of water account for dilutions made in other substances. A mechanism for the memory of alcohol now has to be considered. And what about lactose, from which homeopathic *pillules* are manufactured – how can a solid have 'molecular clusters' imparted to it while still remaining a solid? We also require an explanation for the process of *grafting*, a process first described by the flamboyant Russian, General Korsakoff, in the 1820s[41] and still practised today, where one drop of a homeopathic remedy added to a bottle of plain lactose pillules will supposedly transfer its energy evenly to every other pill in the bottle, turning them into remedies in their own right. Homeopaths tell us the same effect can even be achieved by adding a single potentised pillule to a bottle of ordinary ones in order to potentise the whole lot, a process known as *dry-grafting*.

It is hardly surprising, after all this, that Kate Chatfield, homeopathic teacher and member of the Society of Homeopaths' research ethics committee, when asked in a session of the UK's House of Lords' Select Committee on Science and Technology if it was possible to distinguish one homeopathic remedy from another, felt constrained to answer, 'Only by the label.'[42]

Yet even if the memory of water (or sugar or alcohol) were proven tomorrow there would still be insurmountable obstacles for homeopathy to struggle past before it could be taken seriously by the mainstream.

# Curiouser and curiouser – Provings, The law of similars and the new remedies

As we have seen, homeopaths claim certain properties of the principal ingredients are passed into the remedy as they are succussed and diluted during the process of manufacture. The why and how of this process present grave difficulties for the mainstream credibility of homeopathy.

In the same way that Hahnemann's original *law of infinitesimals* has been taken to extremes in the two centuries since homeopathy was invented, a parallel process of augmentation has also happened to the *law of similars* – the idea that like will cure like.

The testing, or *proving*, of substances still continues, carried out by homeopathic groups on both established and novel base ingredients. These days though provers play safe and sensibly take a greatly diluted 30C preparation rather than the actual base ingredient. As in Hahnemann's day, individuals will take a remedy then record the sensations and symptoms they experience that they feel are attributable to that remedy.

These sensations are then used as the basis for the homeopathic *Materia Medica* (a list of remedies and the symptoms they are used to treat) and the *Repertory* (a list of symptoms alongside suggested remedies that are claimed to address them) which are consulted by practitioners when looking for the *similimum* – the set of symptoms observed in a patient that most closely match those attributed to a specific remedy. It is believed a substance that causes a set of symptoms in a healthy subject will somehow 'cancel out' those same symptoms in a patient who is ill.

Because of their highly subjective nature, provings (or pathogenetic trials as they are sometimes known) are of questionable value, even if the underlying premise was to be accepted. They are generally conducted with the volunteer fully aware of what substance has been taken, so there is no way of a prover knowing which of the, often vague, feelings he or she is experiencing can be attributed to the remedy itself and which are as a result of mundane, everyday changes that would have been experienced anyway.

It's not surprising therefore that provings haven't fared well when investigated objectively. Many trials demonstrate no difference between placebo and homeopathic remedy when taken by healthy volunteers.[43, 44, 45, 46, 47, 48, 49] Revealingly, Professor Harald Walach, the leading homeopathic lecturer and researcher who carried out four of the main studies of provings states, 'The pillar of homeopathy, pathogenetic trials, rests on shaky ground ...' and, after speaking to a number of other homeopaths involved in provings, went so far as to say, 'It seems to be an open secret that true homeopathic symp-toms ... can also be observed with placebo ...'[50] This would seem to make any comparison between the effects of taking a homeopathic remedy and the effects of taking a placebo a rather pointless exercise.

The nature of some types of modern day provings have changed far beyond Hahnemann's original 'test' of a substance by a volunteer.

So-called meditative, or dream provings, often don't involve consuming a material substance at all. Instead they rely on provers in groups or as indi-viduals who will sit and contemplate the remedy in question, after which they will record their thoughts and feelings. Dream provings usually involve the prover placing a remedy under the pillow and then recording any dreams experienced over a period of three nights. After this the impressions of the provers are combined to give an idea what particular condition the remedy may be used to treat.[51, 52]

Having done away with the need to ingest a physical remedy, these new types of provings have opened the doors to a wide variety of bizarre remedies based upon materials that it would be impossible to employ in the normal way. Examples include types of radiation such as that produced by a mobile phone, a computer, a magnetic field or simply colours. Sunbeams, or energy from the moon, the planets Venus and Saturn, and the Milky Way have sup-posedly been captured in various remedies, so too have the north and south poles of a magnet. Natural phenomena such as storms, lightning and the Great Rift Valley have been harnessed and bottled for medicinal purposes, as have shipwrecks, jet-lag and the Berlin Wall.

These *imponderables,* as they are known, have roused the ire of more main-stream homeopaths such as George Vithoulkas, who has condemned them as 'absurd "new ideas" ... that only fanatics of a religious sect could adopt.'[53] To the objective observer, however, they are hardly any less far-fetched than the base ingredients of most of the traditional remedies.

Some of the commonest remedies are based on comfortingly natural or herbal ingredients (although, of course, they contain not a trace of the origi-nal): chamomile, daisy, eyebright, comfrey. Other remedies in the standard homeopathic medicine chest have a less reassuring ring to them – crushed honey bee, snake venom, living spider, putrefied animal tissue. Some wouldn't be out of place in a production of Macbeth – newt, bat, frog, dog, adder, lizard and several varieties of owl.

Small wonder that homeopathic pharmacies prefer to shroud the common names of their remedies behind an obscuring veil of Latin words and abbre-viations. In this way crushed bee becomes the more accessible *Apis mel,* putrefied animal tissue becomes *Pyrogenium*, while the digestive fluid of a live lobster is transformed into the inscrutable *Homarus*.

As an additional complication, nowadays we find remedies prepared, not just from substances claimed to produce similar clinical symptoms to the disease they will be used to treat, but from those bearing a similarity to an aspect of a disease, or which convey a feeling or perception, supposedly related to specific diseases.

This *doctrine of signatures* – where a substance was thought to have the ability to cure a disease that affected something to which it bore a physical resemblance – is a central tenet of modern homeopathy.[54] Thus a yellow flower is supposedly able to combat jaundice, the plant lungwort, having a similar shape to the lungs, is believed to help lung disease and the honey bee is believed to relieve sensations of stinging and itching.

There is of course, no sensible reason why a plant should be able to cure anything solely by virtue of its shape or why a bee, which can inflict a painful sting, should be able to cure similar sensations when taken by mouth as highly dilute medicine or pillules. Power being imparted from physical form, as with the doctrine of signatures, is a variety of sympathetic magic, one of the commonest and most ancient belief systems, dating back to the earliest human communities; purely faith-based and no different from the persistent idea that eating the liver of a lion will bring strength or consuming powdered rhino horn will ensure enhanced sexual potency.

Homeopathy dates from times when the principles of medicine were much different than they are today. It employs starting ingredients, some of which are extremely bizarre, which have no real-world basis as medicines and believes just because an ingredient allegedly produces the signs of or otherwise resembles a disease process it should somehow be able to cure that disease. Homeopathy depends on remedies – based on water, alcohol or lactose – that have been so extremely diluted, even the most convinced homeopath is happy to concede there is no trace of the original ingredient remaining. Yet despite many theories no credible evidence has ever been found for why these chemically neutral remedies are able to retain the properties of the base ingredient, how those properties grow in potency with each dilution, how they then pass into the body or, once they are there, how they manage to cure disease.

Of course, just because a treatment is implausible in the extreme doesn't necessarily mean it can't possibly work. As homeopaths never tire of pointing out, many useful medical interventions proved their worth long before it was discovered exactly how they functioned. In science nothing, not even our most cherished theories, are ever completely certain. The proof of the pudding is, as the expression goes, in the eating. So, never mind the theories, let's have a look at the evidence.

§

## Homeopathy – The evidence

Proponents of homeopathy are very ready to supply copious lists of reports, trials and studies in support of their beliefs. But looking at individual trials isn't always the best way of determining the truth. As we have seen, not all evidence is equal and the results of single papers can be deceptive; it is always possible to cherry-pick the body of evidence and, while ignoring any flaws, find results that suit a preferred position.

For instance, in 2014 a list of some 800 papers was released by UK veterinary homeopaths.[55] The title of the document suggested these were peer-reviewed papers supporting the idea homeopathy works, so they certainly warranted consideration. On inspection, however, results were unimpressive. The list largely contained papers that had an unmistakable risk of bias and questionable methodologies. Some of them found homeopathy to be ineffective or hadn't actually investigated homeopathy at all, and a surprising number of the experiments had required the use and sacrifice of considerable numbers of laboratory animals to arrive at the conclusion that no real conclusion could be made. Several case reports and at least one book review were included that not even the most charitable of reviewers could describe as worthwhile proof. Not one of the papers on the list constituted the 'truth' that was promised by the authors of the list, and the whole exercise speaks volumes for the uncritical attitude of homeopaths to evidence – it seems little has changed since Hahnemann's first credulous acceptance of his experience with Cinchona bark. Similar lists have been published by homeopathic groups in human medicine, with equally disappointing results.[56]

A few veterinary studies have appeared in mainstream, peer-reviewed journals but again are unconvincing. One study of homeopathy in the treatment of skin disease in dogs had only three patients in the critical blinded phase and concluded, 'There is no justification for using the findings reported here to substantiate or repudiate the overall efficacy of homeopathy in either veterinary or human medicine.'[57] Others have shown homeopathy is ineffective whether it is in treating mastitis in cows,[58, 59, 60] skin problems in dogs[61] or diarrhoea and lungworm in calves.[62, 63]

One short communication from 1984, conducted by a leading UK proponent of homeopathy, investigated the effects of homeopathy on still-birth in a group of twenty sows. This was a small study, where no attempt was made at blinding, there was no placebo group and the randomisation process was highly questionable,[64] all of which makes it impossible for any impartial observer to draw any conclusion from the results. This, however, does not stop proponents from invoking it on a regular basis as 'proof' homeopathy is effective.

## The big picture

The best way to properly assess the totality of evidence is to look, not at individual studies, but meta-analyses and systematic reviews that take the results of several randomised, controlled trials and summarise the evidence for a particular claim. Properly performed, such trials are increasingly recognised as a major cornerstone of evidence-based medicine.

A 2007 article in the *Lancet* reports that five large-scale meta-analyses have been conducted in the field of human medicine.[65, 66, 67, 68, 69] They all gave the same result: after excluding methodologically inadequate trials and accounting for publication bias, homeopathy produced no statistically significant benefit over placebo.[70]

The article goes on to suggest placebo treatment may have some (albeit, as the author explains, ethically questionable) clinical benefit in humans. No such benefit will be felt by animal patients, of course.

The database of the Cochrane Library is widely recognised as one of the best resources available for evaluating evidence about the effects of health care interventions.[71] In 2010, six systematic reviews from the database containing references to homeopathy were analysed. The reviews covered the treatment of cancer, attention–deficit hyperactivity disorder, asthma, dementia, influenza and induction of labour. None of them showed homeopathy to have any effect beyond that of placebo.[72] Since then, in a 2012 addition to the database, a team that included some highly experienced homeopathic researchers has also looked at the usefulness of the homeopathic preparation Oscillococcinum® for preventing and treating influenza and influenza-like illness. They concluded 'There was no statistically significant difference between the effects of Oscillococcinum® and placebo.' This review was updated in 2014, the conclusion remained unchanged.[73]

In the lesser canon of veterinary literature by comparison, there has been little in the way of good-quality meta-analyses or systematic reviews of homeopathy. One exception is a systematic review conducted in 2014, notable because of the credentials of the lead author, the same Robert Mathie of the British Homeopathic Association (BHA), who co-authored the Oscillococcinum® review mentioned in the previous paragraph.[74] Out of the eighteen placebo-controlled trials analysed in his veterinary study, only two were considered reliable enough to include. The first found homeopathy had no effect in treating mastitis in cows,[75] while the authors of the second claimed homeopathy had reduced the incidence of diarrhoea (scours) in piglets caused by the bacteria *E. coli*.[76]

This second, supposedly positive, paper is worth looking at more closely. It was published in the journal *Homeopathy* that, for some, might raise questions about impartiality from the very start. According to Dr Mathie's review, it is unclear whether vested interest was present or whether blinding was adequate enough to ensure those involved weren't aware which pigs were receiving placebo and which homeopathy, and the method of randomisation isn't adequately stated, all of which would be seen by many as serious flaws. Furthermore, and not noted in the systematic review, there were critical clinical flaws, most significantly that the authors believed it was possible to judge whether or not a piglet's diarrhoea was caused by *E. coli* solely by the colour of the faeces, something no clinician would ever seriously claim, particularly if they were going to publish research on the subject. All this has led one commentator to conclude, diplomatically, '... the data in this paper are not of high reliability.'[77] Whether Dr Mathie – a first-class researcher but neither a veterinary surgeon nor a doctor of medicine – would have been aware of these clinical shortcomings, can only be guessed.

Despite this one allegedly positive finding though, the final conclusion from the wider review was, '[m]ixed findings ... precluded generalisable conclusions about the efficacy of any particular homeopathic medicine or the impact of individualised homeopathic intervention on any given medical condition in animals.'

Yet, for all the doubts and caveats from the authors, this paper is still presented as positive evidence for homeopathy, with a former president of the British Association of Homeopathic Veterinary Surgeons (BAHVS) claiming, 'This important study affirms that reliable evidence does exist ...'[78] In the face of such unrelenting optimism one can only wonder what, if anything, would constitute *unreliable* evidence.

The following year the same two authors published another analysis of existing trials that had investigated veterinary homeopathy, this time looking at those which had not used a placebo as a control. While this looser approach might have been expected to have produced a more favourable outcome for homeopathy, the final conclusion was no better – none of the trials were considered free enough of bias to be useful, so again it was impossible to draw a meaningful conclusion about homeopathy in animals.[79]

In the last few years even more wide-ranging reviews of the evidence for homeopathy have been conducted.

On two occasions, government bodies have met to consider the appropriateness of funding homeopathic treatment using public money in national health schemes. The scale of these inquiries meant it was possible to take the time to consider a vast amount of clinical, research-based and oral evidence, even including individual comments from concerned members of the public.

In 2010 the UK Parliamentary Science and Technology Committee, after receiving submissions from interested parties, sat for several days, looked at hundreds of pieces of evidence concerning homeopathy and listened to testimonies from homeopathic practitioners, researchers and manufacturers.

Its final report, which ran to a prodigious 275 pages was clear and damning, '. . . the Government should not endorse the use of placebo treatments, including homeopathy. Homeopathy should not be funded on the National Health Service (NHS) and the Medicines and Healthcare products Regulatory Agency (MHRA) should stop licensing homeopathic products . . . The funding of homeopathic hospitals . . . should not continue, and NHS doctors should not refer patients to homeopaths.'[80]

Some years later the Australian National Health and Medical Research Council (NHMRC) conducted a similar review, again considering substantial volumes of evidence from both sides of the argument (much of it the same as that presented in the UK review above). Its conclusions were stark, 'There are no health conditions for which there is reliable evidence that homeopathy is effective. Homeopathy should not be used to treat health conditions that are chronic, serious, or could become serious. People who choose homeopathy may put their health at risk if they reject or delay treatments for which there is good evidence for safety and effectiveness.'[81]

But seemingly regardless of these conclusions, the same pieces of evidence, which still consistently fail to match the claims made of them, continue to be produced by proponents as if they were proof positive for the effectiveness of homeopathy. This came to a head on one occasion shortly after the 2010 UK Parliamentary enquiry, when the BHA, which had been invited to submit evidence, came in for sharp criticism from Members of Parliament and scientists for misrepresenting evidence in ways even the original authors of some of the papers took issue with.[82] This naturally has the effect of making anyone with an interest in the subject extremely wary of taking any allegedly positive evidence presented by homeopathic practitioners at face value.

§

## The rest – Nosodes, sarcodes, isopathy and homeopathic vaccination

Not all remedies of the homeopathic type are made from substances alleged to produce symptoms of disease in healthy volunteers. *Sarcodes* are produced from the tissues of a healthy organ and are claimed to be able to regulate glandular function while *nosodes* are prepared from diseased tissue (pus or cancer, for example) or the causative agent of disease (such as tuberculosis, or parvovirus). Nosodes are employed in a process known as *isopathy* (the *homeo-* part of the word *homeopathy* means 'similar', while the *iso-* part of *isopathy* means 'same'), most controversially for the purposes of *homeoprophylaxis*, often referred to as homeopathic vaccination (see also Chapter Nine, regarding the anti-vaccination movement).

Homeoprophylaxis is a subject of some confusion. Many, particularly non-veterinary, proponents of homeopathy openly advocate the use of nosodes in lieu of vaccination in animals. Veterinary homeopaths, on the other hand, are more guarded about the advice they give, rarely heard to be directly advising nosodes be substituted for conventional vaccines. There is an element of 'wanting to have their cake and eat it' though since at the same time many will hint strongly, in the form of personal experience and anecdotal claims, that it is done while at the same time exaggerating or even fabricating the risks of conventional vaccination. A study involving homeopaths treating human patients in 2003 revealed not a single one of the homeopaths surveyed advised in favour of the vaccination of children to prevent measles, mumps and rubella.[83] To date, no such study has been conducted involving veterinary homeopaths.

There is no credible evidence in mainstream scientific literature demonstrating nosodes have a protective effect against disease and homeopaths themselves concede they don't give rise to antibodies or other conventional evidence of immunity in the way a vaccine does. Anecdotal evidence is unreliable as an indicator of success, as we have seen, especially with something as complex and difficult to interpret as disease control, when levels of exposure, naturally acquired immunity and protection from maternal antibodies will all have confounding effects. This is not to call into question the integrity of people who believe they have had success using nosodes, it's simply that there are many other far more likely explanations for the things they report.

The problem with anecdotal evidence is it's a two-way street, and for every story of an animal being given nosodes then failing to succumb to disease (an outcome that doesn't require nosodes to be effective), there is another where animals that have received nosodes then go on to contract or die from diseases they were supposed to have been protected against (an outcome that indicates nosodes are ineffective). Over the years several such accounts have appeared in the veterinary press.

In one case a team of veterinary surgeons describe a well-meaning owner's devastation as they witnessed an outbreak of parvovirus enteritis unfold in a family of five Shetland sheepdogs. The dogs had supposedly been protected by nosodes sent in the post by an unnamed UK veterinary surgeon, who had misled them into believing they were an 'effective homeopathic vaccine'.[84] In another heartbreaking case a veterinary surgeon describes the death, from clinically confirmed parvovirus infection, of five Lhasa Apso puppies supposedly protected by 'homeopathic vaccines'. The letter ends with a cry of frustration: 'Such meaningless suffering and death due to exploitation of a breeder's ignorance leaves me aghast.'[85]

In another case report mentioned on a veterinary forum and reproduced here with permission, a veterinary surgeon from the south-east of England wrote, 'A small-scale Cairn Terrier breeder was using homeopathic parvovirus vaccine but still getting horrendous episodes of parvovirus enteritis. Eventually I suggested we blood test some "vaccinated" dogs to check their antibody titres. Of course results were all zero. So we vaccinated them properly. Don't know why I didn't think of it sooner!'

As we saw in Chapter Nine, conventional vaccines are highly effective, their mode of action is well known and easy to comprehend, and they have produced dramatic reductions in disease in both animal and human populations. In the rare cases where it is suspected a vaccine may have been associated with an adverse reaction or not to have been protective there is a formal system for reporting such things. None of this is true of nosodes, there is no good quality evidence they have any effect whatsoever, yet many homeopathic veterinary surgeons continue to mislead the public by suggesting they have a place in disease control.

There are even a number of boarding kennels that now advise they will accept cats and dogs that have only received nosodes, rather than science-based vaccinations. Boarding establishments, where large numbers of animals from different backgrounds come together in close proximity, can be a hotbed of diseases such as parvovirus and kennel-cough and a proprietor who doesn't insist on the highest standards of protection is not acting in the best interests of the animals in their care. If you're looking for somewhere for your pets to stay while you jet off for a holiday in the sun then think carefully before entrusting them to this type of establishment in your absence.

## Bach remedies

There is a certain beauty about the flower remedies of Dr Bach. As with homeopathy the remedies are diluted to such a degree no trace of the original substance remains; unlike homeopathy, the original practitioners made no extravagant claims for their ability to cure physical disease.

Dr Edward Bach, born near Birmingham, England, in 1886, was a physician, microbiologist and homeopath who was quite clear science had no place in his system of healing. His remedies were, he said, Divinely revealed. 'No science, no knowledge is necessary...' he wrote in 1933, '... they who will obtain the greatest benefit from this God-sent gift will be those who keep it free from science and free from theories.'[86]

With such emphasis on simplicity it is hardly surprising there hasn't been much in the way of scientific investigation of the Bach Flower Remedies. And there is little doubt the sensitive Dr Bach would have been horrified at one of the few that is to be found and involves the sacrifice of eighteen laboratory rats to investigate the effect on the cardio-vascular system – an effect that practitioners have never claimed.[87]

Bach remedies are made by placing flower heads in open vessels filled with spring water that are then exposed to sunlight. This infusion is serially diluted and combined with brandy to create the final remedy. Originally Dr Bach described twelve remedies (which he called the *Twelve Healers*) and later added further ones, initially referred to as *helpers*, until collating the entire number into a grand total of thirty-eight remedies, each one associated with a specific human state of mind.

They are claimed to treat disturbances of emotional states in humans that, it is claimed, lead to physical disease. The best known of the original twelve is the *rescue remedy*. Prepared originally from the rock rose, now more usually a combination of five infusions, it is believed to help in fearful states. *Cerato*, the remedy prepared from *Ceratostigma*, is claimed to help those who lack self-confidence,[88] while water violet is for those quiet people who like being alone and whose 'peace and calmness is a blessing to those around them'.[89]

Translating such human emotions to animals is an exercise in anthropomorphism and any apparent success from the use of flower remedies in companion species is more likely to depend on modifying the complex interaction between animal and caregiver rather than on any specific individual effect. Dogs and horses in particular have co-evolved with human beings for tens of thousands of years and as such are exquisitely attuned to our moods and feelings. Any veterinary practitioner will recognise cases where anxiety in an owner has led to a similar state of mind in a closely bonded companion animal and where reassuring a worried owner can have a calming effect on that animal. It is easy to appreciate how the administration of a flower remedy to either party in this situation might help promote a mutual improvement in mood and demeanour.

Needless to say, despite a wealth of anecdotes, there is no convincing scientific evidence of any sort indicating Bach Flower Remedies are effective when tested against placebo preparations. And it is quite certain any practitioner true to Dr Bach's original philosophy will be completely unconcerned by this.

## The downside – Where's the harm?

Homeopathic and related remedies are so highly diluted they contain not a trace of the base ingredient used to create them. By taking a homeopathic remedy we, and the animals in our care, are merely ingesting tiny quantities of water, sugar or alcohol; there is little prospect of being directly injured as a result. Yet homeopathy can and does cause real harm.

Conventional medicines have real, well researched, often very powerful effects – when used correctly those effects are beneficial, but occasionally some are undesirable, or even harmful. But they are employed on the basis of informed decision-making, a risk-benefit calculation founded in proven, real world facts. It is simply not possible to have a treatment that has only positive effects and, by the same token, any treatment that never has an adverse effect will never have a positive one either. Large numbers of seriously, even terminally-ill people are treated with conventional medications; palliation, pain relief and symptomatic treatments are used in patients who will inevitably eventually succumb to their illness. As long as homeopathy is mainly confined to the treatment of minor, self-limiting conditions, this will skew the figures to give a false impression of the relative risks of homeopathy and science-based medicine.

Yet the well-understood risks of real medicines are disingenuously used to denigrate the entirety of science-based medical practice and justify the use of homeopathy. This is nothing more than the simplistic *A or B fallacy*: 'Your medicine is bad, so ours must be good.' But whether science-based medicine is good, bad or indifferent has no bearing on the effectiveness of homeopathy; the fact remains, when patients are denied effective medicines in lieu of homeopathy, people (and animals) die.

We have already seen examples of this above – how the use of nosodes, or homeopathic vaccines, has led to illness and death in animals. When homeopathy is used instead of proven medicines to treat disease the consequences too, can be grave. There are a number of websites dedicated to exposing these tragedies in people.[90, 91] Some of the details are harrowing and include cases such as Jacqueline Alderslade, a nurse, who died of asthma after being told by a homeopath to stop her medication; Penelope Dingle, who died in great pain after a homeopath told her she could cure her rectal cancer without the need for conventional medicines or surgery, and Lady Victoria Waymouth, who died of heart failure after being told to stop her medication by a homeopathic doctor. Caroline Lovell died during childbirth when her midwife prescribed rescue remedy instead of calling an ambulance to treat a catastrophic haemorrhage, and actress Sylvia Millecam died of breast cancer after refusing medical treatment in favour of alternative remedies, including homeopathy, on the advice of homeopathic doctors. The toll continues.

Few cases of this sort ever come to light in veterinary medicine. Our animal patients, without the benefit of inquests, coroners' courts and pressure from grieving relatives, depend utterly on the common sense and judgement of their care-givers – us. And when that judgement is lacking or poorly informed there is a price to pay, although in the case of veterinary medicine it is the animal who suffers; owners and veterinary surgeons are rarely called to account for their actions. This 'consulting room conspiracy' ensures that stories of supposed successes are broadcast far and wide, while what any rational person would describe as failures are dismissed with a wealth of excuses – interfering factors (usually conventional medicine or vaccines) the 'healing crisis', homeopathic 'aggravations', or 'poisons leaving the system'.

This last excuse came to light on one of the rare occasions such a case appeared in the veterinary press, where a dog was treated by a veterinary homeopath for acute moist dermatitis – a common condition, easily resolved conventionally, often with only a single treatment but which if left will result in weeping, inflamed and intensely painful skin.[92] The dog presented initially with a small area only an inch or two across, but while the homeopath attended it the situation deteriorated and lesions spread further across the dog's entire head and shoulders and eventually right along its back until, according to a witness, the dog was so badly distressed it became 'depressed and sat rigid in an apparent effort to minimise the pain caused to it by movement'. These symptoms were dismissed by the homeopath as 'the poisons leaving the system', from his perspective this wasn't a deterioration, this was the case going to plan.

In another case taken, with permission, from a veterinary discussion group, a Manchester veterinary surgeon wrote, in 2013:

*'I am feeling a bit heated about the subject of homeopathy right now. Several months ago, I saw a cat with suspected hyperthyroidism where the owner took it to a very well-known holistic/homeopathic vet. He made no diagnostic tests and gave it homeopathic pills and drops to treat the (undiagnosed) hyperthyroidism and "adjust it emotionally".*

*'The owner came back to me a couple of months later. The cat had lost a lot of weight and was a stressed unhappy animal. I did the diagnostic workup, confirmed hyperthyroidism, eliminated kidney failure etc, and outlined the treatment options in great detail. They went off to have a think, decided they did not like the risks of side effects, and went back to the other bloke, who saw it several times after that.*

*'They fairly recently brought back a skeletal animal for euthanasia. "Sadly, the disease was too serious for his individual system to cope. At least we did the best we could for him", said the owners.*

*'A very nice cat with a very treatable disease was made to suffer for an extended period for no good reason. They cried as I put him to sleep. I bit my tongue till it damn near bled!'*

The rationalisations put forward by homeopaths to explain away cases such as this are plentiful, varied and wrong – so much so that some have described homeopathy as not so much a system of medicine as a list of excuses. Homeopathy is little more than a narrative for disease, meaning whatever course a disease treated homeopathically takes – whether it improves, stays the same or gets worse – homeopathy will always have a plausible pretext for why this has happened. This is such a common ploy it is almost impossible to conceive of a situation where a practitioner would admit a remedy simply hadn't worked, far less that homeopathy itself might be ineffective.

Despite the feel-good rhetoric from the majority of homeopaths about 'gentle healing', suffering such as this is actually an integral part of homeopathy. George Vithoulkas, Professor of Homeopathic Medicine, winner of the 'Right Livelihood' Award (known as Alternative Medicine's Nobel Prize) and founder of the International Academy of Classical Homeopathy, describes how the (human) patient must endure: '... if even subtle changes for the better are occurring on the energy or mental/ emotional levels, then the inclination [of the homeopath] will be to wait, even though the patient may be suffering severely ... aggravation of the physical symptoms may become intolerable ... one must wait to the very limit of the patient's endurance. This situation tries the souls of both patient and prescriber.'[93]

In veterinary homeopathy too, similar sentiments are to be found. The Academy of Veterinary Homeopathy (AVH) advises there may be uncomfortable aggravations after your pet takes a homeopathic remedy, 'There may be a discharge or other change ... The problem may be physical, e.g. diarrhoea, eye, ear, nasal or skin discharge, or it may be behavioural, e.g. change in sleeping location, new fears etc. This is healthy and is a sign that your pet is getting rid of accumulated "toxins". It may be difficult to watch, but please interfere with it as little as possible ... **It is very important not to interfere with these symptoms. Doing so will stop the curative process** ...' (emphasis in the original).[94]

This is horribly reminiscent of the old joke where an anxious patient asks the doctor, 'Will it hurt?' to which the doctor replies, happily, 'No, not at all, I won't feel a thing.'

But it is clearly no joke. And while it could be argued if a homeopath and their human patient are happy to enter into a mutual agreement that suffering is good for the soul, or whatever justification they may prefer then that is their decision to make, the same argument cannot be made in veterinary medicine where our patients have no say in the matter and can only trust us to do the best for them.

We have no way of knowing how common the type of cases outlined above might be. In veterinary practice what happens in the consulting room stays in the consulting room; there are simply not the same checks and balances in place as there are in human medicine. Apart from the extremely blunt instrument of animal welfare legislation, designed to prevent deliberate cruelty, animals have little or no protection in cases of damage or injury caused as a result of well-intentioned but misguided alternative treatments. If there were veterinary equivalents of Jacqueline Alderslade, Penelope Dingle, Victoria

225

Waymouth, Caroline Lovell or Sylvia Millecam then no one would ever hear about them.

Well, hardly ever …

In December 2015 articles about veterinary surgeon, Philippa Ann Rodale, a vet who 'specialised in homeopathy', began to appear in the press. Until that time, Mrs Rodale had been a pillar of her local community in the village of Puddletown, in Dorset, England, where she had lived and worked for more than twenty-five years and for which she was eventually honoured by being made a Member of the Most Excellent Order of the British Empire (MBE).

Mrs Rodale was a highly experienced homeopath, respected by her clients. She had trained at the Royal Homeopathic Hospital, London, afterwards being 'deemed to be capable of dealing with homeopathy in animals'. She was a colleague of George MacLeod (1912–1995), who was a Veterinary Fellow of the Faculty of Homeopathy (VetFFHom). A founder member and past president of the BAHVS, MacLeod is widely regarded as one of the most significant figures of modern veterinary homeopathy in the UK, being almost single-handedly responsible for keeping it alive during the middle of the twentieth century. He was a mentor to some high-profile homeopathic veterinary surgeons in practice today, including to Mrs Rodale, and had enough confidence in her abilities to leave her in charge of his practice on several occasions while he was away teaching and giving lectures around the world.[95]

After what was described as an unblemished career of more than forty years, in 2015 a dog, named Dangerous, was brought to Mrs Rodale suffering from a broken spine that she attempted to treat using homeopathic remedies. Ten days after admission, Dangerous was discovered by a member of the public and found to be suffering greatly as a result of his injuries and the lack of effective treatment. The situation was immediately reported to the authorities. Another veterinary surgeon was called to attend but the case was hopeless and Dangerous was put to sleep.[96]

In an undignified end to a long career, Mrs Rodale, amid a flurry of media reports and legal proceedings, was forced to relinquish her membership of the Royal College of Veterinary Surgeons in order to avoid disciplinary action. She was eventually found guilty of causing unnecessary suffering to a dog.

With unseemly haste, the BAHVS moved to distance themselves from Mrs Rodale as soon as reports began to appear. Despite her impeccable homeo-pathic credentials, and being a trusted companion of one of the founding fathers of British homeopathy, a cutting statement appeared on their website pointing out, '... the veterinarian in question is NOT a member of either the BAHVS or The Faculty of Homeopathy and holds NO qualifications in Veterinary Homeopathy' (emphasis in the original).[97] No mention was made about the plight of Dangerous himself or the state of mind of 74 year old Mrs Rodale.

While the desire of homeopathic organisations across the globe to disown the likes of Mrs Rodale is understandable (if heartless), life isn't that simple. When things go too far, homeopathic bodies cannot simply wash their hands and absolve themselves of responsibility by association by means of a few disclaimers in the small print.

The message from professionally qualified homeopaths is that homeopathy is powerful enough to cure cancer, heart disease and congenital abnormalities,[98] yet safe enough to never cause harm. At the same time effective, science-based medicines are alluded to as 'toxic', supposedly associated with fabricated risks such as 'vaccinosis', 'rebound' or 'suppression', and conventional practitioners are caricatured as being motivated only by profit or too lazy to comprehend homeopathy.[99] As long as this rhetoric continues, such professionals have a responsibility they cannot deny when someone takes them at their word and things go wrong, as happened with Dangerous.

§

There are some signs things may be changing for the better however, albeit slowly.

In the field of human health universities, teaching hospitals and health trusts are waking up to the fact they have been teaching or funding a supposed system of medicine with no supporting evidence and many are withdrawing public funding from homeopathy in order to support more deserving areas.[100, 101]

In the veterinary world leading bodies are speaking out against homeopathy and its use in animals. A recent article written on behalf of the International Society of Feline Medicine, British Small Animal Veterinary Association, British Veterinary Association and nine major UK animal charities and welfare groups stated, 'There is no other scientifically proven way of providing immunisation other than vaccination. Homeopathy and "homeopathic vaccines" are not acceptable.'[102]

The British Veterinary Association (BVA), representing the vast majority of UK veterinary surgeons, advises. 'We cannot endorse the use of homeopathic medicines, or indeed any medicine making therapeutic claims, which have no proven efficacy.'[103] The BVA's sister organisation, the Australian Veterinary Association (AVA), is equally direct, '... the veterinary therapies of homeopathy and homotoxicology are considered ineffective therapies ...'[104]

In 2005 the European Board of Veterinary Specialisation (EBVS) unanimously agreed, 'No credit points can be granted for education or training in these so-called supplementary, complementary and alternative treatment modalities ...', while the Swedish Veterinary Association has banned its members from practising homeopathy altogether.[105]

And at the grass roots in the UK profession, a survey conducted in 2013 found, of the 460 veterinary surgeons who responded, 83 per cent felt there were no medical conditions for which homeopathy could be an effective treatment for animals, 78 per cent felt their colleagues should not be able to practise homeopathy using their professional title, and 73 per cent felt pet owners should be asked to sign consent forms prior to treatment commencing to ensure they understood the risks and limitations of using homeopathy in their animals.[106]

In 2016 two campaigns were launched independently in the UK by members of the veterinary profession calling for their governing body, the RCVS, to take action on homeopathy as practised by fellow members. One, the Campaign for Rational Veterinary Medicine, argued the case that, '21st century veterinary treatment should in all cases be based on rational, established scientific principles' and called for restrictions to be imposed on veterinary surgeons who chose to use homeopathy in order to make sure clients were fully informed before embarking on homeopathic treatment.[107] The other campaign went further and, pointing out the use of homeopathy in animals in lieu of science-based medicines 'can lead to unnecessary suffering and even death', called for a complete ban on the use of homeopathy by UK veterinary surgeons.[108] Between them, both campaigns managed to collect nearly 4,000 signatures in support of their positions from concerned members of the public and the veterinary profession itself.

It's not all good news, however, and there is some way to go in the fight for a rational basis to veterinary medicine.

In the UK the RCVS still holds a contradictory stance, emphasising the importance of evidence-based medicine and urging 'normal evidential standards' to be applied to complementary treatments while at the same time maintaining veterinary surgeons should be free to offer homeopathy because it is 'accepted by society' and there is a 'demand from some clients'.[109] The contradiction is obvious when homeopathy is considered alongside other practices that are now effectively (and rightly) banned by the RCVS yet in their time also had a 'demand from some clients', such as tail docking in dogs and the firing of horses.

In the US, a resolution submitted to the American Veterinary Medical Association House of Delegates to the effect that homeopathy was an ineffective therapy and incompatible with evidence-based medicine was defeated, despite being endorsed by a number of veterinary bodies, including the AVMA itself. The outcome was largely for political reasons, as veterinarians fought shy of endorsing a motion that was wrongly felt might have been the beginning of a 'slippery slope', leading to the restriction of freedom to practice in areas other than homeopathy.[110]

In Europe the UK's *Daily Telegraph* investigated a section of the European Union's regulations on organic aquaculture (fish-farming) and reported in April 2015, 'EU orders Britain's organic farmers to treat sick animals with homeopathy.' This move was branded 'scientifically illiterate' by British and Norwegian veterinary surgeons, presumably struggling with the leap of faith required to dose salmon, living in fjords and sea lochs containing billions of gallons of sea water, with a few tiny drops of a homeopathic remedy tipped off the end of the pier.[111] One wag in the UK veterinary press, worried about the wider animal welfare implications of this ruling, announced his intention to get round the legal requirement to use homeopathy by offering his organically-reared livestock a drink of water first, before commencing treatment with effective, science-based medicine.[112]

§

There is a general epistemological principle known as the 'principle of simplicity'. As we discussed in Chapter Three this concept, which has profound relevance not just to science but to everyday experience, is described in the context of homeopathy in a paper published in 2010. Put briefly, the principle states 'given two theories, it is unreasonable to believe the one that leaves significantly more unexplained mysteries'.[113] If the reader is interested in an honest consideration of the reasons science has so far been unable to take homeopathy seriously then a careful reading of this paper will serve as an excellent starting point.

Another commentator on the same subject states 'Principles of parsimony and simplicity mediate the epistemic connection between hypothesis and observations. Perhaps these principles are able to do this because they are surrogates for an empirical background theory ... Once this theory is brought out into the open the principle of parsimony is entirely dispensable.'[114]

In other words, given the implausibility of its fundamentals as described to date, until homeopathy is able to demonstrate its mechanisms of action convincingly and in meaningful terms, the principle of simplicity will always determine that any claim observed results are caused by (rather than merely associated with) homeopathy, remains equally implausible.

Homeopathy is supposedly a powerful, complete, internally consistent system of medicine; it has had more than 200 years to put its house in order and come up with convincing proof. Its supporters claim it can cure some of the worst diseases affecting human and animal – Ebola, HIV/AIDs, cancer, heart failure, arthritis and malaria, to name but a few. Yet the absolute best evidence available shows homeopathy only just manages to outperform a sugar tablet occasionally, on a good day, and in the vast majority of cases it can't even do that.

Contrary to the claims of homeopathic proponents, science understands exactly how homeopathy works. The apparent 'successes' of homeopathy are easy to explain without the requirement for clumsy, contradictory and pseudoscientific theories about mechanisms and modes of action. There is always a more parsimonious explanation that better fits the bill. The truth is, as unpalatable as it may be for some, we simply have no need for homeopathy.

# Manipulation Treatments (Including Chiropractice, Body Work and Energy Medicine)

MANIPULATION therapies are an assortment of different practices with variable, sometimes highly questionable, plausibility and trustworthiness. At one extreme of the spectrum are science-based, *hands-on*, or *body work* practices with impeccable credentials such as physiotherapy, while at the other are the overtly mystic *hands-off* techniques such as Reiki, Therapeutic Touch and Radionics that claim to manipulate, not the physical animal but the purported energy fields that, according to those doing the manipulation, surround and illuminate us all.

In between these two, some practices in this category form a sort of halfway house with elements of *hands-on*, physical manipulation along with a liberal dose of mysticism and spirituality thrown in to cover all bases in both the material and spiritual planes of existence.

§

## Chiropractic

'The "back man" has been part of horsey psyche for centuries'
*Ben Mayes (2015) Vet futures: Changes affecting the equine sector*[1]

Chiropractic is one of the 'big five' types of complementary and alternative medicine by virtue of its popularity and degree of organisation.[2] It is a protected profession, regulated by the Chiropractors Acts 1994 in the UK[3] and by similar legislation in forty-seven other countries including the USA, Canada, Australia, New-Zealand and much of Europe. Chiropractors are authorised to use the title doctor in fourteen countries and physician in four.[4]

231

With these credentials it can come as a surprise to learn there is more to chiropractic than the popular perception that practitioners just treat bad backs. The reality is, as one commentator puts it, 'Chiropractic is rooted in mystical concepts.'[5]

Many (but not all, as we will see) chiropractors, veterinary and human, believe in the power of *The Innate*, a numinous energy force circulating within the body that, it is said, can become occluded by a misaligned spinal column, specifically by a lesion referred to as the vertebral subluxation, or VSL. Practitioners claim the VSL interferes with the regular flow of this force and can result in problems, not just with the back but much more widely in the body. They further believe that correcting it and restoring the force to its rightful pathways can resolve a variety of health problems.

Yet the chiropractic community is a world divided, with practitioners squabbling as they have done since the discipline was first invented over what exactly chiropractic is, what ailments it can address and even the very nature and existence of the one, single lesion that they claim to treat, the vertebral subluxation itself.

## The back story

Chiropractic manipulation was devised by Canadian born Daniel David Palmer (1845–1913), a former school teacher, bee-keeper, fishmonger and magnetic healer with piercing, hypnotic eyes and an enormous bushy beard.

Moving to the USA with his brother, Thomas, in April 1865 at the age of 20, Daniel David (or DD as he is known) was possessed of a determined character and 'the narrow, fierce heart of a prophet'. He initially tried his hand in the already crowded arena of the fashionable art of Magnetic Healing as well as dabbling in phrenology and spiritualism but failed to make an impact. Eventually he decided to go it alone and (with a few ideas he had borrowed from Andrew T. Still, the inventor of osteopathy) start his own school of healing.[6]

The great discovery that led to this decision was made in September 1895 when he made a connection between the onset of deafness and a back disorder in Harvey Lillard, the janitor in the office block where Palmer worked. On examining this gentleman's spine DD found '... a vertebra racked from its normal position'. He reasoned if this was the cause of the problem it might be possible to undo the original damage by replacing the vertebra in the correct position. Thereupon he tells us, using the natural protrusions of the vertebra in question as levers, he 'racked it into position' upon which he reported Mr Lillard's deafness resolved.

His faith in his new technique was further reinforced shortly afterwards when he, once again, identified and realigned a displaced vertebra in a patient suffering heart trouble, giving 'immediate relief'. After these experiences Palmer went on to investigate the cause of other diseases and concluded that 95 per cent of them, from 'Apoplexy ...' to 'Womb (cancer of)' were caused by misalignment of the bones of the spinal column, the so-called vertebral subluxation.[7] This supposed deformity he maintained, caused pressure on and constriction of the nerves as they passed through and between the vertebra, resulting in a 'pinching off' of the flow of *Innate Intelligence*, a spiritual force Palmer believed had to be permitted to flow freely from spine to body organs and back again in order to maintain life and health in its proper balance. The vertebral subluxation is fundamental to the principles and philosophy of chiropractic.

Not burdened with an excess of false modesty, Palmer wrote of himself, 'I am the originator, the Fountain Head of the essential principle that disease is the result of too much or not enough functioning. I created the art of adjusting vertebrae, using the spinous and transverse processes as levers, and named the mental act of accumulating knowledge, the cumulative function, corresponding to the physical vegetative function – growth of intellectual and physical – together, with the science, art and philosophy – Chiropractic ... I have answered the time-worn question – what is life?'[8]

Henceforth DD was referred to as The Discoverer.

Palmer founded the first college of chiropractic that, after a number of different titles, finally settled on the name The Palmer School of Chiropractic (PSC). The intake of students was low in the early years and under DD's governance the enterprise quickly ran into debt. The early movement was beset with splits and schisms. Factions broke away from Palmer's original philosophy and founded rival institutions and practices under an assortment of names – naprapathy, neuropathy, *mixers* and *straights*, the Gonstead school – operating out of a variety of competing colleges. Chiropractors initially rejected the use of X-rays but later came to embrace and profit by them.[9] Many rejected the use of conventional drugs and a substantial number rejected the germ theory of disease.[10]

Nor were divisions confined to different factions of the chiropractic movement, there was family strife too. It seems DD was a difficult father, to say the least. His son, Bartlett Joshua Palmer (known as BJ), who turned out to have a much more shrewd ability when it came to the promotion and marketing of his father's discovery, refers to his father thus, 'To him I owe my earliest teachings which were rough and hard to bear. I considered them entirely too harsh for the crime committed, yet now I can see where thrusting upon my own resources, whether just or unjust, was for the best.'[11] Feuding between father and son was open and widely reported, at one stage they set up rival colleges and slandered one another volubly in their various writings. Things got so bad that when BJ apparently managed to run his father over with his car when he turned up, uninvited, to a celebratory parade in 1913 there were accusations of patricide, although the suspicions were never proven.[12]

Following his father's death, which occurred shortly after the injuries allegedly inflicted by his car, it must have been some consolation to BJ for his loss that he was now able to market and promote the chiropractic movement as he saw fit, without paternal interference. BJ had been educated at the PSC in its earlier years and proved to be a much steadier hand on the rudder of the developing movement, now styling himself The Developer.

Having previously paid off his father's debts and bought out his interests in the college, young Bartlett Joshua went on to take it from strength to strength. He was a marketing genius, even starting a radio station to promote chiropractic (*station WOC* – Wonders Of Chiropractic). He concentrated on the more lucrative practice of training chiropractors rather than treating patients, and supplementing his income with sales of a number of devices such as his *neuro-calometer* (claimed to assist the detection of the VSL, this device was nothing more than a fancy – and pricey – thermometer) that students would have been under considerable pressure to purchase in addition to their far from modest course fees. The result was that BJ made a fortune, eventually becoming a multi-millionaire. One of the principal aphorisms of chiropractic, mentioned in *Chiropractic Briefs Number One*, is 'Health is better than wealth'.[13] BJ must have had some of the healthiest students and patients of the age.

The biggest split in the profession was that between the *straights* and the *mixers*; and it persists to this day. The *straights* believe entirely and exclusively, as DD did, that the VSL is the root of all disease and *Innate Intelligence*, that spiritual entity Palmer likened to God, must be allowed to flow freely if a body is to remain healthy. BJ made much of his claim that his college taught PSU – Pure Straight and Unadulterated – chiropractic. At one point the Palmers, father and son, seriously considered founding chiropractic as a religion (the idea was later abandoned as the chiropractic founding fathers decided religion was superstition, whereas chiropractic was science), and DD compared himself to leading religious figures including Jesus Christ.[14] These chiropractic fundamentalists, the *straights*, still believe spinal manipulation can cure a wide variety of disorders unrelated to the spine, and that conventional medicine, particularly vaccination, is to be avoided wherever possible ('Drugs are a delusive snare,' as Palmer himself put it[15]), some continue to have serious doubts about the germ theory of infectious disease and are happy to promote the concept, originating with chiropractic firebrand and champion of the *straight* cause Dr Fred H. Barge (1933–2003),[16] that germs in the body are akin to 'rats in a dump' – not the cause, but merely a symptom of ill health.[17, 18, 19, 20]

The *mixer* tradition on the other hand stems from the teachings of a chiropractic college set up by lawyer and chiropractor, Willard Carver, in Oklahoma City, not long after the establishment of the original Palmer School.[21] *Mixers* hold that chiropractic can be combined usefully with conventional medical practices – drugs, X-rays, advice on diet, exercise, lifestyle and so on. The divisions between the two approaches are still very real and quite acrimonious at times. *Straights* believe *mixers* have strayed from the true path and are not fit to call themselves chiropractors while the *mixers* believe the *straights* are damaging the profession and hampering mainstream acceptance by clinging to non-scientific, spiritual beliefs and making disproportionate and far-fetched claims.

The big problem for both factions however, the elephant in the room so to speak, is that the principal underpinning of the entire of chiropractic, the vertebral subluxation, does not actually exist – it is a complete fiction.

### In search of a lesion

A joint that subluxates, in the medical sense, is one which has a tendency to pop in and out of place or to partially dislocate. Owners of dogs suffering hip dysplasia for example, may have heard their veterinary surgeon also refer to this condition as a subluxation of the hip joint. But despite no end of investigation using X-rays, MRI scans and dissection, the chiropractic VSL has never been shown to exist, and when different chiropractors have been asked to review the same X-ray or examine the same patient independent of one another no correlation or consistency is found between their interpretations.[22, 23, 24, 25]

The truth is, short of major trauma, vertebrae (the bones of the spine) simply never come out of line in the way chiropractors believe. True, in humans there are problems with posture and curvature of the spine as a consequence of our impractical upright posture but these are addressed by means of exercise and advice regarding a correct carriage, not by popping individual bones back in line. And in patients who have experienced trauma serious enough to genuinely displace vertebrae, while they may suffer distressing symptoms of pain, paralysis and incontinence as a result of damage to the nerve trunks supplying various muscles and sphincters they will most certainly not be found to be at increased risk of the ailments *straight* chiropractors claim to be able to treat and prevent – disease of the internal organs, skin and the immune system. What is more, in these patients it is simply impossible (and would be utterly counterproductive) to 'rack' any displaced vertebrae back in place in the way recommended by *Daddy Chiro* – DD.

Surgical realignment and fixation of broken and dislocated vertebrae is sometimes undertaken where necessary, but is a difficult and risky procedure that cannot be accomplished simply with a flick of the wrist and a few satisfying cracks. The bones of the spine in life (as opposed to in the dry skeletons and diagrams depicted in chiropractic literature) are so tightly bound together with tough ligament and muscle that to move them around independently is an impossible task. A much respected equine medicine and surgery lecturer at Edinburgh University Veterinary College during the 1980s, the fearsome Joe Fraser, never one either to mince his words or to suffer fools gladly, used to say of chiropractors, 'You cannae just move horses' vertebrae around, sonny – not without a bloody sledgehammer!'

This is literally true, one would be far more likely to fracture the vertebral spinous and transverse processes (those 'natural protrusions' DD talked about) using them as levers, than cause any significant and permanent adjustment of the vertebra itself in relation to its neighbours, despite the claims of animal chiropractic organisations to the contrary. One only need review a few of the many videos available on the worldwide web showing attempts by veterinary surgeons and chiropractors to 'realign' the spines of cows and horses to see that absolutely nothing is being achieved, no independent movement of vertebrae one against another is observed, only a vaguely comic Lilliputian pushing and pulling of largely indifferent patients.

There is, of course, one condition where components of the spine could be said to 'come out of line' and that is when a prolapsed intervertebral disc (PIVD, or slipped disc) occurs. Each of the bony vertebrae making up the spinal column is cushioned from its neighbour by a fibrous pad known as the intervertebral disc. This disc is made of a tough outer part, the *annulus fibrosis*, and a soft inner portion, the *nucleus pulposus*. They act as shock absorbers but can with age degenerate to a point where the surrounding *annulus* becomes brittle and may split, allowing the inner pulp to squeeze through, accompanied by local haemorrhage, bruising and swelling, putting pressure on the adjacent spinal cord and causing various degrees of pain and disability – this is a slipped disc. The effect is much like putting a jam doughnut between two house bricks and pressing down hard on the top brick – the jam squirts out from the middle and the doughnut falls apart, making a complete mess everywhere.

Clearly, no matter how much the bricks and doughnut are manipulated and realigned, the jam isn't going to go back whence it came – the doughnut remains an unrecognisable, sticky mess – and the same applies to an intervertebral disc after it has prolapsed. In fact, the more attempts that are made to reconstruct the doughnut by moving the bricks around, the worse the mess gets, and this also is true of chiropractic – there is a real risk in such cases of vigorous spinal manipulation in the form of chiropractic *adjustments* making an already grim situation even worse by causing further damage.

Yet by disingenuously conflating the idea of the non-existent VSL with the painfully real phenomenon of the slipped disc, many chiropractors would have us believe it is possible for chiropractic spinal manipulation to help a slipped disc. Intervertebral discs are portrayed, not as squashy doughnuts, but as firm, homogeneous washers that it is suggested, as with vertebrae, can conveniently be popped back in place with a series of manipulations. Case reports describe dogs, particularly long-backed breeds such as dachshunds or basset hounds, who have developed hindlimb instability following PIVD making a gradual recovery over time while having regular sessions with the local chiropractor. The fact this type of instability will frequently recover in the same way with rest and pain relief alone and without any need to trouble the chiropractor is rarely, if ever, mentioned and, of course, we never see the cases that fail to respond, or those that deteriorate following chiropractic intervention. In the real world fewer than 1 per cent of board-certified veterinary surgeons and neurologists surveyed recommended the use of chiropractic in such cases.[26]

## Reform

Dissent, sometimes heated, continues to split the ranks of chiropractic. The division between *straights* and *mixers* that began back in the days of DD still persists to the extent some practitioners believe unless the issue is resolved it could mean the end of chiropractic as a profession.

Broadly speaking, in the USA the International Chiropractors Association (ICA),[27] founded in 1926 by Palmer, stands for the *straight* school of thought, while the American Chiropractic Association (ACA)[28] represents the *mixers*.[29] On the ICA website, for example, the reader will find the association has been involved in campaigns to limit compulsory childhood vaccination and descriptions of how chiropractic is used allegedly to help in cases unrelated to spinal problems, such as autism; while the ACA broadly restricts its chiropractic advice to treating painful conditions, especially back pain, and has sensible suggestions to offer concerning lifestyle, posture and ergonomics, intended to help readers protect the back.

From the beginning of the twentieth century the American Medical Association (AMA) had been concerned about chiropractic practices including persistent belief in *The Innate* and the continuing use of bizarre diagnostic gadgets and techniques, coupled with sweeping claims that chiropractic was capable of treating virtually every disease known to medicine (including polio) and the stated ambition of chiropractors to act as primary caregivers in the same way as science-based medical practitioners. To combat these antiquated, pre-scientific practices the AMA took legal action against individual chiropractors who practised without a medical licence and otherwise encouraged the medical profession to distance itself from chiropractic. Matters eventually came to a head in a notorious lawsuit, brought against the AMA by the chiropractic community in 1976. The case finally concluded in 1987 when the AMA was found guilty of using underhand tactics to suppress and marginalise chiropractic. The court ruling meant it was no longer possible for medical organisations to pressurise their members into not associating professionally with chiropractors and were obliged to allow chiropractors much more freedom to practice.[30]

Now, four decades later, one section of chiropractors (the *mixers*) fear, having fought tooth and claw in the last century to win the political and legal battle, that by continuing to cling to ideas of *The Innate* and making unsubstantiated claims for chiropractic, they are losing the scientific battle in this century and are at risk of throwing away their new-found freedom. Unless things change, they warn, the profession could go the way the AMA has wanted it to since the 1920s and disappear; without any need for legislative manoeuvring or boycotts.

Some committed *straights* have attempted to sidestep the worrying issue that the lesion that is their entire *raison d'être* doesn't actually exist, by extending and broadening its definition to encompass more vague, less structural terms. One veterinary paper published in 1999 claims rather airily, the VSL is actually 'a dis-relationship of a vertebral segment in association with contiguous vertebrae resulting in a disturbance of normal biomechanical and neurological function', where the 'vertebral segment' in question is extended, for reasons only known to the authors, to encompass not one vertebra but two.[31] Others have gone further and attempted to cloud the issue in the circular logic of metaphysical and spiritual jargon: 'The vertebral subluxation cannot be precisely defined because it is an abstraction, an intellectual construct used ... to explain the success of the chiropractic adjustment ... We cannot isolate the VS in a test tube ... The subluxation is not a thing to be studied.'[32] In other words the VSL exists because chiropractic works and chiropractic works because the VSL exists!

Other, more practical, practitioners have shied away from this kind of bootstrap logic and feel wholesale change is needed if chiropractic is to be taken seriously in the twenty-first century mainstream.

There is evidence, from surveys of chiropractic colleges in North America conducted by Doctor of Chiropractic, David Sikorski, that half of them still remain committed to dogma and teach subjects that are scientifically unsubstantiated. This gives the author cause for concern, and he advises 'chiropractors' quest for greater legitimacy and cultural authority is retarded by this tendency.'[33]

Another survey in the UK found substantial numbers of chiropractors claiming to be able to treat non-spinal conditions including osteoporosis, obesity, hypertension, infertility, infantile colic, otitis media and asthma. As in the USA it was found there was a considerable difference in attitude between members of different chiropractic organisations.[34]

A number of practitioners and professional bodies believe this attitude, along with high-pressure advertising techniques true to the tradition of the original founders of the movement, is undermining the credibility of the profession. One author writes in desperation, 'Chiropractic dogma has strangled us and, if nothing changes, it will be our end.'[35] The European group, the *Société Franco-Européenne de Chiropraxie*, has issued a position statement that advises, 'The teaching of vertebral subluxation complex as a vitalistic construct that claims that it is the cause of disease is unsupported by evidence. Its inclusion in a modern chiropractic curriculum in anything other than an historical context is therefore inappropriate and unnecessary.'[36] The General Chiropractic Council agrees with it and has recently revised its guidelines to practitioners to include the phrase: 'The chiropractic vertebral subluxation complex is an historical concept but it remains a theoretical model. It is not supported by any clinical research evidence that would allow claims to be made that it is the cause of disease.'[37]

Other commentators are even more forthright in their concerns that the practice of chiropractic should move to a more evidence-based footing. Joseph Keating writes of the VSL, 'The widespread assertion of the clinical meaningfulness of this notion brings ridicule from the scientific and health care communities ... The chiropractic subluxation continues to have as much or more political than scientific meaning,'[38] and Donald Murphy of the Rhode Island Spine Centre likens the VSL to '... an albatross around our collective necks that impedes progress ...' Murphy draws a comparison between chiropractic and the profession of podiatry and suggests the former can learn from the latter, who have taken a somewhat unglamorous and arguably otherwise neglected niche area of human health care (foot disorders) and made it their own. He points out podiatrists '... did not invent a "lesion" and a "philosophy" and try to force it on the public. They certainly did not claim that all disease arose from the foot, without any evidence to support this notion. The podiatric medical profession simply did what credible and authoritative professions do – they provided society with services that people actually wanted and needed.' He suggests chiropractors should do the same with regard to back disorders.[39]

Concerns are not new; in 1988 one author and champion of the profession of chiropractic wrote on the subject of reform and acceptance in the modern age. He maintained if chiropractic was to properly and credibly join the ranks of the professions it would have to resolve the issue of 'cultism', submit the VSL to scientific scrutiny in the same way other hypotheses are scrutinised and finally, 'relinquish their claims to be able to treat all kinds of conditions and modify their theory that all illnesses are due to spinal subluxations and that the only appropriate therapy is their removal.'[40]

Boundary disputes over whether chiropractic ought to restrict itself solely to spinal matters or whether it could justifiably claim to be able to treat disease in other parts of the body came to a head in the UK in 2008. In April of that year journalist Simon Singh wrote, in an article in the UK's *Guardian* newspaper, that the British Chiropractic Association (BCA), by maintaining that '... their members can help treat children with colic, sleeping and feeding problems, frequent ear infections, asthma and prolonged crying ...' was 'happily promoting bogus treatments.'[41] The BCA objected to the use of the term 'bogus' and on the basis of this remark Singh was taken to court and sued for an enormous sum by the BCA, perhaps in the hope of repeating the success its US colleagues had gained against the AMA some four decades previously. This time however, the BCA was forced to concede the case and chiropractic organisations were obliged to advise their members to take down their websites and conduct a massive overhaul of their other literature to remove unjustified claims.[42] On the basis of the judgement individual chiropractors faced unprecedented numbers of complaints and fitness to practice charges and the governing body for chiropractors, the General Chiropractic Council (GCC), disowned the claims of the BCA.[43] Times, it seemed, were changing.

Fortunately for our animal patients and despite veterinary practitioners being bombarded with emails and advertisements suggesting there is a fortune to be made by training as a chiropractor (in a six-month period in 2016 I personally received by email no less that sixty-four unsolicited advertisements from the same veterinary chiropractic organisation), veterinary practitioners have not gone quite as far as their colleagues in human practice who claim, quite openly, that subluxations, which only the chiropractor can see, are 'silent killers' and potential patients not yet attending for regular realignments will suffer dire, even fatal, consequences further down the line. This restraint may be as a result of the widespread legal requirement in many regions, including much of Europe and North America, that in the interests of animal welfare a chiropractor may only treat an animal that has been referred to them by a veterinary practitioner.[44]

But animal chiropractic is certainly not immune from far-fetched claims and some practitioners claim, despite a lack of meaningful evidence, the ability to productively treat a wide range of conditions including bowel, liver, skin, ear, thyroid and heart problems as well as seizures and a smorgasbord of behavioural issues. As with chiropractic in humans, there is also a worrying tendency in the veterinary world to advise that long-term prophylactic manipulations are required in order to maintain health. Some advocates, seemingly regardless of the presence or absence of overt clinical problems and certainly without any rational justification, encourage the regular chiropractic manipulation of quite arbitrary groups of dogs including all working dogs; any dog that has played frisbee; any dog that has had a general anaesthetic and, inexplicably, all German Shepherds over 4 years of age.[45]

The lure of the financial returns to be gained from chiropractic 'prophylaxis' is hard to resist for some and the tendency to suggest that spinal manipulation therapy can be used to prevent problems supposedly destined to occur some time in the future or to enhance vague, ill-defined concepts such as *wellness*, quality of life or even *spirituality* in animals is all too common. This self-referential closed circle is the ideal way to ensure caregivers will return (and pay) for treatment again and again, as the chiropractor first diagnoses something he alone can see and then, after the appropriate tweakings, announces an improvement, but one which again only he can see and, what's more, will require repeated manipulations to maintain.

A recent article in the UK's *Guardian* newspaper describes an animal chiropractor doing exactly this as he pronounces on the neck of a horse named Cedric, 'Well out of alignment there. He's not lame, but he's going to go lame if we don't do something about it.'[46] This keenness to treat is sometimes so pronounced one has to wonder whether any animal chiropractor has ever attended a horse whose spine *isn't* out of line.

## Harm from chiropractic

Much has been written elsewhere about the single greatest risk to humans from chiropractic, the cervical arterial dissection (CAD), when sudden and forced manipulations of the head and upper neck by chiropractors causes damage to the major arteries supplying the brain resulting in various complications, from headaches and stiffness to strokes, paralysis or even death.[47, 48, 49, 50] This risk is of such great concern, and the benefits of chiropractic so limited by comparison, that some authors advise referrals should not be made to chiropractors who perform this kind of manipulation[51] and clinical neurologists despair of the 'steady stream of injured patients' provided to the medical profession by the practice of chiropractic.[52]

In animal chiropractic there has been one report of a stroke-like incident in a horse in Sweden that resulted in a malpractice claim. The horse developed signs of neurological disturbances, unsteady gait and difficulty eating and swallowing following a chiropractic adjustment, possibly as a result of damage to the vertebrobasilar artery in the neck. It died of an oesophageal obstruction eighteen months after treatment.[53]

Other reports of injury following chiropractic manipulation in healthy animals are apparently few and far between. Various reasons may account for this difference; smaller animals such as cats and dogs are either rarely in a relaxed enough state or are too agile to allow such extreme movements to be performed, while larger ones – with the unfortunate exception of the case above where damage seems to have been caused by excessive movement of the head relative to the spine – are generally too large and heavily muscled to allow any movement between consecutive vertebrae significant enough to cause harm. The possibility of under-reporting of veterinary adverse events must be considered however, given the much vaunted privacy of the consulting room and, as with other forms of potentially damaging CAVM, the lack in the veterinary world of the checks and balances that serve to protect human patients in such circumstances.

One area of chiropractic where animals are involved is not as patients, but as experimental subjects, a revelation that is surprising considering its claimed gentle and holistic nature. As with homeopathy, there is a significant amount of vivisection employed in research into chiropractic. Cats in particular are much favoured by chiropractic researchers as an experimental model for the human subject and have been dissected and had their spines operated on, fixated and mechanically manipulated over the years in various unsuccessful attempts to demonstrate the nature of the VSL and the effects of chiropractic manipulation.[54, 55, 56, 57, 58, 59, 60, 61]

While vivisection is a necessity in some critical areas of medical research it is a wasteful tragedy to sacrifice laboratory animals in order to attempt to prove a phenomenon even chiropractors admit has consistently failed to materialise in physical form and where clinical evidence is absent.[62, 63]

An underrated risk from chiropractic, as with other types of CAVM is the tendency of practitioners to malign medical advice, thereby running the risk of denying patients essential medical treatment. One study in 2004 found more than a quarter of chiropractors asked advised against childhood and other vaccinations.[64] Some animal chiropractors too are given to denigrating conventional medicines in general and vaccination in particular in ways that run contrary to all the best available evidence for safety and efficacy. While some chiropractors continue to claim, wrongly,[65, 66] that chiropractic is effective in serious, non-spinal conditions such as those listed above this will inevitably leave patients at risk if they are persuaded that chiropractic manipulations can be used instead of rather than alongside conventional medications.

## Veterinary research

Animal chiropractic has been criticised, particularly when it comes to its underlying principles and the relative risks and benefits. One Scandinavian team, led by veterinary surgeon Ragnvi Ekström-Kjellin looked at the websites and curricula of a number of animal chiropractic teaching organisations and found the scientific quality of the courses was 'strikingly low' and often mixed with overt pseudoscience and misleading claims, and that many of the practices that were taught were outside the realm of both science and best practice. Their findings, the authors felt, led to serious questions about the value of animal chiropractic in veterinary practice.[67]

Veterinary research into chiropractic is limited, of questionable quality, and fraught with serious methodological shortcomings.[68, 69, 70] Some commentators demonstrate a woeful ignorance of veterinary matters, in particular the caregiver placebo effect and the many other reasons illness in animals can appear to respond to ineffective treatments (see Chapter Two), and instead fall into the trap of lazily assuming because an animal has improved following adjustment then only the adjustment can be responsible for the improvement.[71]

Orthomanual Therapy was first devised in humans by a Dutch physician and now, as Veterinary Orthomanual Therapy (VOT), has been adapted for use in animal patients. Also claiming to be able to treat patients by means of correcting misaligned vertebrae, the technique appears to all intents and purposes indistinguishable from chiropractic. A study carried out by its chief proponent, the veterinary surgeon who developed the technique for use in animals, looked at VOT when employed alongside conventional treatments (especially exercise restriction) in a group of 261 dachshunds with suspected thoracolumbar intervertebral disc disease (TLDD). The paper claimed, 'Veterinary orthomanual therapy combined with cage rest seems to be effective in treating TLDD in dachshunds and might be considered an acceptable form of non-surgical treatment.'

The authors, however, concede that the great majority of such cases will improve or even resolve completely with cage rest alone and admit the lack of both a control group and any form of diagnostic imaging of the patients under study is a severe (some might say fatal) limitation to any conclusions as to the value of VOT in this distressing and painful condition.

In addition, they fail to mention the point that the supposed vertebral misalignments (graced by them with fanciful names such as *tippers* and *tumblers*) that are claimed to be responsible for or associated with disc disease, although they are illustrated most convincingly in a number of stylised line-drawings that accompany the article, consistently fail to appear on radiographs of actual patients.[72]

Another study that looked at a variety of treatments for the compulsive behavioural condition known as head-shaking in horses found chiropractic to be somewhat less effective than placing a piece of cloth over the muzzle of affected subjects.[73]

One veterinary chiropractor, even after admitting the evidence for the beneficial effects of chiropractic in veterinary practice is limited and there is little agreement on the subject between practitioners, nevertheless went on to demonstrate exactly the sort of faulty, circular reasoning so typical of much that is written on the subject. A group of dogs that the author knew to have urinary tract disorders is described that, after examination by him, he then claimed had vertebral subluxations in similar areas of the spine. His assertion, that this represented 'an association between chiropractic findings in the lumbar region and urinary problems manifesting as retention or incontinence in dogs', is weakened to the point of irrelevance by the clear possibility of observer bias due to the absence of blinding, as the author, to his credit, freely admits.[74] The results might have been more convincing if he had examined a randomly selected group of dogs, some of which had urinary problems, others of which did not, without knowing which was which; or if other chiropractors had been offered the chance to repeat the examination and compared the consistency of results between practitioners. Why this type of control wasn't included as part of the study isn't mentioned.

Only time will tell whether the practice of chiropractic will succeed, as many within its ranks would wish, in casting off the pseudoscientific trappings of mysterious energies and non-existent lesions and focus on what they are widely regarded as doing best, treating bad backs. The stark alternative is, by persisting in these beliefs, one section of the profession is inviting ridicule and incredulity and risks bringing the house down around the ears of everyone else.

The auguries aren't good, however. It's been well over a century since the original split between the *mixers* and the *straights* and, as we have seen, a considerable proportion of chiropractors, human and veterinary, still cling to the untenable concept of the VSL and believe they are capable of treating disorders unrelated to the spine. Furthermore, they persist in carrying out dangerous manipulations for minimal or no benefit at the same time as deriding useful and well-researched medicines.

One suspects it will be some time before *mixers* and *straights* are able to come together and present their mutual profession as one based in science rather than spirituality, and one which is prepared to put its most cherished beliefs to the test and put aside those that are found wanting.

§

## Doggy body work

Chiropractic aside, there is a wider group of body work therapies for animals – mainly dogs and horses but in some cases other species are included – that also involve varying levels of hands-on manipulation of the subject.

245

Different types of therapy provide for different owner expectations, some being distinctly at the leisure end of the spectrum, reflecting a need for owners to feel their pet is occupied and occasionally benefiting from some of the activities they themselves undertake, while others have a more serious intention and are believed to be of benefit to an animal suffering a specific condition.

## Yoga and massage for dogs

Unlikely as it sounds, yoga for dogs is apparently becoming more popular. How this is done varies from practitioner to practitioner but systems such as *Doga* (the sacred bond between dog and owner), and *The Barking Buddha* (Simple Soul Stretches for Yogi and Dogi) seem mainly to involve dog owners practising yoga as usual while their dogs run around the room enjoying themselves in the way dogs do, exhibiting anything from mild frenzy through bemused interest to complete indifference. In response to requests from owners for greater canine participation, one instructor has devised exercises to involve the dogs more directly that, to all appearances, seem simply to consist of owners practising yoga, again in the usual way, only this time while holding their dogs.[75]

Jo-Rosie Haffenden has devised a slightly more serious programme of *Real Dog Yoga* where dogs are themselves required, on a more one to one basis, to do a form of yoga as they are taught to adopt and hold a variety of yoga-type poses: thirty postures, fifteen actions and ten expressions.[76]

Descriptions of numerous other massage and manipulation techniques and systems such as *Galen Myotherapy* for animals of all descriptions but mainly dogs and horses, are to be found widely in books, magazines and on the web. Among the recommended moves are firm to gentle rubbing and stroking motions or rhythmic compressions of the limbs with an open hand. One set of instructions sensibly warns not to attempt anything approaching a deep tissue massage in animals such as might be performed in human athletes as this could cause pain. On the whole, the emphasis is towards gentle, enjoyable strategies aimed at bringing relaxation and enhancing the human–animal bond.

## Tellington Touch

Tellington Touch was first developed by Canadian born horse trainer Lynda Tellington-Jones in the 1980s after studying the Feldenkrais method, invented by Dr Moshe Feldenkrais (1904–1984), which teaches that through minute, repetitive movements participants can enhance their potential and improve flexibility, coordination and mental acuity.

Ms Tellington-Jones began to apply some of the techniques she had learned on horses in the first instance, and later progressed to other species including cats, dogs, cattle and eventually a wide range of more exotic animals, including a killer whale named *Keiko*.

As would be expected given the origins of Tellington Touch, there are influences from other similar systems. Repetitive, passive movements – applied by the practitioner to the subject – are a core component of both Tellington Touch and the Feldenkrais method. Individual Touches are given evocative names that echo the *Asanas* of yoga – yoga has the *cobra*, the *lion* and the *camel*, Tellington Touch has the *python*, the *tiger* and the *llama*; Tellington Touch has *tarantulas pulling the plough*, yoga has both *scorpion* and *plough*.

Tellington Touch comprises different categories of treatment. The basic 'Circular Touches' are small circular movements of the hand employing different degrees of pressure and areas of contact over the body of the animal and are used alongside a series of stylised, stroking movements; gentle pinchings; passive limb manipulation; and the 'belly-lift'. Then there are the 'Leading Exercises', which involve leading dogs and horses using a variety of pieces of equipment including leashes, body wraps and thin, guiding wands over flat ground or, in the third phase (the 'Confidence Course') around and over obstacles in the form of poles, low jumps and other challenges.

By working through the various exercises it is claimed both animal and handler gain an enhanced rapport and greater mutual confidence as both learn to think and cooperate together. The literature contains plenty of straightforward advice about dog and horse behaviour and safety warnings concerning the limitations and risks of training and behavioural modification in animals and in particular has sound advice about what not to do with a dog that is aggressive.

The principal claim of Tellington Touch is that it can help modify animal behaviour and develop and improve the human–animal bond. The philosophy is one of respect and the working together of human and animal to achieve mutually beneficial goals. Nervous horses, aggressive dogs, timid cats and their owners are all reported to have developed relaxed and more confident demeanours as a result of applying the various touches.[77, 78]

# The feel-good factor

These types of activity – doggy yoga, massage, Galen Therapy, Tellington Touch and the like – are a positive experience, providing simple safety precautions are heeded. Regularly touching and handling a dog or horse will ensure a caregiver becomes familiar with what is normal and so be able to more readily identify changes in the form of lumps or painful spots which might require veterinary attention. They are also an effective bonding exercise and likely, in the correct subjects, to have the effect of familiarising a dog or horse with human contact in a low-stress context. Dogs in particular love routine and a regular schedule of stylised touches and strokings as part of a daily programme in a combination of fun, feel-good and frequent health checks will be of great mutual benefit for dog and owner.

This being the case, to suggest such techniques should be scrutinised and tested scientifically would not only be nigh on impossible but would be missing the point (for the record most work published on the veterinary aspects of body work is extrapolated and inferred from the human field[79, 80]). Such activities are fun, they reinforce the animal human bond and it is not beyond the realms of possibility they may help with certain behavioural disorders characterised by wariness, fear, hyperactivity or even aggression if done respectfully, calmly and gently, as advocated by practitioners. By learning some of the recommended approaches it might even be possible to bypass the *school of hard knocks* method of learning and predicting animal behaviour, in a manner that allows more in the way of learning and less in the way of hard knocks, bites and kicks.

And if that was all there was to it then such activities would have no place in this book. Some people though, can't seem to leave things alone; there is a pervasive and irrepressible desire to gild the lily, over-complicate and medicalise simple and common sense-based activities. Consequently, when looking in detail at these practices one finds a perplexing mix of sensible truisms concerning animal behaviour, interspersed with facile, pick and mix pseudoscience, far-fetched New Age puffery and claims about arcane energy fields, all of which presumably is felt adds a degree of credibility, none of which have any evidence behind them.

Unsubstantiated claims about the effect of these techniques on so-called 'cellular-intelligence', or the parasympathetic nervous system, the vagus nerve or 'stress hormones' may be regarded as either entertaining window-dressing or suspect and contrived irritations (particularly when 'vagus' is so frequently misspelled 'Vegas') depending on one's point of view. Even claims about massage reducing blood pressure are unlikely to give rise to problems directly; any veterinary surgeon or nurse who has ever taken a cat's blood pressure or counted a nervous dog's heart rate knows that stress can make an enormous difference to the readings.

It is when practitioners overstep the mark and begin to make overt medical claims that there is a risk of harm. In particular great caution should be exercised with assertions these treatments can relieve the pain of arthritic joints, something for which there is no clear, objective evidence. While many humans suffering arthritis report benefits from massage and gentle manipulation, the same cannot be assumed of animals, who are unlikely to profit in the same way from some of the positive psychological outcomes enjoyed by human patients. Anyone using massage and related techniques to treat painful conditions in animals must be open-minded enough to recognise the tendency in all of us to want to see a companion we love getting better, and how it is possible to believe there has been an improvement even when more objective indicators suggest otherwise.

Furthermore, while it is not too far-fetched an idea that performing massage or passive movements in arthritic animals may help relieve muscle tension around painful joints, it should be borne in mind that damage can be done if such things are performed incorrectly or too vigorously or by someone poorly cognisant of the relevant anatomy and disease processes. These practices should never be used in place of proven treatments and should be performed only after consulting a veterinary surgeon in the first instance or following referral to a chartered animal physiotherapist.

§

## Energy medicine

The final section in this chapter on Manipulation Therapies concerns practices that claim to be able to address, not the fleshly, corporeal aspects of the animal but its higher, spiritual projections. This type of practice encompasses sub-sets of related disciplines including bioenergy healing, Bowen Therapy, Chakra healing, Christian science, distant healing, dowsing, faith healing, intercessory prayer, orgone-energy healing, psionic medicine, psychic healing, Qi-gong, radionics, reiki, shiatsu, spiritual healing, therapeutic touch, vortex healing and zero balancing.

Definitions vary, depending on which author one reads but one thing this hotch-potch of names has in common is that they claim to be able to detect and modify the 'energetic biofields', or 'auras', which we are told surround us at all times in life.

By making this claim, adepts have succeeded in creating a multi-billion dollar, international industry out of an obfuscation – either by accident or design – of two different types of energy, one physical and one abstract, which have been conflated to produce a third, entirely imaginary form.

As every secondary school biology student knows, the body requires energy to exist. We and our animal companions obtain this energy in the form of nutrients such as carbohydrates and fats, which we are then able to store for future use. When required, the chemical energy of those substances is transformed into mechanical energy to enable us to carry out the tasks that are the prerequisites of life – movement, thought, growth, respiration, digestion, reproduction and so on. Many bodily functions (primarily muscular and nervous activity) give off electrical energy as a by-product of this whole process, which can then be quantified in useful ways including the electrocardiogram (ECG), electroencephalogram (EEG) and in electromyography (EMG). So, in a sense, we are indeed surrounded by 'energy fields', but ones that are firmly rooted in the physical world, are well understood and which can be measured using simple equipment.

Then there is another, more abstract type of energy, often referred to as 'vitality'. When we are feeling upbeat and ready to take on life's challenges we say we are 'full of energy'; a jumpy, jittery person might be described as having a lot of 'nervous energy'; while in sombre mood, after having completed a particularly undemanding, repetitive task or just being plain tired, one might be 'lacking in energy'. Even the way we describe our moods, as 'positive' or 'negative', are also ways by which electrical energy is described.

The trick practitioners of energy medicine have performed, and managed to get their followers to believe, is to take the idea of the physical, measurable energy field associated with living creatures and merge it with the second, abstract or subjective concept of energy and come up with the idea they can measure the latter using arcane means, in the same way as we measure the former more conventionally. This is the essence of pseudoscience, a disingenuous confusion of the real and the mystic; a plausible deception stemming entirely from the imaginations of advocates and practitioners.

Most of the practices listed above have a diagnostic element. Practitioners claim to be able to detect disease and illness manifesting as distortions in the *energetic biofield*, using a variety of intermediaries such as pendulums, crystals, dowsing rods, mysterious black boxes or simply through their hands as they are held over the patient. It is claimed by some these disturbances can be felt at considerable distance from the subject.

Treatment is carried out in a reversal of this process, as distortions in the biofield are corrected and (inevitably) 'balanced' by means of further hand-waving or whatever the practitioner's chosen technique or device happens to be, resulting in a restoration of health. This too can supposedly be carried out at considerable physical distance from the patient.

Biofield treatment is in some aspects the pared down core of other forms of CAVM such as homeopathy, acupuncture and chiropractic that claim to be able to manipulate unidentified and undetectable energies. One veterinary practitioner of radionics and *pranamonics* describes them as employing identical energies to acupuncture and homeopathy, but 'cutting out the middle man'. In many ways these practices can be regarded as homeopathy without the pills or acupuncture without the needles.[81]

This concept follows naturally from what is known as the 'non-local' effect of homeopathy – the idea that the supposed action of homeopathic treatment isn't as a result of physical remedies as such, but an energy deriving in part from the process of preparation of the remedy and in part from the practitioner's 'intention to treat', which is independent of physical matter. It has been claimed for instance, most notably by homeopath Jacques Benveniste, that it is possible to render a homeopathic remedy down to a pure energy signature, which can then be sent by email or captured in digital form, ready to be directed towards the patient as required without the need for a physical intermediary such as a lactose pillule or drops of water or alcohol.[82]

# Radionics

Radionics was founded by US physician, Albert Abrams, in the early twentieth century and is principally a type of medical-oriented radiesthesia (dowsing), employing an electrical device known as an *Oscilloclast*, or *black box*, which it is claimed can detect the emanations from patients, often many hundreds of miles away after a connection has been made by means of a 'witness' – a drop of blood, piece of hair or even a photograph.[83] Sometimes a dowsing pendulum is also used in combination with the black box. By adjusting the settings (which radionic jargon refers to as 'rates') on the machine, it is gradually tuned to the patient under scrutiny by manipulating knobs and buttons or sometimes stroking a rubber membrane. By this means any energetic disturbances are mapped out carefully. Once this mapping has been achieved the machine is then switched from 'receive' to 'send' and the energetic waves are broadcast back the way they came to cancel out the anomalies and imbalances suffered by the patient, thus restoring vitality.

Some variations on the *black box* are used that are able to select a homeopathic remedy to do the job of healing. Others will even create the required homeopathic remedy itself from blank lactose tablets placed in a special receptacle in the machine opposite an identical chamber containing the witness with a wire connecting the two. Once the machine is tuned correctly the required healing energy is inserted directly into the tablets, giving them immediate potency, personalised to the patient in question. This claim is naturally impossible to test since no one, not even homeopaths themselves, has reliably demonstrated the ability to tell one homeopathic remedy from another by any means.

The fact that no circuitry ever found in a *black box* has made sense electronically and the devices are often used without being connected to a power source is of no concern to practitioners, who maintain the circuitry is simply a 'channel' for energy, used in the same way as the forked hazel twig of the dowser.[84] One set of instructions, openly available on the internet, describes how it is possible to construct a home-made *black box* from commonplace items including a shoebox, a tin can, the plastic lid from a coffee jar, some wire, screws, three rotary potentiometers with knobs and two quartz crystals. The finished device is apparently most effective when used with the *psionic amplifying helmet*, constructed from tinfoil, wire and magnets, for which assembly instructions are also provided.

When reading much of the literature available on the subjects of radionics and other forms of biofield medicine it becomes difficult to distinguish most of them from religious beliefs. Animal radionics is described by one UK veterinary surgeon and former Dean of the Psionic Medical Society as 'a field of activity where physics and para-physics, science and religion, meet and merge'. He further claims when the radionic practitioner is making a diagnosis he or she 'utilises the principles of dowsing by applying his faculties of extra-sensory perception (ESP) to the problem of detecting disease'. This psychic link, we are told, can be achieved using the *witness*, which connects practitioner and patient via the earth's own energy fields.[85] Other veterinary surgeons go further; one description of the philosophy of *pranamonics* alleges the involvement of spirit-like cosmic energies, originating outside of the patient–practitioner system and moving through the body in a series of connected networks. Readers are cautioned, however, these are not the familiar *chakras* described in humans, since 'in the animal world it appears that the linking of several energy centres into separate circuits, which nevertheless interlink with each other, is the norm'.[86]

One of the greatest proponents of radionics was a chiropractor, Ruth Drown, who like so many others of her calling had 'a love of pseudo-scientific gadgetry' that eventually led to her personally treating some 35,000 patients with her radionic devices and selling many more to others who did the same. She was finally charged with grand theft and taking money under false pretences after failing to notice that three drops of blood presented to her for analysis weren't, as she reported, those of three young sisters about to come down with chicken pox and mumps but were in fact obtained from a selection of farmyard animals.[87]

# Reiki

Reiki is a form of energy healing, supposedly based on ancient Buddhist principles, developed by Dr Usui in Japan in the nineteenth century, which arrived in the US in the 1970s and Europe in the 1980s. Practitioners believe in a universal energy or spirit (a literal translation of the term reiki is *universal life-energy*), which vibrates at different frequencies ranging from the dense, slow vibrations of matter to the fast, pure vibrations of light, consciousness and thought. It is believed Reiki Masters can channel this energy into the patient through their hands in order to bring healing by way of unblocking obstructions in the flow of *Qi*, in the same way an acupuncturist claims to do by the use of needles.

Traditionally this ability was passed directly from Master to apprentice. After an initial process of selection during which both parties would carefully consider the mutual congruence between them, the apprentice would begin a process of charismatic training, absorbing oral histories and learning the rituals of healing. This would take two years or more, until finally the apprentice had become fully 'attuned' to the Master. At this point they were considered to have joined their Master's 'lineage' – a sort of energetic family tree that can be traced back through lines of former Masters – and would be able to practice as full Master in his own right and take on apprentices.

Currently, in the UK it is possible for a student to become a fully-fledged master after studying for two days at a local training college.

This modern day debasement of an apprenticeship process designed not just to impart facts but to bring the novice to full integration, along with other concerns over splits within the Reiki community (currently around twenty different styles of Reiki are practised, some of which claim superiority over the rest), the publication of secret, sacred symbols in books and on the internet, and even attempts to patent Reiki, has given rise to concerns among more traditional practitioners that its core principles and beliefs are no longer properly respected.[88,89]

# The evidence

Firm evidence for any of these practices is pretty thin on the ground; for example, a search for 'veterinary reiki' on the PubMed database comes up blank. A search for 'veterinary radionics' yields a single short communication from 2006 that looked at parasitic worm egg counts in eighty-nine horses studied over a two-year period in three groups given either radionic treatment, conventional worming medication, or left untreated as a control.[90]

Conducted under the auspices of the Confederation of Healing Organisations, this work seems to have built on a similar pilot trial performed in 1987 that, although its findings suggested similar worm burdens in two groups of horses – one treated radionically, the other treated medically – came in for criticism for its lack of control groups and the considerable disparity in management practices between the two groups.[91] The later, 2006, trial controlled for these factors and concluded worm burdens were the same in the groups treated radionically and those not treated at all, while those treated conventionally showed a considerable reduction in infestation.

In human medicine the evidence, while slightly more plentiful, is largely negative in the assessment of energy-based healing practices. Reiki has been found to be 'unproven' in providing relief for painful conditions[92] and a Cochrane review in 2015, after describing the data as 'sparse' (only three papers were found) concluded, 'There is insufficient evidence to say whether or not Reiki is useful for people over 16 years of age with anxiety or depression or both.'[93]

Another study in the *Journal of the Royal Society of Medicine* whose authors included two leading homeopaths, looked specifically at whether it was possible for homeopaths to obtain useful information on disease by employing dowsing methods.[94] The results were described as 'wholly negative', which may have come as a surprise to one veterinary practitioner who claimed, in 2001, to be able to select homeopathic remedies for cases of adrenal gland disease in horses and dogs by using 'radiesthetic principles', which is to say, by dowsing.[95]

One of the most robust and convincing trials conducted on energy therapies was a 1998 paper studying Therapeutic Touch (TT), a technique invented by nurse Dolores Krieger in the 1970s that, ironically, doesn't actually involve any touching. During the study twenty-one TT practitioners of varying levels of experience were asked to determine, under carefully controlled and blinded conditions, over which one of their arms the investigator was holding her hand. The subject and experimenter were shielded from one another by a solid screen, through which the subjects inserted both arms in order to be tested.

TT practitioners claim to be able to not only detect but to interpret and manipulate the so-called *biofield* surrounding every living thing; it is an absolute requirement of the technique that these energy fields be both identifiable and amenable to modification. So it is not unreasonable to expect practitioners who make a living from doing this to be able to tell simply whether a human hand was present or absent as it was held over them.

Unfortunately for the participating practitioners, however, the results obtained in this trial were indistinguishable from chance, no different from those that would have been expected by guessing, and there was no difference in results between practitioners who were more or less experienced. A more comprehensive and damning indictment of *energetic biofields* could not be wished for, despite the *post-hoc* objections and excuses from those who were tested and failed. The fact that the person who designed and carried out the trials was a 9 year old girl doing a project for her fourth grade science fair makes the findings even more astonishing and probably goes a long way to explain why the practitioner subjects were happy to participate in the first place.[96] Whether TT practitioners are now as willing to subject themselves and their art to such telling scrutiny isn't known, but since that time no other trial has ever succeeded in overturning the findings.

There is no question that the so-called *biofield* upon which energy-medicine of all hues depends is anything other than purely imaginary. It is not the same as the mundane emanations from heart, muscle and brain activity that are well understood and measured as a matter of routine in most veterinary clinics across the world. Neither is the invented concept of universal energy, and the idea that our bodies are energy made solid to be confused with Einstein's formula $E=mc^2$. It may be, with sufficient leeway (and providing no one who actually understands particle physics is listening in), that this formula could be taken to suggest that matter and energy are two different states of the same thing but this is light years away from saying, as practitioners of *energy-field* medicine would have it, that matter and energy are somehow interchangeable or that animal and human bodies can be regarded as in any way being 'made of energy', much less that this energy can be manipulated at will for the benefit of the patient. Of course, matter can be converted to energy, as our experience with the atomic weapons programme tells us, but the conversion is considerably more messy and random than practitioners of radionics and therapeutic touch would have us believe and moreover is an irredeemably one-way process.

Although proponents of energy therapies castigate 'those stuck in the time warp of Newtonian physics and wedded to the sacred cow of the double blind trial ...' for their perceived lack of understanding,[97] this is simply, sour grapes; a smokescreen for the inescapable reality that never have any energy fields of the sort described by practitioners been identified by any objective, reliable method, Newtonian, quantum or otherwise.[98] We should have little doubt though, as with other CAVM methodologies, if ever even a hint of such proof offered itself, it would be happily seized upon and all previous misgivings about the scientific method quietly shelved. In the meantime we are simply being asked to take the word of practitioner–advocates with a vested interest in proving, not testing, their claims.

§

## The back man

To return to the epigraph to this section, the 'back man' has indeed been part of horsey psyche for centuries, although, of course, these days it is just as likely to be a 'back woman' who attends.

Regardless of objective evidence or scientific proof there has always been a demand for such things, so much so that the 'back person' is increasingly in demand to attend an ever expanding range of animals including production livestock, the smaller companion animals – cats, dogs and rabbits – and also some exotic and pretty credulity-stretching species including elephants, budgies, lions, tigers, sharks, bears, badgers and buffalo.[99]

This situation seems unlikely to change anytime soon and in many ways it would be a sad day for animals and their various care-givers if it did and this traditional type of treatment was abandoned entirely. There is a note of caution to be struck, however, which this chapter will, with luck, help highlight. If manipulation therapy is being contemplated in an animal you are responsible for, the burden of trust means it is incumbent upon you to ensure the choice of therapist is made carefully. If your preferred practitioner is content to treat minor problems with gentle manipulations, massage or formulaic strokings then little harm is likely to ensue and there may possibly be some benefit to the animal if used sensibly, alongside more science-based treatments.

But if he or she claims to be able to treat your dog's thyroid, or its liver or lung problems or, worse still, a confirmed prolapsed intervertebral disc by means of a chiropractic adjustment or by interrogating and manipulating the so-called biofield, then run a mile. It is you who is being manipulated here, not your animal. You are being bamboozled and asked to believe something that is demonstrably untrue. At best you will be wasting your time and money, at worst you could be doing your animal companion a great disservice by exacerbating pre-existing damage that, if left alone or treated conservatively with rest and pain-relieving medication, may well resolve of its own accord.

Better still, if you or your veterinary surgeon feel animal manipulation is the way to go, seek out the services of a member of the Association of Chartered Physiotherapists in Animal Therapy (ACPAT). Such people are formidably well qualified, having initially studied and qualified in human physiotherapy and then gone on to study veterinary applications in great detail. They are competent, experienced and entirely science-based, will give a truthful and accurate appraisal of any potential problem and work with you, the owner, and the referring veterinary surgeon to come up with a treatment plan that has objective outcomes and can be properly measured in the real world without recourse to mysticism or metaphysics.

# Diagnostics (Including TCM diagnosis, iridology, animal communicators-psychics, applied kinesiology, dowsing, Vega testing)

COMPLEMENTARY and alternative medicine doesn't stop simply at treatments. Many forms of CAM also claim to be able to make diagnoses too. We have already discussed some of these 'diagnostic' techniques, particularly in the chapter on manipulation therapies as we saw how *straight* chiropractors claim to be able to diagnose many forms of disease by examining the spine, and radionics practitioners claim to be able to detect changes in the supposed biofield and thereby diagnose illness caused through disturbances, or imbalances.

Even some homeopaths believe they have the ability to be able to diagnose and decide on an appropriate treatment plan apparently using only intuition. As one veterinary homeopath says, 'Homeopathy is simple. All you have to do in your consultation is perceive something from nature in your patient. You can hear it in their story, see it in their actions, and sometimes you witness it appearing in the space between you and them. That is the remedy they need ...'[1] Whether this apparently unique ability has ever been put to the test by comparing it with other methods isn't made clear. Some homeopaths have also claimed to use dowsing in the same way, although this method has been investigated, including by fellow homeopaths, and no evidence of its usefulness was found.

In this chapter we will explore some of the myriad of other techniques that it is claimed can diagnose illness in patients, although often, as with the treatment, the diagnosis is not one that is recognised by science-based medicine and runs contrary to the way we know the body functions, as we will see.

§

# Traditional Chinese Medicine

Traditional Chinese Medicine (TCM) is covered in Chapters Six and Eight. However, the specifics of its diagnostic claims are worth looking at in more detail.

TCM diagnosis involves superficially similar techniques to Western scientific diagnostics. The problem-oriented approach of scientific medicine to diagnosis involves taking a medical history (for example weight loss, vomiting, thirst, etc), a physical examination, compiling a list of problems discovered, considering the possible diagnoses for these problems in order of probability, then deciding which diagnostic tests to perform in order to narrow the possibilities to one or more specific diagnoses. TCM diagnosis comprises inquiry, inspection, auscultation, olfaction and palpation.

Inquiry is similar to the doctor's or vet's history taking. Inspection involves a visual examination and auscultation involves listening, for example for chest wheeziness, something that most people will be familiar with when a doctor reaches for his stethoscope (as an interesting aside, the stethoscope was invented so that embarrassed nineteenth century doctors did not have to place their ear against a woman's chest). Olfaction is checking for odours, and palpation involves physical examination. However, the variables being assessed in TCM differ greatly from those in the scientific diagnostic process.

For example, while a science-based vet or doctor listens to the heart to assess the presence of murmurs and arrhythmias, part of auscultation in TCM includes listening to the speech. A voice that is too strident or too weak can mean deficiencies or excesses leading to disharmony. Palpation in medicine involves feeling organ shapes, abnormal masses, fluid build-up and pain. Palpation in TCM involves applying pressure to the meridians and assessing the reaction to touch. Pulse taking in medicine and TCM both involve assessment of strength and rate, but a variety of other changes in pulse quality are taken into account in TCM to purportedly give information on the state of various organs.

The problems with TCM diagnosis are numerous. The diagnoses made have no relationship to changes in the real world, and involve diagnosing changes in things, such as *Qi*, that probably don't exist. There is also a poor agreement between different TCM practitioners on the diagnosis when they examine the same patient,[2, 3] which is unsurprising given the subjective nature of the examinations.

The end result of a TCM diagnostic session will not lead to a diagnosis in any meaningful scientific sense. It will not lead to a diagnosis of say meningitis, leptospirosis, or lymphoma. It will instead lead to findings such as an excess or deficiency of yin or yang, liver *Qi* stagnation or deficient spleen system *Qi*. A medical diagnostic pathway may lead to a diagnosis such as renal failure or inflammatory bowel disease, as opposed to made-up conditions such as damp-heat in the gallbladder or cold invasion of the stomach. Note that renal (kidney) failure and inflammatory bowel disease are both scientifically observable and verifiable diagnoses. Renal failure can be quantified by measurement of substances that are excreted from the body by healthy kidneys, such as creatinine, with increases caused by a decrease in glomerular filtration rate or renal function. Inflammatory bowel disease can be physically seen down the microscope when examining biopsies, manifested as stunting of intestinal villi and infiltration with white blood cells. Cold invasion of the stomach can only be diagnosed because a TCM practitioner tells us it is so.

Making the TCM diagnosis allows the TCM practitioner to choose a concoction of herbs that will correct these excesses or deficiencies discovered. However, as the treatment chosen is based upon the faulty diagnostic process, it becomes harder to assess whether TCM is effective for real conditions.

Ayurveda also has its own diagnostic method, which is supposedly aimed at finding the root cause of the disease. This involves assessing the birth type or constitution of the patient, and then using the five senses to assess eight physical parameters: pulse; urine; stools; tongue; speech; touch; vision; appearance. This allows a diagnosis to be performed, which involves assessing imbalances in the three body energies or doshas that are considered to be the source of disease. This leads to the same problem as with TCM – that a diagnostic system based on imaginary body energies will lead to an incorrect or imaginary diagnosis. The selection of treatments will then be based on this flawed diagnosis, making it hard to assess whether Ayurveda is effective.

§

# Iridology

Iridology is a diagnostic technique based on examination of the iris. Different parts of the iris are supposed to correspond to different parts of the body, and abnormalities in the iris relate to pathology in those body parts. Unfortunately, it has been proved that iridology practitioners are unable to differentiate diseases by examining the iris. One study asked iridologists to examine the irises of ninety-five patients who were free of kidney disease and forty-eight with kidney disease. The iridologists were unable to detect which patients had kidney disease.[4] A review of published studies found that there was no evidence to suggest that iridology could detect disease.[5] Despite this, iridology is still popular, and is practised in pets.

§

## Animal communicators and psychics

Pet psychics claim to be able to communicate telepathically with animals, and to be able to inform pet owners of their pet's wishes, feelings and thoughts. A web search reveals websites of many pet psychics who offer services such as communicating with deceased pets, locating lost animals, assisting in the diagnosis of illness, discovering a pet's unknown past, including causes of post-traumatic stress disorder, or just having two-way conversations with pets.

Most animal communicators offer the full range of services, although some specialise. One who specialises in remote healing requests that clients do not contact her about lost pets because she finds their grief upsetting. Those who do offer services for lost pets will offer readings lasting sixty to ninety minutes, sometimes involving a *Google Map* search, with typical prices in the region of £150 in the UK or $180 in Australia. Some animal communicators discuss with the lost pets what is on their mind and negotiate with them to come home. As is usual with alternative medicine and related disciplines, testimonials form the main 'evidence' for benefit, but even the testimonials of success seem extraordinarily weak. One website boasts success from a dog that had been lost for four days, which involved the owner and the psychic visiting some woods, where the psychic was convinced the dog was stuck in a rabbit hole. They called his name and felt he was close, though he did not come. Several hours after the owner returned home, the dog returned. Even more extraordinary was the testimonial regarding a cat that had been missing for seven weeks. The psychic had spent four weeks working with the owners before he returned home, but this is seen as a success for the psychic.

It might be of interest to note here that one of the authors (NT) had the experience where a distressed owner contacted the practice by phone to report her little terrier dog had sadly been missing for some days. While the details were being taken the owner suddenly became distracted and her tone changed – as the receptionist was speaking to her, the dog had simply wandered in through the front door, looking none the worse for his experience. Of course, we can't prove this miracle wasn't due to latent psychic abilities possessed by the member of the practice team who had taken the call but coincidence would seem more likely!

Some psychics claim to offer remote healing. One testimonial on a psychic's website claims that a hands-on veterinary examination revealed that a bladder tumour had shrunk by 30 per cent after a psychic healing session. The testimonial does not note any concurrent conventional treatments given, nor does it take into account the very subjective nature of assessing the size of an abdominal mass by palpation, particularly when located in an organ such as the bladder that naturally varies in size from moment to moment anyway.

Animal psychics seem to employ similar techniques to human psychics in order to impress their clients with a cold reading, i.e. a reading in which the psychic has no prior knowledge of the pet. One video clip, viewed by AG, of a pet psychic's interview with Holly Willoughby and Philip Schofield on ITV's show *This Morning* showed a cold reading performed from a photo of Holly Willoughby's cat. The pet psychic described the cat in vague terms such as gentle and knowing when to seek affection, which Ms Willoughby described as 'spot on'. To his credit Mr Schofield was more sceptical, claiming that he could tell that for himself just by looking at the breed of cat.

Techniques that allow psychics performing cold readings to appear credible include:

- Stating the obvious or the safe, e.g. your dog wants more walks.
- Asking questions, for example, 'Has someone your dog was close to left the home?' If the answer is a yes, it is seen as hit, if not it is just a query.
- Giving vague and generalisable statements, which people will often try to apply to themselves. Derren Brown, the illusionist, performed an amazing trick in which he provided a written cold reading to a group of people, and repeated the trick in different countries. The amazed audience gave the accuracy of the reading as applicable to them with a level up to 90 per cent. It was only afterwards that they found out that he had given exactly the same reading to everyone in the group, and the success of the readings was because the statements he had chosen seemed specific but actually were vague.
- Communicating back to the animals to give the appearance of a two-way conversation.

Animal communicators and psychics can at best be viewed as harmless souls, attempting to give solace to owners of sick, missing or deceased pets.

At worst they can be viewed as frauds, preying on the credulous and vulnerable elements of society, and charging large sums of money for the privilege.

§

## Applied kinesiology

Applied kinesiology is a diagnostic technique that aims to diagnose illness by testing muscle strength. The results of diagnosis are subjective, depending on the practitioner's assessment of strength. Applied kinesiology is sometimes used by chiropractors, but often by other health practitioners too, including vets. As applied kinesiology is hard to perform in animals, surrogate testing is often employed, in which the owner places a hand on their pet, and the practitioner then performs the muscle strength testing on the owner. A double-blinded study and literature review of applied kinesiology found results no better than chance, and also concluded that in other trials that met accepted standards there was no evidence that applied kinesiology could be relied on as a diagnostic tool.[6]

§

## Dowsing

Dowsing or divining is best known as a way of detecting hidden water using a Y-shaped twig. The ability of dowsing to detect water has been disproven scientifically. Dowsing can also be used in medical diagnosis, using a pendulum to cause biofeedback, which the practitioner uses to determine alterations to health. Dowser-healers use their findings to select remedies to correct the body's vibrational energies. There is no evidence of any basis to dowsing. See Chapter Eleven on manipulation treatments for more detail.

§

## Vega testing

Vega testing is one version of an alternative medical technique that is based on an alleged phenomenon called 'Electroacupuncture according to Voll', or EAV. Invented in 1958 by German doctor and acupuncturist Reinhold Voll, the basic EAV device was allegedly able to detect 'energy imbalances' and allergies by means of probes applied by the practitioner to the skin of the patient – so-called electrodermal testing.

Voll claimed this was as a result of the machine's ability to interrogate acupuncture points and meridians but in reality the device is simply a galvanometer – an instrument used for measuring alterations in electrical current and conductivity. Any changes detected by the machine and its successors listed below, far from being measurements of *Qi* as it suffuses the living body, are simply due to a combination of variations in the moistness of the skin, the amount of pressure applied to the probe and wishful thinking.

First developed by Voll in the form of the *Dermatron*, the EAV system was refined by one of his students in the 1970s and marketed as the more commercially successful and better known *Vegatest* device. Since then the range of these types of machine has increased enormously, with computer screens and keyboards taking the place of the original dials and switches. Examples include the Accupath 1000, Asyra, Avatar, BICOM, Bio-Tron, Biomeridian, Computron, CSA 2001, Dermatron, DiagnoMètre, Eclosion and the e-Lybra 8.[7] Some are used by veterinary surgeons to diagnose anything from allergies, organ dysfunction, poisoning, parasite burdens and various infections through to non-specific 'imbalances'. In the USA the FDA has banned the marketing, importation and use of EAV-type machines as medical devices.[8]

Some of these devices have claims that far exceed those of the original Vega machines and practitioners can be heard misleading patients and owners into believing they can work to obtain diagnoses over great distances (using 'radionic principles') or can be used to 'analyse' samples of hair or blood and then to tell the practitioner which homeopathic remedy should be employed to treat the case or even to produce the exact remedy required by imprinting the appropriate 'energy signature' on to blank sugar tablets. There is also a flourishing market in 'off the peg' curative energy signatures conveniently embedded in pendants, discs and keys and even in the form of electronic impulses ready to be downloaded to your MP3 player, PC or smartphone, from where they can be broadcast as required over a 5-mile radius by means of a mini-FM transmitter.[9]

There are no studies that have produced any form of evidence these devices do what practitioners claim. One of the few studies carried out in this field looked at a comparison of the Vegatest electrodermal testing device with the definitive skin-prick test in assessing allergies and found there was no correlation, concluding simply, 'Electrodermal testing cannot be used to diagnose environmental allergies.'[10] Another trial, this time on respiratory allergies, tested 100 volunteers using the electrodermal device DBE 204 and concluded the instrument was incapable of determining whether or not the volunteers had respiratory allergies, even less which ones.[11]

In a more informal test, in 2003 the BBC consumer affairs programme *Inside Out* carried out an undercover investigation of high street retailers using such devices to diagnose allergies in customers, to whom they would then sell the appropriate remedies. Two reporters investigated six shops between them and found none of them could agree about either which allergies were present or the remedies required in order to treat them.[12] The reader could be forgiven for thinking this was a pretty poor track record for devices that currently retail at anything from £10,000 to £15,000 or more.

Dr Stephen Barrett, author of the medical watchdog website *Quackwatch*, hits the nail on the head when he says such devices '... are used to diagnose non-existent health problems, select inappropriate treatment, and defraud insurance companies. I believe that EAV devices should be confiscated and that practitioners who use them are either delusional, dishonest, or both'.[13] Furthermore, he encourages anyone encountering a medical practitioner using such devices to report them to the relevant authorities. In the context of this book this advice should also be extended to veterinary surgeons who employ the same devices, for which there is no evidence of effectiveness, to treat animals who may be in need of science-based treatment that works.

CHAPTER THIRTEEN

# *The Rest*

THE rest of this book has discussed the major complementary and alternative medicine modalities. This chapter gives an overview of some of the more fringe CAM treatments that the authors are aware are used in animals. There is a multitude of other CAM treatments in the human field, some variants of treatments discussed here, some unrelated, and a complete discussion of these is beyond the scope of this book, and not necessarily relevant. As a general principle though, a purported medical treatment that is likely to be ineffective, quackery or outright fraudulent can be recognised by signs such as:

1. Making claims that seem too good to be true. Proponents of a particular alternative medicine often seem to claim benefits in just about any pathology. Claiming a cure for cancer is a particular red flag.
2. Using testimonials and anecdotes instead of proof. As we have seen in Chapter Five, it is easy to be misled by our own in-built biases when evaluating a treatment on uncontrolled studies and case reports.
3. Attacking mainstream medicine. Often alternative treatments are said to be incompatible with conventional medicines. Homeopathy for example, while often touted as being safe because it is complementary, is often recommended to be used instead of conventional medicines, not as well as, because the conventional medicines are said to interfere with the treatment. There also seems to be a culture or philosophy within alternative medicine that denigrates medicine, whether that is because of the naturalistic fallacy, or an increasing distrust of authority and experts.

As I edit this (December 2016), we are in a post-Trump victory, post-*Brexit* world in which analysis of Donald Trump's statements suggest that only 11 per cent of what he says is 'True or Mostly True'[1] and the UK's *Telegraph* newspaper reports Arron Banks, multimillionaire supporter of the campaign for Britain to leave the EU, attributing his campaign's success to the mantra 'facts don't work'.[2]

We have been described as living in a post-factual age, and the echo chambers of social media groups can amplify the lies, half-truths and mistaken beliefs. But it is worth bearing in mind that while we are all entitled to our own beliefs, we are not entitled to our own facts.

§

Other alternative medicine treatments that can be found on the internet claiming efficacy in animals that will not be discussed in this chapter, since they are such minority practices and have next to no evidential basis, include:

*Apitherapy (bee venom and other bee products)*
*Astrology*
*Blood irradiation therapy*
*Chromatherapy (colour therapy)*
*Colloidal silver therapy (note this has been shown to be toxic when given systemically)*
*Cupping therapy*
*Feldenkrais method (see Chapter Eleven, Tellington Touch)*
*Hypnotherapy*
*Light therapy / photonic therapy*
*Manual lymphatic drainage*
*Medical intuitive / clairvoyant*
*Past life therapy*
*Polarity therapy*
*Pranic healing*
*Psychic surgery*
*Qigong*
*Rolfing*
*Thalassotherapy*
*Urine therapy*
*Water cure therapy*

The sheer quantity and variety of these unproven treatments is in itself informative. That there are so many possible forms of alternative medicine, all claiming miraculous efficacy, all without evidence, must surely make it confusing for alternative practitioners to choose a modality. Some alternative practitioners will stick to only one form of alternative medicine, presumably believing it to be the most efficacious, while others incorporate a wide variety of alternative medicines, though how they decide that one pet would benefit from say magnet therapy while another would benefit from crystals is unclear. One UK-based alternative veterinary medicine practitioner offers the following alternative modalities according to his website: homeopathy; acupuncture; herbal treatment; aromatherapy; chiropractic treatment; nutritional advice; laser treatment; ultrasound treatment; back manipulation; Bach flowers; holistic medicine; tissue salts; holistic therapy; integrated medicine; anthroposophical medicines; natural feeding.

It does seem by searching the net that most alternative medical modalities available for people have been tried in animals, and from the comments and testimonials on these pages, that a large number of members of the public put their faith in these remedies.

§

## Energy medicine

Energy medicine involves a vague concept of energy as a life force. Vitalism puts forward the hypothesis that all living material contains something that distinguishes it from non-living material. In the pre-modern West this may be referred to as the vital spark, the soul or the spirit. In the East, the concept relates to *Qi* or *Prana*. Practitioners of energy medicine claim to be able to manipulate the flow of energy in patients in order to cure conditions or improve health. Alternative medicine that incorporate aspects of energy medicine include Traditional Chinese Medicine (TCM), homeopathy, radionics, Ayurveda, essential oil therapy, crystal therapy, magnet therapy, and emotional/spiritual/faith healing. These are discussed further in individual sections relating to those disciplines, particularly in Chapter Eleven.

§

## Auriculotherapy

Auriculotherapy involves stimulation of the external ear to diagnose and treat disease. Stimulation may involve manual pressure, needles, electrical stimulation, lasers and magnets. It can be considered a form of acupuncture (see also Chapter Eight) when needles are used. Although the practice may (or may not) have originated with the ancient Chinese performing acupuncture on the ear, modern auriculotherapy was invented in the 1950s by a neurologist called Paul Nogier, who developed the modality from the now discredited pseudoscience of phrenology. Phrenology involves mapping the skull, with different parts of the skull supposedly corresponding to emotions, thoughts and character, and Nogier extrapolated this to the ear. Since the ear looks like a curled up foetus, he projected a foetal homunculus on to the ear and used this as a basis of mapping the body. The Chinese, during the barefoot doctor era, developed Nogier's theories in accordance with TCM. A modern ear map has points for various anatomical parts such as the appendix and external genitals, as well as points related to specific conditions, such as an asthma point, a haemorrhoids point and a constipation point.

There are no logical, rational, scientific or medical reasons why auriculotherapy might be valid. There are no known anatomical pathways or physiological methods by which the external ear is connected to the body in the way suggested by auriculotherapy practitioners, and even if these were discovered, there is no reason why stimulation of these pathways would be beneficial in treatment or diagnosis of a disease. Rabischong and Terral, in the journal *Medical Acupuncture*, attempt to produce hypotheses that could explain auriculotherapy, but they note many problems with the scientific basis for the discipline, despite concluding that 'it seems no longer possible to doubt the reality of the acupoints and the efficacy of this therapy particularly for addressing pain'.[3]

Fascinatingly, and demonstrating the inherent bias in alternative medicine journals, an editor's note follows this article, responding to the assertion by the authors that there is only one truth, despite different methods of investigation. It reads, 'This viewpoint expressed by the author represents a dualistic, mechanistic Western paradigm as contrasted with the Eastern paradigm that includes the existence of many truths. Another contrast is with modern physics, which posits the existence of multiverses. We wish to present a broad range of perspectives, including those that may differ from those of many proponents of auriculotherapy.'

Regardless of known mechanism, as with all alternative medicines what is important is whether it actually works. There are some studies that appear to show a benefit. For example, one meta-analysis showed a mild improvement in smoking cessation with auriculotherapy compared to controls (although not compared to other smoking cessation strategies), though the conclusions were weak,[4] and the latest Cochrane meta-analysis on acupuncture and related treatments for smoking cessation concluded that although there are possible short-term benefits, there is no unbiased evidence that long-term effects are noted.[5] Another meta-analysis of randomised controlled clinical trials suggested some benefit of auriculotherapy in peri-operative pain,[6] but a more recent systematic review of auricular therapy for chronic pain management in adults found that because of varying results and methodological flaws in studies, it was hard to draw firm conclusions about efficacy.[7]

There is little veterinary evidence for the use of auriculotherapy. Most that exists comes from one person, Jan Still, who performed experimental studies to find the auriculodiagnostic points in dogs, including one study in which the author overdosed five healthy dogs with a laxative to induce acute diarrhoea, and then measured the electrical resistance at various points of the external pinna.[8] Still is also the only author of a veterinary clinical trial of auriculotherapy, which dates back to 1990.[9] In this study, thirty dogs with thoracolumbar disc disease of varying severity had analgesia and anti-inflammatory medication withheld and ear acupuncture was used instead. 50 per cent of dogs recovered completely and 23 per cent improved. Fifty per cent of paralysed dogs failed to recover. No controls were included, and these recovery rates appear to be similar to dogs with thoracolumbar disc disease treated conservatively (i.e. without surgery) reported in neurology texts.

In conclusion, the evidence supporting the use of auriculotherapy in veterinary medicine is very poor, and even in human medicine is weak. It is unlikely to be harmful, but should not be used as a substitute for conventional medicines, for example for pain relief.

§

## Aromatherapy

Aromatherapy uses essential oils with the aim of producing beneficial changes in mental status and physical well-being. More information on essential oils can be found in Chapter Six. Aromatherapy is often administered as a massage, but also by an aromatic bath or by vapourisation. The 2015 report by the Australian government into natural therapies[10] concluded that there is some low-quality evidence to support the use of aromatherapy in anxiety. There is only a single report of the use of aromatherapy in dogs.[11] In this study, thirty-two dogs with a history of travel-induced excitement were exposed to a lavender-based aromatherapy therapy, after initially recording baseline behaviour prior to treatment. The dogs were found to spend

270

significantly less time moving and vocalising and more time sitting and rest-ing when treated with lavender aromatherapy compared to controls.

Safety issues with aromatherapy have been raised in both animals and humans, however.

In a book written by a holistic veterinary surgeon in practice in the UK in the section on aromatherapy the author correctly counsels great caution in oral administration of essential oils in dogs.[12] Yet he goes on to advise oils are applied to dogs' skin in order that 'the energy within the oil … inter-acts with the energy in the patient to produce the healing effect'. What isn't pointed out is that one way or another much of the oil, even when diluted as instructed, will be absorbed by the patient – either ingested directly as it is licked off or absorbed directly through the skin itself, especially if it has not been possible to remove the residue by washing and particularly if the oil has been applied to the 'less hairy' regions of the skin, as advised.

Percutaneous absorption, as it is called, is even more of a problem in cats who have skins thin enough to absorb significant amounts via that route. Once this has occurred cats are then at a further disadvantage as they lack the liver enzymes required to inactivate toxins such as *terpenes* contained within oils such as tea tree oil, citronella, lavender, geranium and mint. *Terpenes*, as the name suggests, are also found in paint stripper in the form of turpentine and are, not surprisingly, toxic. The US-based National Animal Poison Control Centre (NAPCC) lists cases where dermal exposure to oils has caused toxic signs in dogs and cats while in 1998 the *Journal of Veterinary Diagnostics* described a case where three Angora cats, treated topically with oil sold as a flea treatment, developed severe neurological signs and liver damage, with one dying as a consequence.[13]

In the human literature, Posadzki et al identified seventy-one reports of adverse reactions to aromatherapy, including one fatality.[14] The authors of this report concluded that since the evidence for the use of aromatherapy was weak, and that adverse reactions were possible, the use of aromatherapy in any condition was questionable. The same is undoubtedy true of its use in animals.

§

## Low level laser therapy

The use of lasers in medicine is well established, with applications includ-ing surgery and lithotripsy. However, more recently, low-level laser therapy has been introduced as a therapeutic technique. Also known as cold laser therapy, low-level laser therapy is used to treat arthritis, soft tissue injuries and to promote wound healing. A recent systematic review and meta-analysis found evidence for benefit of low-level laser treatment in analgesia for non-specific chronic lower back pain in people, although evidence for an improvement in function was lacking.[15] Another systematic review showed that low-level laser therapy was efficacious in the treatment of neck pain.[16] However, a meta-analysis did not show benefit of this treatment for knee osteoarthritis.[17] In dogs, a prospective study showed an improved time to walking after spinal surgery following the use of low-level laser therapy.[18] The wavelength of light and intensity of the therapy is controversial, and it may be that lasers of the wrong wavelength are ineffective. Nevertheless, there is some evidence for the benefits of low-level laser therapy in the management of certain conditions.

§

## Zero balancing

Zero balancing is a mind–body therapy invented in the early 1970s. As with acupuncturists and chiropractors, zero balancers claim to relieve blockages in the body's energy flow, energy referring to the mystical life force that supposedly suffuses the body but has never been shown to exist. Zero balancing involves finger massage and traction, and some practitioners offer it for pets. Although, as with other massage therapies, dogs can seem to enjoy the experience, there is no evidence that there is any therapeutic effect beyond the benefits achieved by giving a pet a stroke and a cuddle.

§

## Crystal healing

Crystal healing or crystal therapy uses stones or crystals to attempt to effect an improvement in health. Crystals have been reportedly used historically in healing by cultures such as the Mayans, Ancient Greeks, Hawaiian islanders, Native Americans and the Chinese. In modern times, crystals seem to be used most commonly by New Age practitioners, with reference to Hindu tradition. Some crystal healing therapists select crystals by colour and place them at chakras (energy points). As with the meridians of Chinese medicine, these points have not been proven to exist and neither has the mystical energy (prana or life force) that supposedly pervades them. Examples of the purported properties of crystals include amethyst to tune the endocrine system and ward off 'geopathic stress', malachite for asthma, arthritis and epilepsy, and sunstone for gastric ulceration.

Certain crystals are, in fact, able to emit small amounts of electricity when compressed and conversely to deform when electrical charges are applied. These phenomena are known as the *piezo-electric* effect and the *inverse piezo-electric* effect respectively and are useful, for example, in quartz watches. However, there is no evidence of any benefit from crystal therapy. One interesting study took eighty volunteers and graded them for level of belief in the paranormal.[19] Half the volunteers were given a leaflet about crystals to read prior to the experiment, which gave them information about things to expect when touching the crystals, such as feeling warmth in the hands or a tingling feeling. The volunteers then meditated with either a quartz crystal or a fake glass crystal, and then were asked to report their feelings. There was no difference in the reported strength of feelings whether a fake or real crystal was used. However, there was a correlation between prior belief in the power of the crystal and reported sensations, and the group primed with information about crystals also reported stronger feelings than those not primed. It seems from this study that expectation and priming played a significant role in the reported effects of crystals in humans, i.e. any benefits of crystals are likely to be due to the placebo effect.

Pets are unlikely to benefit from expectation or priming, and so are unlikely to receive the same benefit that humans report from receiving crystal therapy. No peer-reviewed evidence benefits of crystal healing could be found on searching PubMed or the CABI abstracts. Nevertheless, amber collars are sold for pets, with claims that their electromagnetic properties and odour repel ticks and fleas, and some holistic vets advertise the use of crystals on their websites as part of their clinical practice.

One UK veterinary surgeon advises that crystals can 'allow a stabilising and healing action to occur' but worryingly, and with no supporting evidence given, advises amethyst is a 'potent pain reliever' and ruby can help in cases of arthritis. He also advocates the use of 'electro-crystal therapy', where flexible tubes of crystals suspended in salt solution are connected to an electrical power source and brought into contact with the animal's body in order to diagnose and treat 'energy imbalances'.[20]

§

## Detox

Ancient Greeks and Romans believed that many diseases were caused by *plethoras* or overabundances in the body, and recommended these be removed by sweating, bloodletting and purging (inducing vomiting and diarrhoea). While these practices have fallen out of favour, except in very specific medical conditions (e.g. bleeding to treat polycythaemia), the modern equivalent is detoxification. Detoxification aims to rid the body of usually unspecified 'toxins', although mercury and other heavy metals are sometimes implicated. It often comes in the form of a celebrity-endorsed fad diet, but also chelation therapy aimed specifically at heavy metal intoxication and colonic irrigation are also used. *Sense About Science* contacted fifteen sellers of detox products in 2009 and found that there was no agreement on the definition of detoxification, that there was little to no evidence to back up claims of benefit, and in fact that mundane things such as brushing and cleaning were being rebranded as detoxification.[21]

Although there is little evidence that detox diets are of any benefit to people, alternative websites recommend detoxification for pets, to treat such conditions as hypothyroidism, cancer, kidney and liver problems. Suggested treatments include herbs, supplements, diets and, in people, substances such as psyllium and bentonite, which, when consumed, artificially bulk the stool to such an extent the false impression is gained of accumulated waste being got rid of via the gut.[22] Searching for evidence for the use of detoxification diets and supplements is complicated by the fact that detoxification (by means of chelation) is an actual medical procedure used, for example, in the treatment of lead poisoning. As with human patients, there appears to be little to no evidence to support the use of detox in pets.

§

## Spiritual and faith healing

Spiritual, or faith healing, emotional healing and distant healing are forms of energy medicine. Spiritual and faith healing can be viewed interchangeably, although technically faith healing takes place within recognised organised religions, while spiritual healing takes place outside those organisations. Distant healing refers to therapies that attempt to heal without touch, using the power of the mind, for example with laying on of hands (of which Tellington Touch is a modern example), or by appeal to a supernatural entity or deity, such as with intercessory prayer (a prayer requesting healing of a third party). Other forms of emotional or spiritual healing such as meditation and mindfulness will not be discussed here, since they are clearly impossible for animals to take part in (although there are some claims to the contrary).

There is likely a strong placebo effect in faith healing. I attended a show by the illusionist Derren Brown, who performed a non-faith healing for the entire audience, using emotive and inspirational words and creative use of the stage lights, and around 100 people within the audience claimed to have received some moderate to dramatic improvement in a medical ailment (I was sadly unaffected, though I think I was fairly healthy anyway!)

A 2000 study showed that 82 per cent of Americans believe that prayer can cure serious illness, and 73 per cent believe that praying for others can cure illness.[23] However, from a theological point of view, intercessory prayer is problematic – is it really the case that an all-loving God should wait to be asked before intervening to provide healing? From an evidentiary point of view, controlled clinical trials have been performed with variable results. Of course, it is impossible to perform truly blinded studies that involve an omniscient, omnipotent God, so it has to be hoped that God played by the rules. Note that most studies of intercessory prayer involved prayer to a Christian God.

One controlled blinded study of the use of intercessory prayer for patients with a cancer showed a small but significant effect of prayer on spiritual and emotional well-being compared to controls.[24] Another randomised, controlled, blinded study of patients in a coronary care unit showed an improvement in a scoring system derived from their medical charts.[25] A Cochrane review of ten randomised controlled trials of intercessory prayer concluded that there was sufficient evidence to justify further research.[26] However, this review was heavily criticised for failing to report that one of the studies was dogged by accusations of fraud, with one of the researchers being subsequently jailed; another of the included trials possibly being satirical rather than serious and for mixing theological and scientific arguments.[27] The commentary on the review discusses the importance of considering a priori and a posteriori likelihoods, meaning that, as with homeopathy, if the a priori (before the study) likelihood of a positive result is very low because of lack of a plausible method, then any a posteriori (after the study) positive results should be treated with caution. Critics stated that this review is not up to the usual standard of Cochrane reviews and have requested it be withdrawn.

Homeopathy is also sold in a form of distant healing. Benveniste, controversial proponent of the theory that water has a memory, also claimed that memory could be transmitted by telephone line. Websites offering distant homeopathy as a service are easily discovered with a web search. One company offers an emergency service distant homeopathy service for emergency treatment for pets in hospital or at home (although only offers the emergency service during weekdays 9am–6pm). It claims it has developed a proprietary system of distant healing based on quantum physics and that it is effective and life-saving. It offers only client testimonials in support of these claims.[28]

A holistic vet describes his experience healing a behavioural problem in a rescue dog using distant Reiki. He connected with the dog and found that his 'energy field was all blown out and scattered'. The various adjustments he made to the dog's energy field included surrounding him with love and colour, directing healing energy under his feet to connect him with the earth, and opened a connection between the owner's heart centre and the dog's centre.[29]

More alarmingly, a non-veterinary healer describes her distant healing of a dog that was not eating or drinking. Rather than seeking veterinary attention, the owner asked the healer to help. She 'checked in on the dog intuitively and sent it distant healing'. Fortunately the dog recovered.[30] Of course, most non-veterinary alternative practitioners put disclaimers on their websites regarding them not replacing veterinary treatment, but this is a classic example of how a probably harmless treatment could nevertheless cause harm due to a delay in seeking effective veterinary treatment.

A systematic review of randomised trials of distant healing concluded that methodologic problems meant that firm conclusions about distant healing could not be drawn, but the number of positive results suggested that it was worthy of further study.[31] However, a follow-up systematic review by one of the same authors taking into account new rigorous studies performed, concluded that the weight of evidence had shifted to distant healing being no more effective than placebo.[32]

Distant healing is likely harmless, but is implausible in the extreme. A cynic may even feel that distant healing is an exercise in making money from clients unable or unwilling to travel to a clinic.

§

## Magnets

Ruminants such as cows can swallow sharp metallic objects that perforate the stomach and lead to an infection around the heart called traumatic pericarditis. Magnets fed to ruminants can trap these objects and prevent them causing damage. Magnets also have a role in diagnostics, in the form of magnetic resonance imaging.

However, other therapeutic claims for magnets are often made. It is easy to find online (and even in some vet practices) magnetic health products in the form for example of collars that claim to help with such conditions as osteoarthritis and parasite prevention. Although it is possible to find studies performed by the companies selling the products that appear to show dramatic effect, there are few peer-reviewed studies. In one study published in *Bioelectromagnetics*, the journal of the Bioelectromagnetics Society a weak effect was found when using a powerful magnetic field to assist the healing in an experimental model of canine osteoarthritis.[33] However, the most important objective results did not reach statistical significance, and furthermore the magnetic field was greatly more powerful than the strength of magnets commonly sold for therapeutic purposes. A study of experimentally induced tendon injuries in rabbits seemed to show an improved in vitro tendon strength after treatment with fibroblast injection and magnet therapy, though it is not clear how much of the improvement was due to the fibroblasts and how much to the magnets.[34] A controlled study of healing in goats with experimentally induced fractures using magnets included in the plaster cast suggested subjectively improved healing.[35] It should be noted that all three of these studies involved inducing injuries in animals in order to assess the effects of a dubious therapeutic modality on healing, and the ethics of this must be considered questionable. Another study to assess the claims that magnetic blankets can improve blood flow and reduce muscular tension and tenderness showed no significant effect on skin temperature, pain thresholds, muscle blood flow or behaviour in healthy horses.[36] Shafford et al, after a study into the use of pulsed electro-magnetic field for analgesia in dogs that had undergone ovariohysterectomy, concluded there was no clear benefit to the treatment.[37]

In the human field, a systematic review of the use of magnets in pain relief concluded that the evidence did not support the therapeutic use of magnets for analgesia, although noted that clinically important effects in the treatment of osteoarthritis could not be ruled out and might warrant further investigation.[38]

In conclusion, any effects of magnets at the strengths typically employed therapeutically are likely to be weak or non-existent, and with current evidence magnets should not be relied upon to provide effective pain relief.

§

## Ozone therapy

Ozone is a form of oxygen, with a molecule comprising three oxygen atoms instead of the usual two, and is therefore a more powerful oxidant than the two-atom form of oxygen. Ozone has antimicrobial properties, and it is also thought to stimulate circulation and the immune response.[39] It has been suggested it may be useful in a wide range of medical and dental treatments. However, it has the potential to be toxic, and increased ozone levels in the air have been associated with increased levels of asthma.[40] The FDA states: 'Ozone is a toxic gas with no known useful medical application in specific, adjunctive, or preventive therapy. In order for ozone to be effective as a germicide, it must be present in a concentration far greater than that which can be safely tolerated by man and animals.'[41]

Ozone is dissolved in a liquid and then injected intravenously or as an enema by alternative practitioners. It can also be injected into body cavities, joints and muscles, and even used to inflate the rectum or vagina. In some cases, blood is taken out of the body and exposed to ozone before being transfused back in.

Ozone has been shown to have antimicrobial effects in vitro,[42] and to inhibit the growth of cancer cells in vitro.[43] Ozone therapy also reduced levels of oxidative stress in a rat model of ischaemia/reperfusion, although not by as much as simple cooling.[44] There is also evidence that ozone therapy reduces fibrosis of the liver due to biliary obstruction,[45] and speeds facial nerve regeneration,[46] both studies being performed in rats.

However, killing cancer cells and bacteria in a test tube or a rat is only an initial basis for further research. Lots of things kill cancer cells and bacteria, including bleach and boiling. In vivo research is necessary to assess whether a treatment is effective and safe in real situations.

There are a few good quality systematic reviews of ozone therapy. One systematic review suggested that ozone therapy was beneficial for lower back pain, but noted there were no placebo-controlled trials and that multiple concurrent therapies and lack of a precise diagnosis limited the power of the study to assess an effect.[47] A systematic review of the effectiveness and cost-effectiveness of ozone for the treatment of dental caries concluded that 'the current evidence base for HealOzone is insufficient to conclude that it is a cost-effective addition to the management and treatment of occlusal and root caries'.[48] A Cochrane review of ozone therapy for the treatment of foot ulcers in diabetes mellitus concluded that there was insufficient evidence to draw firm conclusions.[49] A systematic review in dentistry concluded that promising in vitro findings had not been replicated in vivo.[50] However, some single controlled studies show some promise. For example, a controlled study of ozone therapy (given by rectal insufflation) as an adjunctive treatment in coronary artery disease showed improved haemostatic and oxidative stress indices. No side effects were observed.[51] A case series showed some promise of rectal ozone therapy improving the symptoms of radiation-induced haemorrhagic proctitis.[52]

Veterinary conditions for which ozone therapy have been recommended include cancer, autoimmune disease and skin wounds, as well as supposedly potentiating homeopathy, acupuncture and chiropractic.[53] A training course in ozone therapy for vets is offered by the American Academy of Ozonotherapy. Veterinary research on ozone therapy is sparse. One study appeared to show an improvement in outcomes of sheep with retained placentae or after manual obstetric interventions using intrauterine ozone therapy.[54] Intrarectal ozone has been suggested to be as effective a pain relief as meloxicam in one controlled study.[55] Percutaneous ozone administration appeared to shrink herniated intervertebral discs in dogs, although as this was a small uncontrolled study, the natural progression of the condition may have been responsible for this effect.[56]

Is ozone therapy safe? Generally, the treatment appears safe,[57] if somewhat unpleasant (although it is said by proponents to be non-invasive, I'm not sure I would apply that term to rectal insufflation). Risks include fatality due to gas embolisation[58] and meteorism – a gassy swelling of the abdomen.[59] Although meteorism is reported as transient, the anatomy of dogs leaves them prone to the fatal gastric dilatation volvulus syndrome when gas accumulates in the stomach, and while there are no reports of this associated with ozone therapy, it must be at least a theoretical risk.

In conclusion, ozone therapy appears to be another of those frustrating alternative therapies that has biological plausibility, but is associated with some (probably small) risk, and for which evidence for clinical applications remains uncertain and/or contradictory. Until further evidence is provided, the use of ozone therapy must be considered experimental.

§

# Hopi ear candling

Ear candles, or 'cones' are made from a hollow tube of cloth that is impregnated with waxes and often fragrant materials such as honey and herbs, sealed at one end and open at the other. Practitioners advocate inserting the narrow end into the ear canal and then lighting the wider, open end while it is held in place for up to ten minutes and allowed to burn down. It is claimed this can remove wax and debris from the ear canal as well as having other, more widespread effects, from reducing stress and anxiety to relieving colds, flu and sinusitis to improving asthma and even 'cleansing' the lymphatic system.

To demonstrate the effectiveness of the technique, users will cut open used candles along their length to display what they claim is ear wax inside, drawn out by the candle. But burning candles while they are not in contact with the body results in the same effect, making it clear the debris is simply accumulations of melted and partly burned wax from the candle itself, which conveniently resembles ear wax in both colour and consistency.

Even a brief search of the literature available from practitioners reveals a wide range of contradictions in the world of ear candling. Many claim the flame has the effect of creating a vacuum along the tube, allowing ear wax to be sucked out, using the compelling analogy of a chimney venting noxious soot and smoke away. Others state with conviction no sucking is involved and in fact the candles merely 'stimulate' the ear to get rid of the wax itself. Yet others claim the idea these candles remove wax is a complete myth and they are supposed only to relax the user.

Some advocates insist protective plates of card or tinfoil are used in order to prevent injury from dripping wax and hot ash while others are quite indignant that no wax ever drips from these devices and there is no risk. Some prefer the use of a specific brand of candle (although which one varies from person to person) while others stress the supposed origin of the practice among the Hopi people of North America and maintain the only effective candles are the ones obtained direct 'from the reservation'.

Even the idea these candles are an ancient practice used by the Hopi is hotly contested, not least by the Hopi themselves, who seem justifiably embarrassed at their fabricated and spurious connection with this dubious therapy and have taken steps to have their tribal name removed from marketing material.

The American Academy of Otolaryngology–Head and Neck Surgery (AAO-HNS) tells us, 'There are no controlled studies or other scientific evidence that support the safety and effectiveness of these devices for any of the purported claims or intended uses …'[60] Only one study seems to have been published and, after taking measurements, its authors concluded that no vacuum was produced and no ear wax removed by the candles.[61] In addition they noted in some cases wax was actually deposited by the candles into the ear canal, rather defeating the object. They also surveyed 122 otolaryngologists and identified twenty-one injuries to the ears of patients who had used ear candles. Their final conclusion: 'Ear candles have no benefit in the management of cerumen [ear wax] and may result in serious injury.'

Given the implausibility and risks of this technique you may be surprised to learn that some advocate its use in animals, particularly dogs. There are websites and videos available online describing how to perform ear candling on pets and extolling its usefulness in ear infections and other conditions. It is claimed also to relax stressed animals. Once again the false argument is made that it must work because animals don't experience the placebo effect (see Chapter Five). No proper studies have been performed to investigate the effects of ear candling in dogs or any other non-human species.

Ear infections in dogs can be serious and painful and ear candling will have no benefit in such cases. Indeed, even if you manage to avoid causing direct injury by burning or hot wax, it is likely that simply by inserting a candle into the infected, inflamed ear canal of a dog you will make things worse by causing greater damage and pushing debris further down into the ear canal, towards the eardrum. There are no conceivable circumstances that would warrant the use of this technique in animals.

§

## The treatment of pyometra

Pyometra literally means 'pus in the womb' and is a condition commonly seen by veterinary surgeons in practice, usually affecting bitches. Although the clinical signs are as a result of infection, the underlying problem is a hormonal one that affects the uterus in such a way as to predispose it to invasion by harmful bacteria. Once established, however, the infection quickly leads to serious illness as a result of sepsis and toxic shock and causes damage to other organs of the body, particularly the kidneys. The condition is serious and life-threatening and treatment options are limited.

Up to fairly recently the only option was to surgically remove the uterus and ovaries in a procedure known as ovaro-hysterectomy (or spaying) while giving the appropriate supportive treatment such as intravenous fluid therapy, antibiotics and anti-inflammatory and pain-relieving medication. While this is still the preferred means of treatment some veterinary surgeons will nowadays occasionally opt for an intensive medical regime instead, involving hormonal and antibacterial treatments, which can resolve the signs of pyometra if managed carefully, often in a hospital environment. This more conservative treatment is carried out in the knowledge there are risks, firstly of treatment failure or secondly of the problem resurfacing later, at the time of the next season, or 'heat'. It can also be a painful experience for the bitch depending on the drugs used, and suitable analgesia will be required.

So it was particularly distressing to discover the advice, from certain quarters of the alternative medical community, that surgery for pyometra can not only be avoided but is actually counter-productive. A variety of treatments are recommended by CAVM practitioners for pyometra including the homeopathic remedies aconite, sepia, Nux Vomica (strychnine), arsenic and rescue remedy; herbal remedies and other supplements including turmeric, vitamin C, sodium bicarbonate and cider vinegar.

One website tells us surgery is 'never curative' and will only result in so-called suppression or bottling up of the infection,[62] while another informs readers that once pyometra is confirmed and there is vomiting, inappetence, depression, excess thirst, a copious purulent vaginal discharge and convincing signs on X-ray and blood count, then it is time for surgery, *or* urgent treatment with so-called herbal antibiotics.[63] In fact no responsible veterinary surgeon would suggest even real antibiotics on their own to treat this condition. While they are helpful when stabilising a patient prior to surgery, they are unlikely to effect a cure as they will make little or no impression on the volumes of pus present in the reproductive tracts of affected bitches.

In fairness, some sources with an alternative bent will offer good advice along the lines that this condition should be seen by a veterinary surgeon. But such advice is often undermined by the suggestion that alternative remedies can be tried initially and only when the affected bitch becomes weak, thin, off her food or the discharge becomes particularly offensive should she be taken to the vet. What isn't mentioned is that by this time she is likely to be so weak from shock, dehydration and multiple organ damage as to make surgery even more risky than it would have been in the first place. There is also a risk in delaying treatment that the uterus could burst, resulting in the pus escaping directly into the abdomen itself, something that will have profound long-term consequences including adhesions and damage to other organs even if the bitch is fortunate enough to survive the surgery.

Such advice is, to put it mildly, both irresponsible and highly dangerous. Claims of so-called miracle cures of pyometras should be taken with an extremely large pinch of salt and in light of all that is written in the chapters in the first part of this book – did the patient actually have pyometra in the first place or was it a misdiagnosis by a vet or self-diagnosis by the owner;

were any other conventional treatments being given concurrently with the alternative remedies that we are not being told about for reasons of 'clarity', just how long did the alleged improvement last? Ask yourself all these questions carefully and with an open mind, because the chances of a bitch surviving a pyometra without conventional medical and surgical treatment and support are vanishingly small.

It bears repeating that any claims CAVM alone can treat pyometra in a bitch are irresponsible and dangerous, and likely to put animal lives at risk by delaying effective treatment. If you have an unspayed bitch (or, occasionally cat) who is showing any of the signs above (even if there is no actual discharge) then you should contact a veterinary surgeon about her as a matter of urgency.

# *Conclusion*

'Everybody wants to believe it, that's what makes it so clever, a lie that's preferable to the truth.'

*Sherlock Holmes, to Dr Watson*

As 2016 draws to a close and this book nears completion we learn the Oxford Dictionary has just announced its international word of the year. That word is 'post-truth', an adjective defined as 'relating to or denoting circumstances in which objective facts are less influential in shaping public opinion than appeals to emotion and personal belief'. The use of the word has spiked this year 'in the context of the EU referendum in the United Kingdom and the presidential election in the United States'.[1]

There are signs we have entered a 'post-truth' era not only in politics, but in science and medicine too where it seems, perversely, that the support of evidence or expert opinion is for some more a reason to reject than to accept ideas. Conversely it appears if a message, no matter how far-fetched, is repeated often enough and with sufficient heart-warming spin (or perhaps written in very large letters on the side of a bus[2]) there is no limit to what will be believed. Sentiment threatens to triumph over reason, charisma over careful consideration.

One of the leading campaigners in favour of *Brexit* (Britain's exit from the EU), Michael Gove MP, captured the mood perfectly. When faced with informed opinion that contradicted his view he responded, most memorably, 'I think people in this country have had enough of experts.'[3]

And the same too can be said for purveyors of CAVM, who operate in a murky world of nods and winks, slippery half-truths and insinuations, twisted facts and groundless fears, all wrapped up with a little pop-science and presented with a smiling countenance. Inconvenient counter-arguments are dismissed as conspiracy and those presenting them denigrated as stooges of the pharmaceutical industry. Poor-quality evidence is presented time and again until the whole thing becomes, in the words of Sherlock Holmes, 'a lie that is preferable to the truth'.[4] Recall the story of Bedford, where the role of anti-cancer drugs was left out of the account of a homeopathic 'cure for cancer', and the list of 800 papers from the BAHVS, which claimed to prove the effectiveness of homeopathy but did nothing of the sort; think back to the scaremongering of the anti-vaccination and raw food lobbies. None of that was the truth, but it is what many worried, vulnerable people are desperate to believe.

When considering Complementary and Alternative Veterinary Medicine it is vital to get at the facts behind the myths and the 'post-truth' rhetoric before entrusting ourselves and our animals to its care. And this includes both the promises and dire warnings from those who profit by it.

Let's have a look at those promises and warnings by reviewing some of the themes we've covered so far and a few new ones as well, to discover just how they stand up to scrutiny.

## Things CAVM practitioners would like us to believe are true:

### *Myth 1 – CAVM can help fight the overuse of antibiotics*

Wrong! The answer to the overuse of antibiotics is to use fewer antibiotics, not to use an ineffective alternative therapy instead.

There are serious and legitimate concerns over increasing numbers of bacteria resistant to common antibiotics, and the overuse of drugs generally. These are important issues that are being addressed, but the solution will lie in scientific study, judicious use and education of both practitioner and patient about when pharmacological treatment is indicated and when it isn't. We should all be doing our best to reduce the unnecessary use of drugs and prepare to be critical if they are used in questionable situations. But some CAVM practitioners go beyond legitimate criticism and display a blanket disdain for science-based drugs of almost any kind, regardless of merit.

### *Myth 2 – CAVM is good for animal welfare*

Wrong! Animal welfare is not served by substituting effective medicines with ineffective ones.

There is little argument that a lot can be done in farming to enhance welfare and reduce disease rates by lowering stocking densities, improving animal housing and opting for slower growth rates and lower milk yields, thus reducing production pressures on livestock. Unfortunately some farming systems encourage an over-reliance on drugs as a quick fix – a sticking plaster as it were, to make up for shortcomings in animal management and husbandry. Giving antibiotics to a batch of calves with pneumonia, for instance, may seem easier in the short-term than going to the trouble and expense of altering calf sheds to provide better ventilation.

But some, particularly organic guidelines, go too far and not only encourage sensible improvements in husbandry but promote homeopathy as a viable alternative to science-based medicine as well. As we have seen, the use of homeopathy in preference to science-based medicine is a legal requirement for such systems in the EU.

This raises serious ethical and welfare questions and undermines improvements made elsewhere, as organic farmers are put under pressure to delay the administration of essential, science-based medication for fear of draconian and costly milk and meat withdrawal times while at the same time they are falsely reassured that homeopathy will do the job just as well.

### *Myth 3 – CAVM practitioners are more compassionate and empathic*

Wrong! If your veterinary surgeon appears uncaring or distant that's not because they have failed to comprehend CAVM, it's because they're not doing their job properly.

Veterinary surgeons and animal owners are all different, and in veterinary practice it can be difficult to cater for every need. Some caregivers will want everything possible done for an animal patient, regardless of cost and inconvenience, others will resist even the most basic forms of treatment, opting for purely palliative care, symptomatic treatment or even euthanasia at an early stage in the development of an illness. Who is to say which approach is better, but the answer is most certainly not to condemn any disagreement as a fault of 'conventional medicine', at worst it is an incompatibility between a vet and an owner.

If your vet or doctor isn't treating you with respect or giving you the time you need or seems to be too interventionist, or not interventionist enough, the answer is to do something about it – speak to your vet, tell them of your concerns and try to get things changed. If all else fails, move to a different veterinary practice. But don't assume things will be any better with a practitioner of CAVM.

On the other hand, just because someone seems pleasant and listens and treats you in the way you want to be treated doesn't mean they are a good veterinary surgeon. They may well be, but it is by no means guaranteed; sometimes the good practitioner is the one who explains the difficult things, the truth you may not want to believe. Vets can't be all things to all people all of the time but most of us are good people and have the best interests of owner and animal at heart.

## *Myth 4 – CAVM practitioners are 'holistic'*

Wrong! All good vets are 'holistic' and treat the whole animal.

Claims from practitioners of CAVM to have a monopoly on 'holistic' treatment are bogus. No veterinary surgeon, no matter how specialised, will ever confine themselves to treating just one part of an animal – a single organ or an isolated injury – to the exclusion of the rest. To do so would be absurd and extremely difficult. It is the whole animal that is ill, not just one part of it. So a cat with an overactive thyroid gland will not only receive treatment to reduce thyroid activity but also medication to support the heart, and nutrition to counteract weight loss while further controlling the production of thyroid hormone. Any later changes in health status will always be viewed in light of this pre-existing condition, so regular health checks and the monitoring of organs such as heart and kidney will be carried out, or at least discussed with the owner. A cow with mastitis won't just get a course of antibiotics, a good vet will also consider the incidence in the herd and look at any predisposing factors that might help reduce the numbers of future cases. A lame dog will not only have the affected leg thoroughly examined but everything else as well to rule out the possibility of a more generalised problem such as arthritis, infection, spinal disease, growth or nutritional problems. A good vet will always consider age, weight, breed, levels of exercise, diet and lifestyle in any diagnosis.

When a practitioner of CAVM says they are 'holistic' this is often code for the claim they treat things that only they are able to see – the *subluxation* of the chiropractor, the *vital force* of the homeopath or the acupuncturist's *Qi*. None of these actually exist and claiming to treat them doesn't mean one is practising holistically. In many ways CAVM practitioners are less 'holistic' than their conventional colleagues. Is it holistic to believe for instance, as *straight* chiropractors do, that 95 per cent of diseases originate from one cause only, the VSL; is making a diagnosis by dowsing or by claiming to detect the *biofield* over vast distances really treating the whole animal?

### *Myth 5 – CAVM is no different from plenty of other medical practices that have limited scientific support*

Wrong! Much of CAVM isn't only non-evidence-based, it is non-rational.

It is common to hear proponents of CAVM claim (incorrectly[5]) that hardly any medical or surgical interventions have a proper evidence base to support them. But even if such a claim were true would this mean CAVM was no different from other medical treatments that haven't been subject to the 'gold-standard' double-blind placebo-controlled trial (DBPCT)? The answer is a resounding 'NO!'

As we saw in Chapter Three, many mainstream treatments are so obviously effective there has never been a requirement to perform a DBPCT to verify their use. The same cannot be said for CAVM interventions; although practitioners claim consistent and unmistakable results in the consulting room, this effect vanishes when subject to even the most basic of independent analyses.

A distinction must be made between what might be called 'plausible' forms of CAVM, such as Western herbal medicine including the use of supplements and nutraceuticals, and 'implausible' forms, such as acupuncture, homeopathy, *straight* chiropractic and radionics. 'Plausible' CAVM claims a conventional mode of action in the same way mainstream pharmaceuticals work – interaction between molecules, cell-membrane-bound receptors and so on. To that extent it could be said the jury is still out, and despite a deal of shaky evidence for many of the claims, getting the occasional positive result in trials isn't beyond the bounds of possibility (although, of course, at that point whatever compound was being tested would no longer be alternative or complementary, but simply medicine).

The problem comes with the 'implausible' forms of CAVM that claim mechanisms of action that defy all attempts at rational, scientific explanation (quantum mechanics included). Putting themselves outside the purview of science in this way means these particular types of CAVM have effectively renounced the real world. They are not only non-science-based, they are non-rational and are thus in an altogether different league from so far unproven medical practices or even 'plausible' forms of CAVM.

Incidentally, this exposes a vulnerability in the otherwise laudable aims of Evidence-Based Veterinary Medicine (EBVM) where every treatment under scrutiny is given a level playing field from the outset, regardless of any *a priori* merit or plausibility. Faith-healing and homeopathy are, in the first instance, treated with the same seriousness as antibiotic and hormone therapies regardless of the fact the former have no basis in the real world and rely only on mystical explanations. Negative or inconclusive trials are met with calls for further research rather than a realisation that in some cases enough is enough and further testing would be a waste of resources.[6]

## *Myth 6 – CAVM is safe*

Wrong! As we saw in Chapter Four, if a treatment has no 'side effects' it can have no actual effects; and when CAVM is used instead of real medicine it is dangerous.

Any real drug will have an effect on the body, that is how it works. Some of those effects are desirable, others less so. Which is which depends on what the aims of treatment are, the dose given and the constitution of the patient, including the existence of concurrent problems. In this way science-based medicines are given only after careful consideration of the risks and benefits. There is no such thing as a 'side effect', there are only 'effects' that may be more or less desirable in different circumstances. Only in the fantasy world of CAVM belief is it possible to have treatments that have powerful beneficial effects yet are utterly safe. This is nothing more or less than a pipe dream, life just isn't that simple.

If a vaccine has poor efficacy or is causing unacceptable adverse reactions, or a drug seems to be causing undesirable effects the answer for the manufacturer is to do more research and improve the vaccine, and for the practitioner it is to have a think, consult a textbook or other expert opinion and come up with an alternative drug, not to switch to ineffective nosodes or homeopathic remedies instead.

With prescription drugs comes accountability. Every drug on the market has been through rigorous laboratory tests and clinical trials both before and after being put on the market. Once a drug is launched this continues, with practitioners, both veterinary and human medical, obliged to report any suspected adverse reactions to the authorities so a database can be built up and guidelines for use modified. If there are a lot of similar reactions for the same product then questions will be asked and in some cases a drug may be withdrawn from the market.

No such system exists in the world of CAVM. If there was, for instance, a homeopathic equivalent of Thalidomide, we'd never hear about it.

This one-sided scaremongering by proponents of both CAM and CAVM over both expert opinion and the risks of science-based medicines is lampooned in an article in the UK's *Telegraph* newspaper that highlights the disturbing fact that almost every commercial airliner that crashed had a qualified pilot at the controls. This is shocking, the article continues, clearly there is a major association between qualified pilots and fatal airline crashes.[7] The logic is inescapable, but do we hear about groups of angry protestors campaigning to have qualified pilots banned and replaced with aircrew trained in complementary and alternative piloting skills? Clearly not. The answer to problems with air traffic safety is to improve aircraft design and piloting skills; banning pilots would be ridiculous. By the same token, neither should we replace proven, tried and tested medicines with ineffective and largely unregulated complementary and alternative ones.

### Myth 7 – CAVM is natural; drugs, pet foods and vaccines contain chemicals

Wrong! Everything contains 'chemicals', including CAVM remedies themselves.

As we have seen this 'nature is best' argument is a fallacy. In reality everything around us in nature – the air we breathe, the food we eat – is made of 'chemicals'. There is nothing inherently bad about 'chemicals', the term is entirely neutral, but those opposed to modern medicines and commercial pet foods will try to convince us there is by rattling off lists of ingredients in a way that suggests because some of them are described using long, unfamiliar terms they must be bad for us. But again, the answer here is not to fall for the line that because something has a scientific-sounding name it must therefore be 'artificial' and bad for us and our animals.

This aversion has even been given its own name, chemophobia, a blanket irrational fear of chemicals for some and a powerful marketing tool for others. It is epitomised in the mantras of various self-appointed holistic food gurus such as, 'If you can't pronounce it, don't eat it,' and, 'There is just no acceptable level of any chemical to ingest, ever.'[8]

The specious nature of this argument is exposed as nothing more than scaremongering when we consider for example the seeds, or pseudo-grains, of the plant *Chenopodium quinoa*, a member of the family Amaranthaceae and pretty unpronounceable by any standards. They are further damned since they also contain chemicals, a coating of bitter-tasting *saponins*, toxic glycosides that destroy blood cells, are used as laundry detergents[9] and which, unless removed by processing, produce quantities of soapy foam when boiled.[10] So, being both unpronounceable and containing toxic chemicals one might expect these tiny seeds to be reviled by food gurus and chemo-phobics everywhere. Yet *Quinoa* ranks among the latest, most fashionable 'superfoods' around today, lauded as 'one of the healthiest and most nutri-tious foods on the planet'[11] and dubbed the 'miracle grain of the Andes'. So popular has Quinoa become that demand from affluent consumers in the developed world has increased to the point where mass cultivation is now causing great hardship for indigenous peoples in its region of origin, the South Americas, as land that once produced a wide diversity of crops is now turned over to stark monoculture and locals can no longer afford to buy what was once a nutritious and easily accessible staple food.[12]

It is possible to make anything sound bad if is described using suffi-ciently loaded terms. The secretion from modified mammalian sweat glands, squeezed out and collected in bottles – sounds disgusting, but you put it on your cornflakes every morning; it's just another way of describing milk. And what about taking a big bite from a juicy reproductive organ – anyone who has ever eaten an apple has done this! A well-informed campaign group has recently highlighted the fact that tap water contains up to $10^6$ parts per million of the industrial solvent *dihydrogen monoxide* (DHMO), a chemical known to be associated with malignant cancers and which is responsible for the deaths of thousands of people every year. Hundreds of members of the public have signed petitions to have it banned and it is even possible to buy a 'Ban DHMO' T-shirt to help promote the cause.[13] Does this mean we should be refusing to drink tap water until DHMO is removed, or lobbying the authorities to take action? No, it turns out DHMO is another name for $H2O$ – *dihydrogen monoxide* is ordinary water and the DHMO website is an entertaining and enlightening spoof.

The answer to concerns over 'chemicals' is don't get mad, get smart and think for yourself. Find out more about science and about what these sub-stances are first, before joining vociferous, agenda-driven lobby groups just because their names sound strange or worrying.

### *Myth 8 – CAVM has plenty of scientific evidence to back up its claims*

Wrong! The only evidence presented in favour of CAVM is weak and unconvincing.

Proponents of CAVM and homeopathy in particular claim there are hundreds, even thousands, of papers, trials and studies that support their position. But when this so-called evidence is examined closely it is always, every single time, found to be deficient. Studies are discovered to be weak, underpowered or published in journals with a vested interest, or they don't give the results CAVM proponents pretend they do. Studies whose results are inconclusive or call for further research are regarded by believers, not as evidence of no effect, but as positive proof.

The American Institute of Homeopathy has recently produced a list of 6,000 papers it claims supports homeopathy.[14] In a previous chapter we considered a similar list of 800 papers presented by the British Association of Homeopathic Veterinary Surgeons. This is an astronomical number of studies, far more than have been carried out in support of any other single medical intervention. Think about it – homeopathy is supposedly entirely safe and simple – if the supporting evidence for effectiveness really was that overwhelming then no conspiracy could possibly be big or sophisticated enough to keep it quiet and every single practitioner of any form of medicine on the planet would be using it almost exclusively, not just a tiny minority of homeopaths.

The only conclusion, after reading some of the great lists of papers published on various pro-CAVM websites, is either the people who posted the lists haven't read them themselves, or they are hoping that no one else will, because they most certainly do not show what is claimed. And as for anecdotes – stories of miracle cures – anyone who has read this far will know why, although they are powerful illustrations, they cannot be used as proof for the effectiveness of anything as unlikely as CAVM. No matter how many of them you read or how entertaining, surprising or moving they are, the plural of anecdote isn't data.

§

The section above has dealt with the myths those marketing CAVM would like us to believe. So far in this book we have discussed a number of other facts that people who make a living from CAVM find uncomfortable and would like us to overlook in favour of propaganda and personal preference. Let us look at a summary – the things we actually know to be true.

## Things CAVM practitioners would prefer us not to know:

Fact 1 – In the past, treatments now known to be ineffective were accepted as mainstream. Large numbers of people believing a treatment works doesn't mean it does.

Fact 2 – There are well understood reasons why intelligent, otherwise rational, people can believe a treatment is effective when it isn't.

Fact 3 – Animals will recover from chronic, serious, even apparently life-threatening injuries and diseases in the most unlikely cases, with minimal or no treatment.

Fact 4 – With the exception of Western herbal medicine, no form of complementary and alternative veterinary medicine has a mechanism of action or effectiveness that has been externally validated. The active ingredients in Western herbal medicines act in the same way as conventional drugs but are in a much cruder form with variable concentrations and unreliable, occasionally harmful effects.

Fact 5 – CAVM can cause harm to animals – to patients either directly or by delaying or preventing effective treatment, and to experimental animals used to test treatments already known to be ineffective. Both authors of this book were surprised to discover the level of vivisection employed during laboratory studies into CAM and CAVM.

Fact 6 – The various CAVM treatments are mutually incompatible. Herbal remedies fall in strength with dilution while homeopathic remedies supposedly get stronger; chiropractors believe diseases are caused by misalignment of the spinal column; homeopaths believe a cure can be achieved by restoring the balance of the all-pervasive *vital essence*; acupuncturists believe disease is caused by blockages in the flow of *Qi* that can be relieved by needling, while radionics practitioners prefer to believe diseases can be managed by manipulating electro-magnetic waves given off by patients who don't even have to be on the same continent to effect a diagnosis and treatment.

Yet despite this many CAVM practitioners happily embrace multiple practices, oblivious to the obvious contradictions.

§

Having got thus far the reader should now appreciate there is nothing CAVM claims that cannot easily be explained by ordinary means. When this is considered alongside the lack of regulation and accountability accompanying the use of CAVM one thing becomes crystal clear, CAVM is an unnecessary embellishment, a lucrative exercise in smoke and mirrors. While on occasion appearing to offer hope and consolation to owners, these are mere illusions;

CAVM brings no benefit to the individual animal, its net effect is harmful and it has no place in the treatment of animals.

And if anyone ever tries to convince you of the idea that Complementary and Alternative Medicine must work because it is supposedly effective in animals, the authors would sincerely hope you are now sufficiently informed to put them right. You might even consider buying them a copy of this book!

# References

## Preface

Boissel, J. P., Cucherat, M., Haugh, M. and Gauthier, E. (1996) 'Critical literature review on the effectiveness of homoeopathy: overview of data from homoeopathic medicine trials', In: *Homoeopathy Medicine Research Group: report to the European Commission Directorate General XII: science, research and development*, Brussels, pp. 195–210.

Kleijnen, J., Knipschild, P. and ter Riet, G. (1991) 'Clinical trials of homoeopathy', *British Medical Journal*, vol. 9, no. 302, pp. 316–323.

Linde, K. et al (1997) 'Are the clinical effects of homoeopathy placebo effects? A meta-analysis of placebo-controlled trials', *Lancet*, vol. 350, no. 9081, pp. 834–843.

Linde, K. and Jonas, W. (2005) 'Are the clinical effects of homoeopathy placebo effects?', *Lancet*, vol. 366, no. 9503, pp. 2081–2082.

§

## Chapter One – What Is Complementary and Alternative Veterinary Medicine?

01] American Veterinary Association (AVMA), *Guidelines for Complementary and Alternative Veterinary Medicine* [Online]. Available at https://www.avma.org/About/Governance/Documents/2014W_2013W_Resolution3_Attch2.pdf (Accessed 24 October 2015).

02] British Small Animal Veterinary Association (BSAVA) (2013) *Position Statement: Complementary and alternative therapies* [Online]. Available at https://www.bsava.com/Resources/Veterinary-resources/Position-statements/Complementary-therapies

03] Barnes, P. M., Powell-Griner, E., McFann, K., and Nahin, R. L. (2004) 'Complementary and Alternative Medicine Use Among Adults: United States, 2002', *Advance Data From Vital and Health Statistics*, no. 343, p. 1 [Online].

Available at https://nccih.nih.gov/sites/nccam.nih.gov/files/news/camstats/2002/report.pdf (Accessed 4 April 2017).

04] House of Lords Science and Technology Select Committee (2000) *6th Report of Session 1999–2000 – Complementary and Alternative Medicine* [Online]. Available at www.publications.parliament.uk/pa/ld199900/ldselect/ldsctech/123/12301. htm (Accessed 10 September 2016).

05] Kaptchuk, T. J and Eisenberg, D. M (2005) 'A Taxonomy of Unconventional Healing Practices' in Lee-Treweek, G., Heller, T., Spurr, S., MacQueen, H. and Katz, J. (eds) *Perspectives on Complementary Medicine: A Reader*, Abingdon, Routledge, Taylor and Francis/Milton Keynes, The Open University, p. 9.

06] Cormack, J. R. (1851) 'Miscellaneous Intelligence', *London Journal of Medicine*, vol. 3, no. 34, p. 963.

07] Saks, M. (2003) 'Bringing together the orthodox and alternative in health care', *Complementary Therapies in Medicine*, vol. 11, pp. 142–145.

08] Roberts, M. J. D. (2009) 'The Politics of Professionalization: MPs, Medical Men, and the 1858 Medical Act', *Medical History*, vol. 53, no. 1, pp. 37–56.

09] Junod, S. W. (2000) 'An alternative perspective: Homeopathic drugs, Royal Copeland, and federal drug regulation', *Food and Drug Law Journal*, vol. 55, no 1, pp. 161–183.

10] Saks, M. (2005) 'Political and Historical Perspectives' in Heller, T., Lee-Treweek, G., Katz, J., Stone, J. and Spurr, S. (eds) *Perspectives on Complementary and Alternative Medicine*, Abingdon, Routledge, Taylor and Francis/Milton Keynes, The Open University, p. 61.

11] Heller, T. and Spur, S. (2005) 'Introduction' in Heller, T., Lee-Treweek, G., Katz, J., Stone, J. and Spurr, S. (eds) *Perspectives on Complementary and Alternative Medicine*, Abingdon, Routledge, Taylor and Francis/Milton Keynes, The Open University, p. xiii.

12] Astin, J. A., (2000) 'The characteristics of CAM users: a complex picture', in Kelner, M., Wellman, B., Pescosolido, B. and Saks, M. (eds) *Complementary and Alternative Medicine: Challenge and Change*, London, Harwood Academic Publishers, p. 104.

§

## Chapter Two – Why CAVM Appears to Work in Animals

01] Coulter, H. L. (1980) *Homoeopathic Science and Modern Medicine*, Berkeley, North Atlantic Books, p. 90.

02] Adams, P. (1996) *Natural Medicine for the Whole Person*, Shaftesbury, Element Books Ltd, p. 12.

03] Koehler, G. (1986) *The Handbook of Homoeopathy*, Wellingborough, Thorson's Publishing Group, p. 28.

04] Henriques, M. (2016) *How a dog's mind can easily be controlled* [Online]. Available at www.bbc.com/earth/story/20161017-why-animals-experience-the-placebo-effect-much-like-we-do (Accessed 24 November 2016).

05] Beyerstein, B. (1997) 'Why Bogus Therapies Seem to Work', *Skeptical Inquirer*, vol. 21, no. 5 [Online]. Available at www.csicop.org/si/show/why_bogus_thera pies_seem_to_work (Accessed 16 September 2016).

06] Porter, V. (1997) *Country Tales – Old Vets*, Newton Abbot, David & Charles, p. 157.

07] Allen, J. (2015) 'Petco pulls dog "calming" medicine with 13 per cent alcohol after outcry, petition from customers', *7News*, 19 January [Online]. Available at www.thedenverchannel.com/lifestyle/pets/petco-pulls-dog-calming-medi cine-with-13-percent-alcohol-after-outcry-petition-from-customers01162015 (Accessed 16 September 2016).

08] US Food and Drugs Administration (FDA) (2009) *Warnings on Three Zicam Intranasal Zinc Products*, [Online], Available at www.fda.gov/ForConsumers/ ConsumerUpdates/ucm166931.htm (Accessed 14 September 2016).

09] Cracknell, N. R. and Mills, D. S. (2008) 'A double-blind placebo-controlled study into the efficacy of a homeopathic remedy for fear of firework noises in the dog (*Canis familiaris*)', *The Veterinary Journal*, vol. 177, pp. 80–88.

10] Hahnemann, S. (1983 [1921]) *Organon of Medicine*, 6th edn (trans. J. Kunzli, A. Naude and P. Pendleton) London, Orion, p. 30.

11] Whitehead, M., Chambers, D., Taylor, N., Jessop, M., Gough, A., Atkinson, M., Hyde, P., McKenzie, B. and Guthrie, A. (2016) 'Homeopathy and cancer', *Veterinary Record*, vol. 179, pp. 78–79.

12] Wada, M., Hasegawa, D., Hamamoto, Y., Asai, A., Shouji, A., Chambers, J., Uchida, K. and Fujita, M. (2016) 'A canine case with cystic meningioma showing miraculous reduction of the cystic lesion' *Journal of Veterinary Medical Science*, vol. 78, no 1 pp. 101–104.

§

## Chapter Three – What Is Science and Why Does it Matter?

01] Coulter, H. L. (1980) *Homoeopathic Science and Modern Medicine*, Berkeley, North Atlantic books, p. 155.

02] Gregory, A. (2001) *Eureka! The Birth of Science*, Duxford, Icon Books Ltd, pp. 13–16.

03] Roberts, J. (ed.) (2005) *The Oxford Dictionary of the Classical World*, Oxford, Oxford University Press, pp. 36, 474 and 746.

04] Stone, J. (1996) 'Regulating complementary medicine: standards not status', *British Medical Journal*, vol. 312, pp. 1492–1493.

05] *Richard Dimbleby Lecture: Science, Delusion and the Appetite for Wonder* (1996) BBC 1, 12 November. [Dawkins later expanded on the ideas expressed in this lecture in his 1998 book *Unweaving the Rainbow*, published by Penguin Ltd.]

06] Medawar, P. in Singh, S. and Ernst, E. (2008) *Trick or Treatment? Alternative Medicine on Trial*, London, Random house, p. 87.

07] Offit, P. (2013) *Killing us softly: The Sense and Nonsense of Alternative Medicine*, London, Fourth Estate, pp. 134–135.

08] Conzemius, M. and Evans, R. (2012) 'Caregiver placebo effect for dogs with lameness from osteoarthritis', *Journal of the American Veterinary Medical Association*, vol. 241, no. 10, pp. 1314–1319.

09] Smith, G. C. and Pell, J. P. (2003) 'Parachute use to prevent death and major trauma related to gravitational challenge: systematic review of randomised controlled trials', *British Medical Journal*, vol. 327, pp.1459–1461.

10] Cardwell, J. M. (2008) 'An overview of study design', *Journal of Small Animal Practice*, vol. 49, pp. 217–218.

11] Rawlins, M. D. (2008) 'De testimonio: On the evidence for decisions about the use of therapeutic interventions (The Harveian Oration)', *Lancet*, vol. 372, pp 2152–2161.

12] Holmes, M. and Cockroft, P. (2004) 'Evidence-based veterinary medicine 3. Appraising the evidence', *In Practice*, vol. 26, pp. 154–164.

13] Alternative Veterinary Medicine Centre (2007) *Prejudice against Homeopathy* [Online]. Available at www.alternativevet.org/prejudice.htm (accessed 23 May 2015).

14] Bunge, M. (2009) 'The Philosophy behind Pseudoscience', in Frazier, K (ed.) *Science under Siege*, Amherst, Prometheus Books, pp. 235–251.

15] Anon (1991) 'Unproven methods of cancer management. Laetrile', *CA: A Cancer Journal for Clinicians*, vol. 41, no. 3, pp. 187–192.

16] Sehon, S. and Stanley, D. (2010) 'Evidence and simplicity: why we should reject homeopathy', *Journal of Evaluation in Clinical Practice*, vol. 16, no. 2, pp. 276–281.

17] Stone, J. and Katz, J. (2005) 'Can complementary and alternative medicine be classified?' in Heller, T., Lee-Treweek, G., Katz, J., Stone, J. and Spurr, S. (eds) *Perspectives on Complementary and Alternative Medicine*, Abingdon, Routledge, Taylor and Francis/Milton Keynes, The Open University, p. 36.

18] Saks, M. (2005) 'Political and Historical Perspectives' in Heller, T., Lee-Treweek, G., Katz, J., Stone, J. and Spurr, S., (eds) *Perspectives on Complementary and Alternative Medicine*, Abingdon, Routledge, Taylor and Francis/Milton Keynes, The Open University, p. 76.

19] Benson, O. and Stangroom, J. (2007) *Why Truth Matters*, London, Continuum, p. 41.

20] Novella, S. (2003) *'Alternative Engineering': A Postmodern Parable* [Online]. Available at www.quackwatch.org/01QuackeryRelatedTopics/alteng.html (Accessed 10 September 2016).

21] Fisher, P. and Scott, D. L. (2001) 'A randomized controlled trial of homeopathy in rheumatoid arthritis', *Rheumatology*, vol. 40, pp. 1052–1055.

22] Baerlein, E. and Dower, L. G. (1980) *Healing With Radionics: The Science of Healing Energy*, Wellingborough, Thorsons Publishers Ltd. [As a footnote to this final section, although it isn't mentioned anywhere in the textbook, it is possible the paragraph in question refers to a study by biologist, Dr Frank A. Brown who supposedly found that live oysters transferred to his laboratory adapted their feeding times to the local phases of the moon, rather than to tidal movements at their place of origin. The study seems never to have been formally peer-reviewed or published, no version of it is available online and its most popular application is as an aid to anglers when trying to ensure a good day's fishing, not the 'science' of radionics. There is no suggestion of any 'interconnection which makes radionic therapy possible', and it seems even anglers are sceptical of its real world usefulness.]

§

## Chapter Four – When Thinking Goes Wrong

01] Bennett, B., (2015) *Logically Fallacious, the Ultimate Collection of Over 300 Logical Fallacies*, Academic Edition, Sudbury MA, Archieboy Holdings.

02] Galad, B. S., Li, W., Grady, S. et al (2015) 'Administration of thimerosal-containing vaccines to infant rhesus macaques does not result in autism-like behavior or neuropathology', *Proceedings of the National Academy of Sciences USA*, vol. 112, no.40, pp 12498–12503.

03] Safeminds (2016) *About Safeminds* [Online], Available at www.safeminds.org/about-2 (Accessed 7 October 2016).

04] Woodmansey, D. (2016) 'BVA concern at low profits in most practice', *Veterinary Times*, 14 September [Online]. Available at https://www.vettimes.co.uk/news/bva-concern-at-low-profits-in-most-practices (Accessed 21 December 2016).

05] Brogan, R. J. and Mustaq, F. (2015) 'Acupuncture-induced pneumothorax: the hidden complication', *Scottish Medical Journal*, vol. 60, no. 2, pp. e11–13.

06] Ariely, D., (2009) *Predictably Irrational*, Glasgow, HarperCollins.

07] Kahneman, D. (2011) *Thinking Fast and Slow*, London, Penguin.

08] Li, M. and Chapman, G. B. (2009) '"100 per cent of anything looks good": the appeal of one hundred per cent ', *Psychonomic Bulletin and Review*, vol. 16, no. 1, pp. 156–162.

09] Perneger, T. V. and Agoritsas, T. (2011) 'Doctors and patients' susceptibility to framing bias: a randomized trial', *Journal of General Internal Medicine*, vol. 26, no. 12, pp. 1411–1417.

10] Bornstein, B. H. and Emler, A. C. (2001) 'Rationality in medical decision making: a review of the literature on doctors' decision-making biases', *Journal of Evaluation in Clinical Practice*, vol. 7, no. 2, pp. 97–107.

11] Kiviniemi, M. T. and Rothman, A. J. (2006) 'Selective memory biases in individuals' memory for health-related information and behavior recommendations', *Psychology and Health*, vol. 21, no. 2, pp. 247–272.

12] Krems, J. F. and Zierer, C. (1994) 'Are experts immune to cognitive bias? Dependence of "confirmation bias" on specialist knowledge', *Zeitschrift fur Experimentelle und Angewandte Psychologie*, vol. 41, no. 1, pp. 98–115.

13] Institor, H. (2014) *Why are cats immune to chemtrails?* [Online], Available at http://harddawn.com/why-are-cats-immune-to-chemtrails (Accessed 30 April 2016).

14] Goldacre, B. (2013) *Bad Pharma*, London, Fourth Estate.

15] Gough, A. and Murphy, K. (2015) *Differential Diagnosis in Small Animal Medicine*, 2nd edn, Oxford, Wiley-Blackwell.

§

## Chapter Five – But We Just Know it Works!

01] British Association of Homeopathic Veterinary Surgeons (2012) *Successful Case* [Online]. Available at: www.bahvs.com/cured-cancer-case-2 (Accessed 22 October 2016).

02] Gregory, P. (2014) 'EBM "formalisation" of vet decisions', *Veterinary Times*, vol. 44, no. 24, p. 31.

03] Gregory, P. (2003) 'Homoeopathy "doesn't need proof"', *Veterinary Times*, vol. 33, no. 22, pp. 7–8.

04] Jewell, G. (2000) 'Comments on practising complementary and alternative modalities', *Canadian Veterinary Journal*, vol. 41, p. 351 [Online]. Available at: www.ncbi.nlm.nih.gov/pmc/articles/PMC1476254/pdf/canvetj00017-0009c. pdf (Accessed 29 March 2015).

05] Academy of Veterinary Homeopathy (2014) *Homeopathic treatment resolves cat's fears and vomiting after eating* [Online]. Available at http://theavh.org/home opathic-treatment-resolves-cats-fears-and-vomiting-after-eating (Accessed 30 March 2015).

06] Whole Dog Journal (2008) *Healing Your Canine with Energy Medicine and Holistic Dog Care Techniques* [Online]. Available at www.whole-dog-journal. com/issues/11_2/features/Energy-Medicine-and-Holistic-Dog-Care_16006-1. html (Accessed 30 March 2015)

07] Dowding, O. (2008) *Homeopathy on the farm – if homeopathic success is all in the patient's mind, how does this work for animals?* [Online]. Available at www.the-cma.org.uk/cma_images/Oliver%20Dowding%20Presentation%20homeopa thy%20conference%2018%206%2008.pdf (Accessed 16 April 2017).

08] Griffith, S. (2009) 'Flower power for orphaned elephants', *Veterinary Nursing Times*, vol. 9, no. 2, p. 8.

09] Mcbride, W. G. (1961) 'Thalidomide and congenital abnormalities', *Lancet*, vol. 278, no. 7216, p. 1358.

10] Preston, J. M. (1983) 'Adverse reactions to unapproved applications', *Veterinary Record*, vol. 112, no. 12, p. 286.

11] Gilovich, T. (1993) *How We Know What Isn't So*, New York, The Free Press, Chapter 6, pp. 88–111.

12] Conzemius, M. G. and Evans, R. B. (2012) 'Caregiver placebo effect for dogs with lameness from osteoarthritis', *Journal of the American Veterinary Association*, vol. 241, no. 10, pp. 1314–1319.

13] RCVS Knowledge (2015) *History of the veterinary profession* [Online]. Available at: https://knowledge.rcvs.org.uk/heritage-and-history/history-of-the-veterinary-profession (Accessed 1 April 2015).

14] Thornton J. T. (1976) 'Methylene Blue treatment for downer cows', *Modern Veterinary Practice*, vol. 57, no. 12, p.1023.

15] Dun, F. (1901) *Veterinary Medicines*, 10ᵗʰ edn, MacQueen, J (ed). Edinburgh, David Douglas, p. 52.

16] Anon (1828) 'Phrenology – Its Utility and Importance in Animals', *Farrier and Naturalist*, vol. 1, pp. 34–35. See: http://rcvsknowledgelibraryblog.org/2014/04/28/eclipse-and-his-equine-bumps (Accessed 1 April 2015).

17] Greenstone, G. (2010) 'The history of bloodletting', *British Columbia Medical Journal*, vol. 52, no. 1, p. 12–14.

18] Silver, I. A. (1988) 'The firing of man and animals', *Veterinary History*, vol. 5, no. 4, pp. 124–129.

19] Clayton Jones, D. G. (1992) 'Firing or the actual cautery', *Equine Veterinary Education*, vol. 4, no. 6, pp. 313–316.

20] Hayward, M. and Adams, D. (2001) *The firing of horses – A review for the Animal Welfare Advisory Committee of the Australian Vet Association* [Online]. Available at www.gungahlinvet.com.au/petcare-info/publications/the-firing-of-horses.pdf (Accessed 1 April 2015).

21] Dean, G. (2012) 'Phrenology and the grand delusion of experience', *Skeptical Inquirer*, vol. 36 no. 6, pp. 30–38 [Online]. Available at: www.csicop.org/si/show/phrenology_and_the_grand_delusion_of_experience (accessed 1 April 2015)

22] Dun, F. (1901) *Veterinary Medicines*, p. 51.

23] Silver, I. A. (1988) 'The firing of man and animals', *Veterinary History*.

24] Preece, R. (2004) 'Veterinary Bloodletting and the Status of Animals', *Veterinary History*.

25] Greenstone, G. (2010) 'The history of bloodletting', *British Columbia Medical Journal*.

26] Silver, I. A. (1988) 'The firing of man and animals', *Veterinary History*.

27] Dean, G. (2012) 'Phrenology and the grand delusion of experience', *Skeptical Inquirer*.

28] Arenas, C., Peña, L., Granados-Soler, J. L. and Pérez-Alenza, M. D. (2016) 'Adjuvant therapy for highly malignant canine mammary tumours: Cox-2 inhibitor versus chemotherapy: a case–control prospective study', *Veterinary Record*, vol. 179, no. 5, p. 125.

29] For example: Muranushi, C., Olsen, C. M., Pandeya, N. and Green, A. C. (2015) 'Aspirin and Nonsteroidal Anti-Inflammatory Drugs Can Prevent Cutaneous Squamous Cell Carcinoma: a Systematic Review and Meta-Analysis', *Journal of Investigative Dermatology*, vol. 135, pp. 975–983.

§

# Chapter Six – Herbs and Supplements

01] Solecki, R. S. (1975) 'Shanidar IV, a Neanderthal Flower Burial in Northern Iraq', *Science*, vol. 190, no. 4217, pp. 880–881.

02] van Tellingen, C. (2007) 'Pliny's pharmacopoeia or the Roman treat', *Netherlands Heart Journal* , vol. 15, no. 3, pp. 118–120.

03] Speed, M. P., Fenton, A., Jones, M. G., Ruxton, G. D. and Brockhurst, M. A. (2015) 'Coevolution can explain defensive secondary metabolite diversity in plants', *The New Phytologist*, vol. 208, no. 4, pp. 1251–1263.

04] Liu, J. P., Yang, M., Liu, Y., Wei, M. L. and Grimsgaard, S. (2006) 'Herbal medicines for treatment of irritable bowel syndrome', *Cochrane Database of Systematic Reviews 2006*, Issue 1, Art. No.: CD004116 [Online] DOI: 10.1002/14651858. CD004116.pub2 (Accessed 28 January 2017).

05] Liu, Z. L., Xie, L. Z., Zhu, J., Li, G. Q., Grant, S. J. and Liu, J. P. (2013) 'Herbal medicines for fatty liver diseases', *Cochrane Database of Systematic Reviews 2013*, Issue 8, Art. No.: CD009059 [Online] DOI: 10.1002/14651858.CD009059.pub2 (Accessed 28 January 2017).

06] Cameron, M., and Chrubasik, S. (2013) 'Topical herbal therapies for treating osteoarthritis', *Cochrane Database of Systematic Reviews 2013*, Issue 5, Art. No.: CD010538 [Online] DOI: 10.1002/14651858.CD010538 (Accessed 28 January 2017).

07] Arnold, E., Clark, C. E., Lasserson, T. J. and Wu, T. (2008) 'Herbal interventions for chronic asthma in adults and children', *Cochrane Database of Systematic Reviews 2008*, Issue 1, Art. No.: CD005989 [Online] DOI: 10.1002/14651858. CD005989.pub2 (Accessed 28 January 2017).

08] Abenavoli, L., Capasso, R., Milic, N. and Capasso, F. (2010) 'Milk thistle in liver diseases: past, present, future', *Phytotherapy Research*, vol. 24, no. 10, pp. 1423–1432.

09] Skorupski, K. A., Hammond, G. M., Irish, A. M., Kent, M. S., Guerrero, T. A., Rodriguez, C. O. and Griffin, D. W. (2011) 'Prospective randomized clinical trial assessing the efficacy of Denamarin for prevention of CCNU-induced hepatopathy in tumor-bearing dogs', *Journal of Veterinary Internal Medicine*, vol. 25, no. 4, pp. 838–845.

10] Au, A.Y., Hasenwinkel, J. M. and Frondoza, C. G. (2013) 'Hepatoprotective effects of S-adenosylmethionine and silybin on canine hepatocytes in vitro', *Journal of Animal Physiology and Animal Nutrition*, vol. 97, no. 2, pp. 331–341.

11] Reichling, J., Schmökel, H., Fitzi, J., Bucher, S. and Saller, R. (2004) 'Dietary support with Boswellia resin in canine inflammatory joint and spinal disease', *Schweizer Archiv fur Tierheilkunde*, vol. 146, no. 2, pp. 71–79.

12] Ernst, E. and Huntley, A. (2000) 'Tea tree oil: a systematic review of randomized clinical trials', *Forschende Komplementarmedizin und Klassische Naturheilkunde*, vol. 7, no. 1, pp. 17–20.

13] Hammer, K. A., Carson, C. F., Riley, T. V. and Nielsen, J. B. (2006) 'A review of the toxicity of *Melaleuca alternifolia* (tea tree) oil', *Food and Chemical Toxicology*, vol. 44, no. 5, pp. 616–625.

14] Jepson, R. G. and Craig, J. C. (2008) 'Cranberries for preventing urinary tract infections', in Jepson, R. G. (ed.) *Cochrane Database of Systematic Reviews 2008*, Issue 1, Art. No.: CD001321 [Online] DOI: 10.1002/14651858.CD001321.pub4 (Accessed 28 January 2017).

15] Ernst, E. (2004) 'Risks of herbal medicinal products', *Pharmacoepidemiology and Drug Safety*, vol. 13, no. 11, pp. 767–771.

16] Charlton, A. (2004) 'Medicinal uses of tobacco in history', *Journal of the Royal Society of Medicine*, vol. 97, no. 6, pp. 292–296.

17] Ernst, E. (2003) 'Cardiovascular adverse effects of herbal medicines: a systematic review of the recent literature', *Canadian Journal of Cardiology*, vol. 19, no. 7, pp. 818–827.

18] Valdivia-Correa, B., Gómez-Gutiérrez, C., Uribe, M. and Méndez-Sánchez, N. (2016) 'Herbal Medicine in Mexico: A Cause of Hepatotoxicity. A Critical Review', *International Journal of Molecular Sciences*, vol. 17, no. 2, p. 235.

19] Chaudhary, T., Chahar, A., Sharma, J. K., Kaur, K. and Dang, A. (2015) 'Phytomedicine in the Treatment of Cancer: A Health Technology Assessment', *Journal of Clinical and Diagnostic Research*, vol. 9, no. 12, p. XC04–XC09.

20] Izzo, A. A., Hoon-Kim, S., Radhakrishnan, R. and Williamson, E. M. (2016) 'A Critical Approach to Evaluating Clinical Efficacy, Adverse Events and Drug Interactions of Herbal Remedies', *Phytotherapy Research*, vol. 30, no. 5, pp. 691–700.

21] Vickers, A., Zollman, C. and Lee, R. (2001) 'Herbal medicine', *The Western Journal of Medicine*, vol. 175, no. 2, pp. 125–128.

22] Ozdemir, M., Aktan, Y., Boydag, B. S., Cingi, M. I. and Musmul, A. (no date) 'Interaction between grapefruit juice and diazepam in humans', *European Journal of Drug Metabolism and Pharmacokinetics*, vol. 23, no. 1, pp. 55–59.

23] Bailey, D. G. and Dresser, G. K. (2004) 'Interactions between grapefruit juice and cardiovascular drugs', *American Journal of Cardiovascular Drugs*, vol. 4, no. 5, pp. 281–297.

24] Colombo, D., Lunardon, L. and Bellia, G. (2014) 'Cyclosporine and Herbal Supplement Interactions', *Journal of Toxicology*, 2014, pp. 1–6.

25] Chan, T. Y. K. (2016) 'Herbal Medicines Induced Anticholinergic Poisoning in Hong Kong', *Toxins*, vol. 8, no. 3, p. 80.

26] Chan, T. Y. K. (2016) 'Aconitum Alkaloid Poisoning Because of Contamination of Herbs by Aconite Roots', *Phytotherapy Research*, vol. 30, no. 1, pp. 3–8.

27] Zamir, R., Hosen, A., Ullah, M. O. and Nahar, N. (2015) 'Microbial and Heavy Metal Contaminant of Antidiabetic Herbal Preparations Formulated in Bangladesh', *Evidence-based Complementary and Alternative Medicine: eCAM*, p. 243593.

28] Posadzki, P., Watson, L. and Ernst, E. (2013) 'Contamination and adulteration of herbal medicinal products (HMPs): an overview of systematic reviews', *European Journal of Clinical Pharmacology*, vol. 69, no. 3, pp. 295–307.

29] Martins, R. R., Duarte Farias, A., Russel Martins, R. and Gouveia Oliveira, A. (2016), 'Influence of the use of medicinal plants in medication adherence in elderly people', *International Journal of Clinical Practice*, vol. 70, pp. 254–260.

30] Safire, W. (n.d.) *The Way We Live Now On Language* [Online], Available at www.fimdefelice.org/p2417.html (Accessed 13 April 2016).

31] Advisory Committee on Borderline Substances (2012) *Appendix 6: products which will not be considered by the ACBS* [Online] Available at www.gov.

uk/government/uploads/system/uploads/attachment_data/file/358665/
Appendix6.pdf (Accessed 20 April 2016).

32] Mato, J. M. and Lu, S. C. (2007) 'Role of S-adenosyl-L-methionine in liver health and injury', *Hepatology*, vol. 45, no. 5, pp. 1306–1312.

33] Guo, T., Chang, L., Xiao, Y. and Liu, Q. (2015) 'S-adenosyl-L-methionine for the treatment of chronic liver disease: a systematic review and meta-analysis', *PloS one*, vol. 10, no. 3, p. e0122124.

34] Rutjes, A. W., Nüesch, E., Reichenbach, S. and Jüni, P. (2009) 'S-Adenosylmethionine for osteoarthritis of the knee or hip', *Cochrane Database of Systematic Reviews 2009*, Issue 4, Art. No.: CD007321 [Online] DOI: 10.1002/14651858.CD007321.pub2 (Accessed 28 January 2017).

35] Imhoff, D. J., Gordon-Evans, W. J., Evans, R. B., Johnson, A. L., Griffon, D. J. and Swanson, K. S. (2011) 'Evaluation of S-adenosyl l-methionine in a double-blinded, randomized, placebo-controlled, clinical trial for treatment of presumptive osteoarthritis in the dog', *Veterinary Surgery*, vol. 40, no. 2, pp. 228–232.

36] Henrotin, Y., Marty, M. and Mobasheri, A. (2014) 'What is the current status of chondroitin sulfate and glucosamine for the treatment of knee osteoarthritis?', *Maturitas*, vol. 78, no. 3, pp. 184–187.

37] Müller-Fassbender, H., Bach, G. L., Haase, W., Rovati, L. C. and Setnikar, I. (1994) 'Glucosamine sulfate compared to ibuprofen in osteoarthritis of the knee', *Osteoarthritis and Cartilage*, vol. 2, no. 1, pp. 61–69.

38] McAlindon, T. E., LaValley, M. P., Gulin, J. P. and Felson, D. T. (2000) 'Glucosamine and chondroitin for treatment of osteoarthritis: a systematic quality assessment and meta-analysis', *Journal of the American Medical Association*, vol. 283, no. 11, pp. 1469–1475.

39] Cibere, J., Kopec, J. A., Thorne, A., Singer, J., Canvin, J., Robinson, D. B., Pope, J., Hong, P., Grant, E. and Esdaile, J. M. (2004) 'Randomized, double-blind, placebo-controlled glucosamine discontinuation trial in knee osteoarthritis', *Arthritis and Rheumatism*, vol. 51, no. 5, pp. 738–745.

40] Towheed, T., Maxwell, L., Anastassiades, T. P., Shea, B., Houpt, J., Welch, V., Hochberg, M. C. and Wells, G. A. (2005) 'Glucosamine therapy for treating osteoarthritis', in Towheed, T. (ed.) *Cochrane Database of Systematic Reviews 2005*, Issue 2, Art. No.: CD002946 [Online] DOI: 10.1002/14651858.CD002946.pub2 (Accessed 28 January 2017).

41] Bausell, R. B. (2007) *Snake Oil Science*, Oxford, Oxford University Press, pp. 251–252.

42] Clegg, D. O., Reda, D. J., Harris, C. L., Klein, M. A., O'Dell, J. R., Hooper, M. M., Bradley, J. D., Bingham, C. O., Weisman, M. H., Jackson, C. G., Lane, N. E., Cush, J. J., Moreland, L. W., Schumacher, H. R., Oddis, C. V., Wolfe, F., Molitor, J. A., Yocum, D. E., Schnitzer, T. J., Furst, D. E., Sawitzke, A. D., Shi, H., Brandt, K. D., Moskowitz, R. W. and Williams, H. J. (2006) 'Glucosamine, Chondroitin Sulfate, and the Two in Combination for Painful Knee Osteoarthritis', *New England Journal of Medicine*, vol. 354, no. 8, pp. 795–808.

43] D'Altilio, M., Peal, A., Alvey, M., Simms, C., Curtsinger, A., Gupta, R. C., Canerdy, T. D., Goad, J. T., Bagchi, M. and Bagchi, D. (2007) 'Therapeutic

Efficacy and Safety of Undenatured Type II Collagen Singly or in Combination with Glucosamine and Chondroitin in Arthritic Dogs', *Toxicology Mechanisms and Methods*, vol. 17, no. 4, pp. 189–196.

44] Conzemius, M. G. and Evans, R. B. (2012) 'Caregiver placebo effect for dogs with lameness from osteoarthritis', *Journal of the American Veterinary Medical Association,* vol. 241, no. 10, pp. 1314–1319.

45] Laverty, S., Sandy, J. D., Celeste, C., Vachon, P., Marier, J.-F. and Plaas, A. H. K. (2005) 'Synovial fluid levels and serum pharmacokinetics in a large animal model following treatment with oral glucosamine at clinically relevant doses', *Arthritis and Rheumatism,* vol. 52, no. 1, pp. 181–91.

46] Higler, M. H., Brommer, H., L'Ami, J. J., de Grauw, J. C., Nielen, M., van Weeren, P. R., Laverty, S., Barneveld, A. and Back, W. (2014), 'The effects of three-month oral supplementation with a nutraceutical and exercise on the locomotor pattern of aged horses', *Equine Veterinary Journal,* vol. 46, pp. 611–617.

47] Leung, A. Y. (2006) 'Traditional toxicity documentation of Chinese Materia Medica – an overview', *Toxicologic Pathology,* vol. 34, no. 4, pp. 319–326.

48] Levinovitz, A. (2013) *Chairman Mao Invented Traditional Chinese Medicine* [Online] Available at www.slate.com/articles/health_and_science/medical_examiner/2013/10/traditional_chinese_medicine_origins_mao_invented_it_but_didn_t_believe.html (Accessed 24 June 2016).

49] Manheimer, E., Wieland, S., Kimbrough, E., Cheng, K. and Berman, B. M. (2009) 'Evidence from the Cochrane Collaboration for Traditional Chinese Medicine Therapies', *The Journal of Alternative and Complementary Medicine,* vol. 15, no. 9, pp. 1001–1014.

50] Hu, J., Zhang, J., Zhao, W., Zhang, Y., Zhang, L. and Shang, H. (2011) 'Cochrane Systematic Reviews of Chinese Herbal Medicines: An Overview', *PLoS one,* J. H. Verbeek (ed.), vol. 6, no. 12, p. e28696.

51] Coghlan, M. L., Maker, G., Crighton, E., Haile, J., Murray, D. C., White, N. E., Byard, R. W., Bellgard, M. I., Mullaney, I., Trengove, R., Allcock, R. J. N., Nash, C., Hoban, C., Jarrett, K., Edwards, R., Musgrave, I. F. and Bunce, M. (2015) 'Combined DNA, toxicological and heavy metal analyses provides an auditing toolkit to improve pharmacovigilance of traditional Chinese medicine (TCM)', *Scientific reports,* vol. 5, p. 17475.

52] Hu, J., Zhang, J., Zhao, W., Zhang, Y., Zhang, L. and Shang, H. (2011) 'Cochrane Systematic Reviews of Chinese Herbal Medicines: An Overview', *PLoS one.*

53] Still, J. (2003) 'Use of animal products in traditional Chinese medicine: environmental impact and health hazards', *Complementary Therapies in Medicine,* vol. 11. no. 2, pp. 118–122.

54] Liu, Z., Jiang, Z., Fang, H., Li, C., Mi, A., Chen, J., Zhang, X., Cui, S., Chen, D., Ping, X., Li, F., Li, C., Tang, S., Luo, Z., Zeng, Y. and Meng, Z. (2016) 'Perception, Price and Preference: Consumption and Protection of Wild Animals Used in Traditional Medicine', *PloS one,* vol.11, no. 3, p. e0145901.

55] Save the Rhino (2016) *Poaching for Rhino Horn* [Online], Available at https://

www.savetherhino.org/rhino_info/threats_to_rhino/poaching_for_rhino_horn (Accessed 27 April 2016).

56] Ellis, R. (2005) *Poaching for traditional Chinese medicine*, in *Save the rhinos: European Association of Zoos and Aquaria (EAZA) Rhino Campaign 2005/6*, pp. 91–95 [Online], Available at www.rhinoresourcecenter.com/pdf_files/117/1175860939.pdf (Accessed 20 January 2017).

57] Tsai, L. E. (2008) *Detailed Discussion of Bears Used in Traditional Chinese Medicine* [Online], Animal Legal and Historical Center, Michigan State Universtiy College of law. Available at www.animallaw.info/article/detailed-discussion-bears-used-traditional-chinese-medicine (Accessed 8 January 2017).

58] Thorat, S. P., Rege, N. N., Naik, A. S., Thatte, U. M., Joshi, A., Panicker, K. N., Bapat, R. D. and Dahanukar, S. A. (1995) 'Emblica officinalis: a novel therapy for acute pancreatitis – an experimental study', *Hepatic, Pancreatic and Biliary Surgery*, vol. 9, no. 1, pp. 25–30.

59] Nammi, S., Gudavalli, R., Babu, B. S. R., Lodagala, D. S. and Boini, K. M. (2003) 'Possible mechanisms of hypotension produced 70 per cent alcoholic extract of *Terminalia arjuna* (L.) in anaesthetized dogs', *BMC Complementary and Alternative Medicine*, vol. 3, no. 1, p. 5.

60] Sinyorita, S., Ghosh, C. K., Chakrabarti, A., Auddy, B., Ghosh, R. and Debnath, P. K. (2011) 'Effect of Ayurvedic mercury preparation Makaradhwaja on geriatric canine – a preliminary study', *Indian Journal of Experimental Biology*, vol. 49, no. 7, pp. 534–539.

61] Gupta, R., Ingle, N. A., Kaur, N., Yadav, P., Ingle, E. and Charania, Z. (2015) 'Ayurveda in Dentistry: A Review', *Journal of International Oral Health*, vol. 7, no. 8, pp. 141–143.

62] Kessler, C. S., Pinders, L., Michalsen, A. and Cramer, H. (2015) 'Ayurvedic interventions for osteoarthritis: a systematic review and meta-analysis', *Rheumatology International*, vol. 35, no. 2, pp. 211–232.

63] Saper, R. B., Phillips, R. S., Sehgal, A., Khouri, N., Davis, R. B., Paquin, J., Thuppil, V. and Kales, S. N. (2008) 'Lead, mercury, and arsenic in US and Indian-manufactured Ayurvedic medicines sold via the internet', *Journal of the American Medical Association*, vol. 300, no. 8, pp. 915–923.

64] Centers for Disease Control and Prevention (CDC) (2012) 'Lead poisoning in pregnant women who used Ayurvedic medications from India – New York City, 2011–2012', *Morbidity and Mortality Weekly Report*, vol. 61, no. 33, pp. 641–646.

65] Breeher, L., Mikulski, M. A., Czeczok, T., Leinenkugel, K. and Fuortes, L. J. (2015) 'A cluster of lead poisoning among consumers of Ayurvedic medicine', *International Journal of Occupational and Environmental Health*, vol. 21, no. 4, pp. 303–307.

66] Carson, C. F., Hammer, K. A. and Riley, T. V. (2006) '*Melaleuca alternifolia* (Tea Tree) oil: a review of antimicrobial and other medicinal properties', *Clinical Microbiology Reviews*, vol. 19, no. 1, pp. 50–62.

67] Carson, C. F., Cookson, B. D., Farrelly, H. D. and Riley, T. V. (1995) 'Susceptibility of methicillin-resistant *Staphylococcus aureus* to the essential oil of

*Melaleuca alternifolia*', *Journal of Antimicrobial Chemotherapy*, vol. 35, no. 3, pp. 421–424.

68] Cox, S. D., Mann, C. M., Markham, J. L., Bell, H. C., Gustafson, J. E., Warmington, J. R. and Wyllie, S. G. (2000) 'The mode of antimicrobial action of the essential oil of *Melaleuca alternifolia* (tea tree oil)', *Journal of Applied Microbiology*, vol. 88, no. 1, pp. 170–175.

69] Carson, C. F., Hammer, K. A. and Riley, T. V. (2006) 'Melaleuca alternifolia (Tea Tree) oil: a review of antimicrobial and other medicinal properties', *Clinical Microbiology Reviews*.

70] Dryden, M. S., Dailly, S. and Crouch, M. (2004) 'A randomized, controlled trial of tea tree topical preparations versus a standard topical regimen for the clearance of MRSA colonization', *Journal of Hospital Infection*, vol. 56, no. 4, pp. 283–286.

71] Russell, M. (1999). 'Toxicology of tea tree oil', In Southwell, I. and Lowe, R. (eds.) *Tea tree: the genus Melaleuca, vol. 9*, Amsterdam, Harwood Academic Publishers, p. 191–201.

72] Hammer, K. A., Carson, C. F. and Riley, T. V. (1999) 'Influence of organic matter, cations and surfactants on the antimicrobial activity of *Melaleuca alternifolia* (tea tree) oil in vitro', *Journal of Applied Microbiology*, vol. 86, no. 3, pp. 446–452.

73] Kawakami, E., Washizu, M., Hirano, T., Sakuma, M., Takano, M., Hori, T. and Tsutsui, T. (2006) 'Treatment of prostatic abscesses by aspiration of the purulent matter and injection of tea tree oil into the cavities in dogs', *Journal of Veterinary Medical Science*, vol. 68, no. 11, pp. 1215–1217.

74] Reichling, J., Fitzi, J., Hellmann, K., Wegener, T., Bucher, S. and Saller, R. (2004) 'Topical tea tree oil effective in canine localised pruritic dermatitis – a multi-centre randomised double-blind controlled clinical trial in the veterinary practice', *Deutsche Tierarztliche Wochenschrift*, vol. 111, no. 10, pp. 408–414.

75] Weseler, A., Geiss, H. K., Saller, R. and Reichling, J. (2002) 'Antifungal effect of Australian tea tree oil on *Malassezia pachydermatis* isolated from canines suffering from cutaneous skin disease', *Schweizer Archiv fur Tierheilkunde*, vol. 144, no. 5, pp. 215–221.

76] Villar, D., Knight, M. J., Hansen, S. R. and Buck, W. B. (1994) 'Toxicity of melaleuca oil and related essential oils applied topically on dogs and cats', *Veterinary and Human Toxicology*, vol. 36, no. 2, pp. 139–142.

77] Khan, S. A., McLean, M. K. and Slater, M. R. (2014) 'Concentrated tea tree oil toxicosis in dogs and cats: 443 cases (2002–2012)', *Journal of the American Veterinary Medical Association*, vol. 244, no. 1, pp. 95–99.

78] Tanen, D. A., Danish, D. C., Reardon, J. M., Chisholm, C. B., Matteucci, M. J. and Riffenburgh, R. H. (2008) 'Comparison of oral aspirin versus topical applied methyl salicylate for platelet inhibition', *The Annals of Pharmacotherapy*, vol. 42, no. 10, pp. 1396–1401.

79] Batista, L. C. D. S. O., Cid, Y. P., De Almeida, A. P., Prudêncio, E. R., Riger, C. J., De Souza, M. A. A., Coumendouros, K. and Chaves, D. S. A. (2016) 'In vitro efficacy of essential oils and extracts of *Schinus molle* L. against *Ctenocephalides felis*', *Parasitology*, vol. 143, no. 5, pp. 627–638.

80] Song, C.-Y., Nam, E.-H., Park, S.-H. and Hwang, C.-Y. (2013) 'In vitro efficacy of the essential oil from *Leptospermum scoparium* (manuka) on antimicrobial susceptibility and biofilm formation in *Staphylococcus pseudintermedius* isolates from dogs', *Veterinary Dermatology*, vol. 24, no. 4, pp. 404–408, e87.

81] Blaskovic, M., Rosenkrantz, W., Neuber, A., Sauter-Louis, C. and Mueller, R. S. (2014) 'The effect of a spot-on formulation containing polyunsaturated fatty acids and essential oils on dogs with atopic dermatitis', *Veterinary Journal*, vol. 199, no. 1, pp. 39–43.

82] Low, S. B., Peak, R. M., Smithson, C. W., Perrone, J., Gaddis, B. and Kontogiorgos, E. (2014) 'Evaluation of a topical gel containing a novel combination of essential oils and antioxidants for reducing oral malodor in dog', *American Journal of Veterinary Research*, vol. 75, no. 7, pp. 653–657.

83] Genovese, A. G., McLean, M. K. and Khan, S. A. (2012) 'Adverse reactions from essential oil-containing natural flea products exempted from Environmental Protection Agency regulations in dogs and cats', *Journal of Veterinary Emergency and Critical Care*, vol. 22, no. 4, pp. 470–475.

84] Henley, D. V., Lipson, N., Korach, K. S. and Bloch, C. A. (2007) 'Prepubertal Gynecomastia Linked to Lavender and Tea Tree Oils', *New England Journal of Medicine*, vol. 356, no. 5, pp. 479–485.

85] Rodriguez, E. and Wrangham, R. (1993) 'Zoopharmacognosy: The Use of Medicinal Plants by Animals', in *Phytochemical Potential of Tropical Plants*, Boston, Springer US, pp. 89–105.

86] Milan, N. F., Kacsoh, B. Z. and Schlenke, T. A. (2012) 'Alcohol consumption as self-medication against blood-borne parasites in the fruit fly', *Current Biology*, vol. 22, no. 6, pp. 488–493.

87] Simone-Finstrom, M. D. and Spivak, M. (2012) 'Increased resin collection after parasite challenge: a case of self-medication in honey bees?', *PloS one*, vol. 7, no. 3, p. e34601.

88] Suárez-Rodríguez, M., López-Rull, I. and Garcia, C. M. (2013) 'Incorporation of cigarette butts into nests reduces nest ectoparasite load in urban birds: new ingredients for an old recipe?', *Biology Letters*, vol. 9, no. 1, p. 20120931.

89] Sueda, K. L. C., Hart, B. L., Cliff, K. D., Alenza, D. P., Rutteman, G. R., Pena, L., Beynen, A. C., Cuesta, P., Andersone, Z., Andersone, Z., Ozolins, J., Beaver, B. L., Berschneider, H. M., Fontanarrosa, M. F., Vezzani, D., Basabe, J., Eiras, D. F., Franson, J. C., Jorgenson, R. D., Boggess, E. K., Greve, J. H., Freeman, L. M., Michel, K. E., Gobar, G. M., Kass, P. H., Gosling, S. D., Vazire, S., Srivastava, S., John, O. P., Hart, B. L., Hart, B. L., Hosmer, D. W., Lemeshow, S., Houpt, K. A., Huffman, M. A., Canton, J. M., Huffman, M. A., Page, J. E., Sukhdeo, M. V. K., Gotoh, S., Kalunde, M. S., Chandrasiri, T., Towers, G. H. N., Janson, C., Wist, M., Kim, H. L., Gerber, G. S., Patel, R. V., Hollowell, C. M., Bales, G. T., Kirkpatrick, C. E., Lindsay, S. R., McCobb, E. C., Brown, E. A., Damiani, K., Dodman, N. H., Overall, K. L., Papageorgiou, N., Vlachos, C., Sfougaris, A., Tsachalidis, E., Plumb, D. C., Ramirez-Barrios, R. A., Barboza-Mena, G., Munoz, J., Angulo-Cubillan, F., Hernandez, E., Gonzalez, F., Escalona, F., Reips, U., Rhodes, S. D., Bowie, D. A., Hergenrather, K. C.,

Stahler, D. R., Smith, D. W., Guernsey, D. S., Thorne, C. and Wrangham, R. (2008) 'Characterisation of plant eating in dogs', *Applied Animal Behaviour Science*, vol. 111, vols 1–2, pp. 120–132.

§

## Chapter Seven – Raw Feeding

01] Pion, P. D., Kittleson, M. D., Rogers, Q. R. and Morris, J. G. (1987) 'Myocardial failure in cats associated with low plasma taurine: a reversible cardiomyopathy', *Science*, vol. 237, no. 4816, pp. 764–768.

02] US Food and Drug Adminstration (2016) *Recalls and Withdrawals* [Online], Available at www.fda.gov/animalveterinary/safetyhealth/recallswithdrawals (Accessed 11 January 2017).

03] Billinghurst, I. (n.d.) *Meet Dr Billinghurst* [Online], Available at www.barfworld.com/html/dr_billinghurst/meet.shtml (Accessed 11 January 2017).

04] Billinghurst, I. (2012) *Give Your Dog a Bone*, Bathurst, New South Wales, Warrigal Publishing.

05] Lonsdale, T. (1995) 'Periodontal disease and leucopenia', *Journal of Small Animal Practice*, vol. 36, no. 12, pp. 542–546.

06] Lonsdale, T. (2001) *Raw Meaty Bones*, New South Wales, Rivetco Pty Ltd.

07] Lonsdale, T. (n.d.) *Why not 'BARF'?* [Online], Available at www.rawmeaty-bones.com/petowners/whynotBARF.php (Accessed 11 January 2017).

08] Billinghurst, I. (2012) *Give Your Dog a Bone*.

09] Lonsdale, T. (2001) *Raw Meaty Bones*.

10] Pitcairn, R. and Pitcairn, S. (2005) *Dr Pitcairn's complete guide to natural health for dogs and cats*, 3rd edn, Emmaus PA, Rodale Inc.

11] US Food and Drug Administration (2015) *Food and Drug Administration/Center for Veterinary Medicine Report on the Risk from Pentobarbital in Dog Food* [Online], Available at www.fda.gov/AboutFDA/CentersOffices/OfficeofFoods/CVM/C VMFOIAElectronicReadingRoom/ucm129131.htm (Accessed 17 March 2016).

12] Wortinger, A. (2005) 'Nutritional myths', *Journal of the American Animal Hospital Association*, vol. 41, no. 4, pp. 273–276.

13] Rumbeiha, W. and Morrison, J. (2011) 'A review of class I and class II pet food recalls involving chemical contaminants from 1996 to 2008', *Journal of Medical Toxicology*, vol. 7, no. 1, pp. 60–66.

14] Bischoff, K, and Rumbeiha, W.K. (2012) 'Pet food recalls and pet food contaminants in small animals', *Veterinary Clinics of North America: Small Animal Practice*, vol. 42, no. 2, pp. 237–250.

15] Gorrel, C. (1998) 'Periodontal disease and diet in domestic pets', *Journal of Nutrition*, vol. 128, no. 12 (Suppl), pp. 2712S–2714S.

16] Marx, F. R., Machado, G. S., Pezzali, J. G., Marcolla, C. S., Kessler, A. M., Ahlstrøm, Ø. and Trevizan, L. (2016) 'Raw beef bones as chewing items to reduce dental calculus in Beagle dogs', *Australian Veterinary Journal*, vol. 94, nos. 1–2, pp. 18–23.

17] Harvey, C., Serfilippi, L. and Barnvos, D. (2015) 'Effect of Frequency of Brushing Teeth on Plaque and Calculus Accumulation and Gingivitis in Dogs', *Journal of Veterinary Dentistry*, vol. 32, no. 1, pp. 16–21.

18] Quest, B. W. (2013) 'Oral health benefits of a daily dental chew in dogs', *Journal of Veterinary Dentistry*, vol. 30, no. 2, pp. 84–87.

19] Roudebush, P., Logan, E. and Hale, F. A. (2005) 'Evidence-based veterinary dentistry: a systematic review of homecare for prevention of periodontal disease in dogs and cats', *Journal of Veterinary Dentistry*, vol. 22, no. 1, pp. 6–15.

20] Pavlović, D., Gomerčić, T., Gužvica, G., Kusak, J. and Huber, Đ. (2007) 'Prevalence of dental pathology in wolves (*Canis lupus L.*) in Croatia', *Veterinarski Arhiv*, vol. 77, no. 3, pp. 291–297.

21] Carlsen, M. H., Halvorsen, B. L., Holte, K., Bøhn, S. K., Dragland, S., Sampson, L., Willey, C., Senoo, H., Umezono, Y., Sanada, C., Barikmo, I., Berhe, N., Willett, W. C., Phillips, K. M., Jacobs, D. R. and Blomhoff, R. (2010) 'The total antioxidant content of more than 3100 foods, beverages, spices, herbs and supplements used worldwide', *Nutrition Journal*, vol. 9, no. 1, p. 3.

22] Spitze, A. R., Wong, D. L., Rogers, Q. R. and Fascetti, A. J. (2003) 'Taurine concentrations in animal feed ingredients; cooking influences taurine content', *Journal of Animal Physiology and Animal Nutrition*, vol. 87, nos. 7–8, pp. 251–262.

23] Gagné, J. W., Wakshlag, J. J., Center, S. A., Rutzke, M. A. and Glahn, R. P. (2013) 'Evaluation of calcium, phosphorus, and selected trace mineral status in commercially available dry foods formulated for dogs', *Journal of the American Veterinary Medical Association*, vol. 243, no. 5, pp. 658–666.

24] Ahlstrøm, Ø., Krogdahl, A., Vhile, S. G. and Skrede, A. (2004) 'Fatty Acid composition in commercial dog foods', *The Journal of Nutrition*, vol. 134, no. 8 (Suppl), pp. 2145S–2147S.

25] Kerr, K. R., Beloshapka, A. N., Morris, C. L., Parsons, C. M., Burke, S. L., Utterback, P. L. and Swanson, K. S. (2013) 'Evaluation of four raw meat diets using domestic cats, captive exotic felids, and cecectomized roosters', *Journal of Animal Science*, vol. 91, no. 1, pp. 225–237.

26] Singleton, C., Wack, R. and Larsen, R. S. (2012) 'Bacteriologic and nutritional evaluation of a commercial raw meat diet as part of a raw meat safety program', *Zoo Biology*, vol. 31, no. 5, pp. 574–585.

27] Dillitzer, N., Becker, N. and Kienzle, E. (2011) 'Intake of minerals, trace elements and vitamins in bone and raw food rations in adult dogs', *British Journal of Nutrition*, (S1), pp. S53–56.

28] Kawaguchi, K., Braga, I. S., Takahashi, A., Ochiai, K. and Itakura, C. (1993) 'Nutritional secondary hyperparathyroidism occurring in a strain of German shepherd puppies', *Japanese Journal of Veterinary Research*, vol. 41, nos. 2–4, pp. 89–96.

29] Schlesinger, D. P. and Joffe, D. J. (2011) 'Raw food diets in companion animals: a critical review', *The Canadian veterinary journal*, 52(1), pp. 50–54.

30] Kölle, P. and Schmidt, M. (2015) '[Raw-meat-based diets (RMBD) as a feeding principle for dogs]', *Tierarztliche Praxis. Ausgabe K, Kleintiere / Heimtiere*, vol. 43, no. 6, p. 409–419.

31] Viviano, K. R., Lavergne, S. N., Goodman, L., Vanderwielen, B., Grundahl, L., Padilla, M. and Trepanier, L. A. (2009) 'Glutathione, cysteine, and ascorbate concentrations in clinically ill dogs and cats', *Journal of Veterinary Internal Medicine*, vol. 23, no. 2, pp. 250–257.

32] Lutz, S., Sewell, A. C., Bigler, B., Riond, B., Reusch, C. E. and Kook, P. H. (2012) 'Serum cobalamin, urine methylmalonic acid, and plasma total homocysteine concentrations in border collies and dogs of other breeds', *American Journal of Veterinary Research*, vol. 73, no. 8, pp. 1194–1199.

33] Czerwonka, M., Szterk, A. and Waszkiewicz-Robak, B. (2014) 'Vitamin B12 content in raw and cooked beef', *Meat Science*, vol. 96, no. 3, pp. 1371–1375.

34] Dillitzer, N., Becker, N. and Kienzle, E. (2011) 'Intake of minerals, trace elements and vitamins in bone and raw food rations in adult dogs', *British Journal of Nutrition*.

35] Strøm, P. C. and Arzi, B. (2014) 'Diagnostic imaging in veterinary dental practice. Complicated crown-root fracture of the mesial root of left mandibular 1st molar in a dog', *Journal of the American Veterinary Medical Association*, vol. 245, no. 12, pp. 1335–1337.

36] Chandler, M. (2014) 'The Raw Meaty Bones Diet?', proceedings of the *British Small Animal Veterinary Congress*, Birmingham, 3–6 April.

37] Marks, S. L., Rankin, S. C., Byrne, B. A. and Weese, J. S. (2011) 'Enteropathogenic Bacteria in Dogs and Cats: Diagnosis, Epidemiology, Treatment, and Control', *Journal of Veterinary Internal Medicine*, vol. 25, no. 6, pp. 1195–1208.

38] Plessas, I. N., Jull, P. and Volk, H. A. (2013) 'A case of canine discospondylitis and epidural empyema due to Salmonella species', *Canadian Veterinary Journal*, vol. 54, no. 6, pp. 595–598.

39] Philbey, A. W., Brown, F. M., Mather, H. A., Coia, J. E. and Taylor, D. J. (2009) 'Salmonellosis in cats in the United Kingdom: 1955 to 2007', *Veterinary Record*, vol. 164, no. 4, pp. 120–122.

40] Stiver, S. L., Frazier, K. S., Mauel, M. J. and Styer, E. L. (2003) 'Septicemic salmonellosis in two cats fed a raw-meat diet', *Journal of the American Animal Hospital Association*, vol. 39, no. 6, pp. 538–542.

41] Marks, S. L., Rankin, S. C., Byrne, B. A. and Weese, J. S. (2011) 'Enteropathogenic Bacteria in Dogs and Cats: Diagnosis, Epidemiology, Treatment, and Control', *Journal of Veterinary Internal Medicine*.

42] Penny, D., Henderson, S. M. and Brown, P. J. (2003) 'Raisin poisoning in a dog', *Veterinary Record*, vol. 152, no. 10, p. 308.

43] Axelsson, E., Ratnakumar, A., Arendt, M.-L., Maqbool, K., Webster, M. T., Perloski, M., Liberg, O., Arnemo, J. M., Hedhammar, A. and Lindblad-Toh, K. (2013) 'The genomic signature of dog domestication reveals adaptation to a starch-rich diet', *Nature*, vol. 495, no. 7441, pp. 360–364.

44] Torin, D. S., Freeman, L. M. and Rush, J. E. (2007) 'Dietary patterns of cats with cardiac disease', *Journal of the American Veterinary Medical Association*, vol. 230, no. 6, pp. 862–867.

45] Joffe, D. J. and Schlesinger, D. P. (2002) 'Preliminary assessment of the risk of

Salmonella infection in dogs fed raw chicken diets', *Canadian Veterinary Journal*, vol. 43, no. 6, pp. 441–442.

46] Weese, J. S., Rousseau, J. and Arroyo, L. (2005) 'Bacteriological evaluation of commercial canine and feline raw diets', *Canadian Veterinary Journal*, vol. 46, no. 6, pp. 513–516.

47] Strohmeyer, R. A., Morley, P. S., Hyatt, D. R., Dargatz, D. A., Scorza, A. V. and Lappin, M. R. (2006) 'Evaluation of bacterial and protozoal contamination of commercially available raw meat diets for dogs', *Journal of the American Veterinary Medical Association*, vol. 228, no. 4, pp. 537–542.

48] Morley, P. S., Strohmeyer, R. A., Tankson, J. D., Hyatt, D. R., Dargatz, D. A. and Fedorka-Cray, P. J. (2006) 'Evaluation of the association between feeding raw meat and *Salmonella enterica* infections at a greyhound breeding facility', *Journal of the American Veterinary Medical Association*, vol. 228, no. 10, pp. 1524–1532.

49] Leonard, E. K., Pearl, D. L., Finley, R. L., Janecko, N., Peregrine, A. S., Reid-Smith, R. J. and Weese, J. S. (2011) 'Evaluation of pet-related management factors and the risk of Salmonella spp. carriage in pet dogs from volunteer households in Ontario (2005–2006)', *Zoonoses and Public Health*, vol. 58, no. 2, pp. 140–149.

50] Finley, R., Ribble, C., Aramini, J., Vandermeer, M., Popa, M., Litman, M. and Reid-Smith, R. (2007) 'The risk of salmonellae shedding by dogs fed salmonella-contaminated commercial raw food diets', *Canadian Veterinary Journal*, vol. 48, no. 1, pp. 69–75.

51] Finley, R., Reid-Smith, R., Ribble, C., Popa, M., Vandermeer, M. and Aramini, J. (2008) 'The occurrence and antimicrobial susceptibility of salmonellae isolated from commercially available canine raw food diets in three Canadian cities', *Zoonoses and Public Health*, vol. 55, nos. 8–10, pp. 462–469.

52] Lefebvre, S. L., Reid-Smith, R., Boerlin, P. and Weese, J. S. (2008) 'Evaluation of the risks of shedding salmonellae and other potential pathogens by therapy dogs fed raw diets in Ontario and Alberta', *Zoonoses and Public Health*, vol. 55, nos. 8–10, pp. 470–480.

53] Lenz, J., Joffe, D., Kauffman, M., Zhang, Y. and LeJeune, J. (2009) 'Perceptions, practices, and consequences associated with foodborne pathogens and the feeding of raw meat to dogs', *Canadian Veterinary Journal*, vol. 50, no. 6, pp. 637–643.

54] Jenkins, D. J., Lievaart, J. J., Boufana, B., Lett, W. S., Bradshaw, H. and Armua-Fernandez, M. T. (2014) '*Echinococcus granulosus* and other intestinal helminths: current status of prevalence and management in rural dogs of eastern Australia', *Australian Veterinary Journal*, vol. 92, no. 8, pp. 292–298.

55] Olkkola, S., Kovanen, S., Roine, J., Hänninen, M.-L., Hielm-Björkman, A. and Kivistö, R. (2015) 'Population genetics and antimicrobial susceptibility of canine campylobacter isolates collected before and after a raw feeding experiment', *PloS one*. vol. 10, no. 7, p. e0132660.

56] Nilsson, O. (2015) 'Hygiene quality and presence of ESBL-producing *Escherichia coli* in raw food diets for dogs', *Infection Ecology & Epidemiology*, vol. 5, p. 28758.

57] Naziri, Z., Derakhshandeh, A., Firouzi, R., Motamedifar, M. and Shojaee Tabrizi, A. (2016) 'DNA fingerprinting approaches to trace Escherichia coli sharing between dogs and owners', *Journal of Applied Microbiology*, vol. 120, no. 2, pp. 460–468.

58] de Brito, A. F., de Souza, L. C., da Silva, A. V. and Langoni, H. (2002) 'Epidemiological and serological aspects in canine toxoplasmosis in animals with nervous symptoms', *Memorias do Instituto Oswaldo Cruz*, vol. 97, no. 1, pp. 31–35.

59] Mitchell, S., Bell, S., Wright, I., Wall, R., Jeckel, S., Blake, D., Marshall, P., Andrews, C., Lee, M. and Walsh, A. (2016) 'Tongue worm (Linguatula species) in stray dogs imported into the UK', *Veterinary Record*, vol. 179, no. 10, pp. 259–260.

60] Köhler, B., Stengel, C. and Neiger, R. (2012) 'Dietary hyperthyroidism in dogs', *Journal of Small Animal Practice*, vol. 53, no. 3, pp. 182–184.

61] Zeugswetter, F. K., Vogelsinger, K. and Handl, S. (2013) 'Hyperthyroidism in dogs caused by consumption of thyroid-containing head meat', *Schweizer Archiv fur Tierheilkunde*, vol. 155, no. 2, pp. 149–152.

62] Sontas, B. H., Schwendenwein, I. and Schäfer-Somi, S. (2014) 'Primary anestrus due to dietary hyperthyroidism in a miniature pinscher bitch', *Canadian Veterinary Journal*, vol. 55, no. 8, pp. 781–785.

63] Broome, M. R., Peterson, M. E., Kemppainen, R. J., Parker, V. J. and Richter, K. P. (2015) 'Exogenous thyrotoxicosis in dogs attributable to consumption of all-meat commercial dog food or treats containing excessive thyroid hormone: 14 cases (2008–2013)', *Journal of the American Veterinary Medical Association*, vol. 246, no. 1, pp. 105–111.

64] Lopes, F. M., Gioso, M. A., Ferro, D. G., Leon-Roman, M. A., Venturini, M. A. F. A. and Correa, H. L. (2005) 'Oral fractures in dogs of Brazil—a retrospective study', *Journal of Veterinary Dentistry*, vol. 22, no. 2, pp. 86–90.

65] Schlesinger, D. P. and Joffe, D. J. (2011) 'Raw food diets in companion animals: a critical review', *The Canadian veterinary journal*.

66] Strohmeyer, R. A., Morley, P. S., Hyatt, D. R., Dargatz, D. A., Scorza, A. V. and Lappin, M. R. (2006) 'Evaluation of bacterial and protozoal contamination of commercially available raw meat diets for dogs', *Journal of the American Veterinary Medical Association*.

67] Raw Fit Pet (2013) *Survey Results* [Online], Available at http://rawfitpet.wix site.com/rawfitpet/survey-results (Accessed 11 January 2017).

68] American Veterinary Medical Association AVMA (n.d.) Raw or Undercooked Animal-Source Protein in Cat and Dog Diets [Online], Available at www.avma. org/KB/Policies/Pages/Raw-or-Undercooked-Animal-Source-Protein-in-Cat-and-Dog-Diets.aspx (Accessed 11 January 2017).

69] American Animal Hospital Association AAHA (2011) *Raw Protein Diet* [Online], Available at www.aaha.org/professional/resources/raw_protein_diet. aspx (Accessed 11 January 2017).

70] British Small Animal Veterinary Association BSAVA (2014) *Companion Animal Nutrition* [Online], Available at www.bsava.com/Resources/Veterinary-resources/Position-statements/Companion-animal-nutrition (Accessed 11 January 2017).

71] Canadian Veterinary Medical Association CVMA (2012) *Raw food diets for*

313

*pets—Canadian Veterinary Medical Association and Public Health Agency of Canada joint position statement* [Online], Available at www.canadianveterinarians. net/documents/raw-food-diets-for-pets (Accessed 11 January 2017).

72] World Small Animal Association WSAVA (2011) *Nutritional Assessment Guidelines* [Online], Available at www.wsava.org/sites/default/files/JSAP%20 WSAVA%20Global%20Nutritional%20Assessment%20Guidelines%20 2011_0.pdf (Accessed 11 January 2017).

73] Buff, P. R., Carter, R. A., Bauer, J. E. and Kersey, J. H. (2014) 'Natural pet food: a review of natural diets and their impact on canine and feline physiology', *Journal of Animal Science*, vol. 92, no. 9, pp. 3781–3791.

74] Bosch, G., Hagen-Plantinga, E. A. and Hendriks, W. H. (2015) 'Dietary nutrient profiles of wild wolves: insights for optimal dog nutrition?', *British Journal of Nutrition*, vol. 113, Suppl 1, pp. S40–54.

75] Inoue, M., Hasegawa, A., Hosoi, Y. and Sugiura, K. (2015) 'A current life table and causes of death for insured dogs in Japan', *Preventive Veterinary Medicine*, vol. 120, no. 2, pp. 210–218.

§

## Chapter Eight – Acupuncture

01] Fulder, S. (1998) 'The basic concepts of alternative medicine and their impact on our views of health', in Lee-Treweek, G., Heller, T., Spurr, S., MacQueen, H. and Katz, J. (eds) *Perspectives on Complementary and Alternative Medicine: A Reader*, Abingdon, Routledge/The Open University, p 5.

02] Kavoussi, B. (2009) 'The untold story of acupuncture', *Focus on Alternative and Complementary Therapies*, vol. 14, no. 4, pp. 276–286.

03] Encyclopedia Britannica (2016) *Xia Dynasty – Chinese History* [Online]. Available at www.britannica.com/topic/Xia-dynasty (Accessed 9 April 2016).

04] Bynum, W. (2008) *The History of Medicine: A Very Short Introduction*, Oxford, Oxford University Press, pp. 6–7.

05] Schoen, A. M. (ed) (1994) *Veterinary Acupuncture: Ancient Art to Modern Medicine*, Goleta, American Veterinary Publications, p. 1.

06] Association of British Acupuncturists (ABVA) (n.d.) *What is Acupuncture?* [Online]. Available at www.abva.co.uk/pet-owner-area/what-is-acupuncture (Accessed 15 April 2017).

07] Lin, J. and Panzer, R. (1994) 'Use of Chinese herbal medicine in veterinary science: History and perspectives', *Revue Scientifique et Technique*, vol. 13, no. 2, pp. 425–432.

08] Gaynor, J. S. (2005) 'Therapeutic Use of Acupuncture for Pain Control', in Ettinger, S. J. and Feldman, E. C. (eds) *Textbook of Veterinary Internal Medicine: Diseases of the Dog and Cat*, 6th edn, St. Louis, Elsevier Saunders, p. 533.

09] Day, C. E. I. (2004) 'Alternative Medicine', in Andrews, A. H., Blowey, R. W., Boyd, H. and Eddy, R. G. (eds) *Bovine Medicine Diseases and Husbandry of Cattle*, 2nd edn, Oxford, Blackwell Science, p. 1091.

10] Unschuld, P. U. (1985) *Medicine in China: A History of Ideas*, Berkeley, University of California Press, p. 2.

11] Ramey, D., Imrie, R. H. and Buell, P. D. (2001) 'Veterinary Acupuncture and Traditional Chinese Medicine: Facts and Fallacies', *Compendium on Continuing Education*, vol 23, no. 2, pp. 188–193.

12] Schwartz, C. (1996) *Four Paws, Five Directions: A Guide to Chinese Medicine for Cats and Dogs*, Berkely, Celestial Arts Publishing, p. v.

13] Concon, A. A. (1979) 'Energetic concepts of classical Chinese acupuncture American', *Journal of Acupuncture*, vol. 7, no. 1, pp. 41–47.

14] Imrie, R. H., Ramey, D. W., Buell, P. D., Ernst, E. and Basser, S. P. (2001) 'Veterinary Acupuncture and Historical Scholarship: Claims for the Antiquity of Acupuncture', *The Scientific Review of Alternative Medicine*, vol. 5, no 3, pp. 135–141.

15] Jaggar, D. (1994) 'History and Concepts of Veterinary Acupuncture', in Schoen, A. M. (ed) (1994) *Veterinary Acupuncture: Ancient Art to Modern Medicine*, Goleta, American Veterinary Publications, p. 5.

16] White, S. S. (1994) 'Acupuncture of Horses in China', in Schoen, A. M. (ed) *Veterinary Acupuncture: Ancient Art to Modern Medicine*, Goleta, American Veterinary Publications, p. 581.

17] University of Pennsylvania Museum of Archaeology and Anthropology collections (2016) *Relief: object no. C395* [Online]. Available at www.penn.museum/collections/object/167942 (Accessed 26 October 2016).

18] Jaggar, D. (1994) 'History and Concepts of Veterinary Acupuncture', in Schoen, A. M. (ed) (1994) *Veterinary Acupuncture: Ancient Art to Modern Medicine*, p. 13.

19] Ramey, D., Imrie, R. H. and Buell, P. D. (2001) 'Veterinary Acupuncture and Traditional Chinese Medicine: Facts and Fallacies'.

20] Lin, J. and Panzer, R. (1994) 'Use of Chinese herbal medicine in veterinary science: History and perspectives'.

21] Jaggar, D. (1994) 'History and Concepts of Veterinary Acupuncture', in Schoen, A. M. (ed) (1994) *Veterinary Acupuncture: Ancient Art to Modern Medicine*, p. 13.

22] Buell, P. D., May, T. and Ramey, D. (2010) 'Greek and Chinese horse medicine: deja vu all over again', *Sudhoffs Archiv*, vol 94, no. 1, pp. 31–56.

23] Jaggar, D. (1994) 'History and Concepts of Veterinary Acupuncture', in Schoen, A. M. (ed) (1994) *Veterinary Acupuncture: Ancient Art to Modern Medicine*, p. 14.

24] Ramey, D., Imrie, R. H. and Buell, P. D. (2001) 'Veterinary acupuncture and Traditional Chinese Medicine: Facts and Fallacies'.

25] Ramey, D. W. (2000) 'Do acupuncture points and meridians actually exist?', *Compendium on Continuing Education*, vol. 22, no. 12, pp. 1132–1136.

26] White, S. S. (1994), in Schoen, A. M. (ed) *Veterinary Acupuncture: Ancient Art to Modern Medicine*, p. 584.

27] Lindley, S. (as Scott) (2001) 'Developments in Veterinary Acupuncture', *Acupuncture in Medicine*, vol. 19, no. 1, pp. 27–31.

28] Lindley, S. (as Scott) (2001) 'Developments in Veterinary Acupuncture'.

29] Kavoussi, B. (2009) 'The untold story of acupuncture'.

30] Unschuld, P. U. (1998) *Chinese Medicine* (trans. N. Wiseman), Brookline, Massachusetts, Paradigm Publications, p106–107.

31] Ramey, D. W. (2000) 'Do acupuncture points and meridians actually exist?'.

32] Ramey, D. and Buell P. D. (2004) 'A true history of acupuncture', *Focus on Alternative and Complementary Therapy*, vol. 9, no. 4, pp. 269–273.

33] Kavoussi, B. (2009) 'The untold story of acupuncture'.

34] Walker, J. (2013) *How to Cure the Plague and Other Curious Remedies*, London, British Library, p. 66–67.

35] Jaggar, D. (1994) 'History and Concepts of Veterinary Acupuncture', in Schoen, A. M. (ed) (1994) *Veterinary Acupuncture: Ancient Art to Modern Medicine*, p. 13.

36] Unschuld, P. U. (1998) *Chinese Medicine*, p11–22.

37] Kavoussi, B. (2009) 'The untold story of acupuncture'.

38] Ramey, D. and Buell P. D. (2004) 'A true history of acupuncture'.

39] Christie, D. (1914) *Thirty years in Moukden 1883–1913: Being the Experiences and Recollections of Dugald Christie, C.M.G.*, London, Constable and Company Ltd.

40] Bivins, R. (2007) *Alternative Medicine? A History*, Oxford, Oxford University press, pp. 69–73 and 122–131.

41] Unschuld, P. U. (1998) *Chinese Medicine*, p. 110.

42] Reston, J. (1971) 'Now, about my operation in Peking', *New York Times*, 26 July, pp. 1 and 6.

43] Kavoussi, B. (2009) 'The untold story of acupuncture'.

44] Beyerstein, B. L. and Sampson, W. (1996) 'Traditional Medicine and Pseudoscience in China: A Report of the Second CSICOP Delegation (Part 1)', *Skeptical Inquirer Magazine*, vol 20, no. 4, July/August 1996 [Online]. Available at www.csicop.org/si/show/china_conference_1 (Accessed 1 February 2016).

45] Bauer, M. (2004) 'An Interview with Dr Paul Unschuld, Part One', *Acupuncture Today*, vol. 5, no. 7.

46] Kavoussi, B. (2009) 'The untold story of acupuncture'.

47] Xinnong, C. (ed) (1987) *Chinese Acupuncture and Moxibustion*, 1996 reprint, Beijing, Foreigh Languages Press, Foreword and p. xv.

48] Unschuld, P. U. (1998) *Chinese Medicine*, p 1.

49] Keng H. C. and T'ao N. H. (1980) 'Evaluation of Acupuncture Anesthesia Must Seek Truth from Facts', in Unschuld, P.U. (1985) *Medicine in China, A History of Ideas*, Berkeley, University of California Press, pp. 360–366.

50] Bauer, M. (2004) 'An Interview with Dr Paul Unschuld, Part One'.

51] Kavoussi, B. (2009) 'The untold story of acupuncture'.

52] Jourdan, A. (2016) 'China to consolidate drug market, promote traditional medicines', *Reuters*, 15 February [Online]. Available at http://uk.reuters.com/article/us-china-pharmaceuticals-idUKKCN0VO07S (Accessed 15 April 2017).

53] Unschuld, P. U. (1998) *Chinese Medicine*, p 2.

54] Xinhua (2006) 'Traditional Chinese medicine losing out to western drugs: online survey', *People's Daily Online* 30 October [Online]. Available at http://en.people.cn/200610/30/eng20061030_316501.html (Accessed 6 November 2016).

55] Kimm, J. (2015) 'Acupuncture and herbal medicine use in animals', *Companion*, June, pp. 22–25.

56] Bauer, M. (2004) 'An Interview with Dr Paul Unschuld, Part One'.

57] Simon, J., Guiraud, G., Esquerre, J. P., Lazorthes, Y. and Guiraud, R. (1988) 'Acupuncture meridians demythified. Contribution of radiotracer methodology', *Presse Medicale*, vol. 17, no. 26, pp. 1341–1344.

58] Lazorthes, Y., Esquerré. J. P., Simon, J., Guiraud, G. and Guiraud, R. (1990) 'Acupuncture meridians and radiotracers', *Pain*, vol. 40, no. 1, pp. 109–112.

59] Ramey, D.W. (2000) 'Do acupuncture points and meridians actually exist?'.

60] Sung, B., Kim, M. S., Lee, B-C., Ahn, S-H., Hwang, S-Y. and Soh, K-S. (2010) 'A cytological observation of the fluid in the primo-nodes and vessels on the surfaces of mammalian internal organs', *Biologia*, vol. 65, no. 5, pp. 914–918.

61] Ramey, D. W. (2000) 'Do acupuncture points and meridians actually exist?'.

62] Moroz, A. (1999) 'Issues in acupuncture research: The failure of quantitative methodologies and the possibilities for viable, alternative solutions', *American Journal of Acupuncture*, vol. 27, pp. 95–103.

63] Molsberger, A. F., Manickavasagan, J., Abholz, H. H., Maixner, W. B. and Endres, H. G. (2012) 'Acupuncture points are large fields: The fuzziness of acupuncture point localization', *European Journal of Pain*, vol. 16, pp. 1264–1270.

64] Lindley, S. (2006) 'Veterinary acupuncture: a Western, scientific approach', *In Practice*, vol. 28, no. 9, pp. 544–547.

65] Gough, A. (2011) 'Complementary and Alternative Veterinary Medicine: Controversy and Criticism', *Veterinary Times* [Online]. Available at www.vet-times.co.uk/article/complementary-and-alternative-vet-medicine-controversy-and-criticism (Accessed 5 November 2016). [A copy of this interview can be found in the appendix].

66] Moroz, A., Freed, B., Tiedemann, L., Bang, H., Howell, M. and Park, J. J. (2013) 'Blinding Measured: A Systematic Review of Randomized Controlled Trials of Acupuncture', *Evidence-based Complementary and Alternative Medicine*, vol. 2013, Article ID 708251 [Online]. doi.org/10.1155/2013/708251 (Accessed 6 November 2016).

67] Moroz, A. (1999) 'Issues in acupuncture research: The failure of quantitative methodologies and the possibilities for viable, alternative solutions'.

68] Resch, K. L. and Ernst, E. (1995) ['Proving the effectiveness of complementary therapy. Analysis of the literature exemplified by acupuncture']-[Article in German], /*Fortschritte der Medizin*/, vol. 113, no. 5, pp. 49–53.

69] Ernst, E. and White, A. R. (1997) 'A review of problems in clinical acupuncture research', *American Journal of Chinese Medicine*, vol. 25, no. 1, pp. 3–11.

70] Bullock, M. L., Kiresuk, T. J., Sherman, R. E., Lenz, S. K., Culliton, P. D., Boucher, T. A. and Nolana, C. J. (2002) 'A large randomized placebo controlled study of auricular acupuncture for alcohol dependence', *Journal of Substance Abuse Treatment*, vol. 22, no. 2, pp. 71–77.

71] Goddard, G., Karibe, H., McNeill, C. and Villafuerte, E. (2002) 'Acupuncture and sham acupuncture reduce muscle pain in myofascial pain patients', *Journal of Orofacial Pain*, vol. 16, no. 1, pp. 71–76.

72] Gaw A. C., Chang L. W. and Shaw, L. C. (1975) 'Efficacy of acupuncture on osteoarthritic pain. A controlled, double-blind study', *New England Journal of Medicine*, vol. 293, no. 8, pp. 375–378.

73] Hielm-Bjorkman, A., Raekallio, M., Kuusela, E., Saarto, E., Markkola, A. and Tulamo, R. M. (2001) 'Double-blind evaluation of implants of gold wire at acupuncture points in the dog as a treatment for osteoarthritis induced by hip dysplasia', *Veterinary Record*, vol. 149, no. 15, pp. 452–456.

74] Yuan, J., Purepong, N., Kerr, D. P., Park, J., Bradbury, I. and McDonough, S. (2008) 'Effectiveness of Acupuncture for Low Back Pain: A Systematic Review', *Spine*, vol. 33, no. 23 pp. E887-E900.

75] Habacher, G., Pittler, M. H. and Ernst, E. (2006) 'Effectiveness of acupuncture in veterinary medicine: A systematic review', *Journal of Veterinary Internal Medicine*, vol. 20, no. 3, pp. 480–488.

76] Lindley, S. (2006) 'Veterinary acupuncture: a Western, scientific approach'.

77] Lindley, S. (2014) 'Perspectives: Acupuncture for dogs', *Companion*, June, pp. 8–12.

78] Iff, I. (2015) 'Novel Pain Management Options: Acupuncture', *BSAVA.com* [Podcast]. 10 April. Available at www.bsavalectures.com/audio_files/congress2015/Hall%2007/Isabelle%20Iff%2001.mp3 (Accessed 5 November 2016).

79] Sanderson, R. O., Beata, C., Flipo, R. M., Genevois, J. P., Macias, C., Tacke, S., Vezzoni, A. and Innes, J. F. (2009) 'Systematic Review of the Management of Canine Arthritis', *Veterinary Record*, vol. 164, no. 14, pp. 418–424.

80] Jaeger, G. T., Larsen, S., Søli, N. and Moe, L. (2007) 'Two years follow-up study of the pain-relieving effect of gold bead implantation in dogs with hip-joint arthritis', *Acta Veterinaria Scandinavica*, vol. 23, no. 49, p. 9.

81] Hielm-Bjorkman, A., Raekallio, M., Kuusela, E., Saarto, E., Markkola, A. and Tulamo, R. M. (2001) 'Double-blind evaluation of implants of gold wire at acupuncture points in the dog as a treatment for osteoarthritis induced by hip dysplasia'.

82] Lie, K. I., Jæger, G., Nordstoga, K. and Moe, L. (2001) 'Inflammatory response to therapeutic gold bead implantation in canine hip joint osteoarthritis', *Veterinary Pathology*, vol. 48, no. 6, pp. 1118–1124.

83] Robinson, N. (2008) Gold Bead Implants – Medicine or Malpractice [Online] Available at https://www.onehealthsim.org/gold-bead-implants-medicine-or-malpractice (Accessed 6 November 2016).

84] Moffet, H. H. (2009) 'Sham acupuncture may be as efficacious as true acupuncture: a systematic review of clinical trials', *Journal of Alternative and Complementary Medicine*, vol. 15, no. 3, pp. 213–216.

85] Enblom, A. (2008) *Dissertation on Health Sciences Thesis No. 1088: Nausea and vomiting in patients receiving acupuncture, sham acupuncture or standard care during radiotherapy*, thesis for doctoral degree, Linköping, Linköping University Faculty of Health Sciences, p. 2.

86] Linde, K., Streng, A., Jürgens, S., Hoppe, A., Brinkhaus, B., Witt, C., Wagenpfeil, S., Pfaffenrath, V., Hammes, M. G., Weidenhammer, W., Willich,

S. N. and Melchart, D. (2005) 'Acupuncture for Patients With Migraine: A Randomized Controlled Trial', *Journal of the American Medical Association*, vol. 293, no. 17, pp. 2118–2125.

87] Kaptchuk, T. J., Kelley, J. M., Conboy, L. A., Davis, R. B., Kerr, C. E., Jacobson, E. E., Kirsch, I., Rosa N Schyner, R. N., Bong Hyun Nam, B. H., Nguyen, L. T. Park, M., Rivers, A. L., McManus,C., Kokkotou, E., Drossman, D. A., Goldman, P. and Lembo, A. J. (2008) 'Components of placebo effect: randomised controlled trial in patients with irritable bowel syndrome', *British Medical Journal*, vol. 336, pp. 999–1003.

88] Chae, Y., Lee, I. S., Jung, W. M., Park, K., Park, H. J. and Wallraven, C. (2015) 'Psychophysical and neurophysiological responses to acupuncture stimulation to incorporated rubber hand', *Neuroscience Letters*, vol. 591, pp. 48–52.

89] Colquhoun, D. and Novella, S. P. (2013) 'Acupuncture Is Theatrical Placebo', *Anesthesia and Analgesia*, vol. 116, no. 6, pp. 1360–1363.

90] Jaeger, G. T., Larsen, S. and Moe, L. (2005) 'Stratification, blinding and placebo effect in a randomized, double blind placebo-controlled clinical trial of gold bead implantation in dogs with hip dysplasia', *Acta Veterinaria Scandinavica*, vol. 46, nos. 1–2, pp. 57–68.

91] Muñana, K. R., Zhang, D. and Patterson, E. E. (2010) 'Placebo effect in canine epilepsy trials', *Journal of Veterinary Internal Medicine*, vol. 24, no. 1, pp. 166–170.

92] Conzemius, M. and Evans, R. (2012) 'Caregiver placebo effect for dogs with lameness from osteoarthritis', *Journal of the American Veterinary Medical Association*, vol. 241, no. 10, pp 1314–1319.

93] Ernst, E. (2006) 'Acupuncture – a critical analysis', *Journal of Internal Medicine*, vol. 259, no. 2, pp 125–137.

94] Melzack, R. and Wall, P. D. (1969) 'Pain mechanisms: a new theory', *Science*, vol. 150, no. 3699, pp. 971–979.

95] Iff, I. (2015) 'Novel Pain Management Options: Acupuncture'.

96] Lindley, S. (2006) 'Veterinary acupuncture: a Western, scientific approach'.

97] Moffet, H. H. (2009) 'Acupuncture: Will Ugly Facts Kill the Beautiful Theories', *Journal of Alternative and Complementary Medicine*, vol. 15, no. 12, pp. 1263–1264.

98] Lundeberg, T., Lund, I., Näslund, J. and Thomas, M. (2008) 'The Emperors sham—wrong assumption that sham needling is sham', *Acupuncture in Medicine*, vol. 26, no. 4, pp. 239–242.

99] Lindley, S. (2006) 'Veterinary acupuncture: a Western, scientific approach'.

100] Gough, A. (2011) 'Complementary and Alternative Veterinary Medicine: Controversy and Criticism'.

101] Colquhoun, D. and Novella, S. P. (2013) 'Acupuncture Is Theatrical Placebo'.

102] Moffet, H. H. (2009) 'Acupuncture: Will Ugly Facts Kill the Beautiful Theories'.

103] Lindley, S. (as Scott) (2001) 'Developments in Veterinary Acupuncture'.

104] McGlone, F. (2008) 'British Association Festival of Science: The importance of touch and the pleasure of stroking', *Guardian* [Podcast]. 18 September. Available at https://www.theguardian.com/science/audio/2008/sep/16/pleasurable. stroking.francis.mcglone

§

## Chapter Nine – The Anti-Vaccination Movement

01] Centre for Disease Control CDC (2013) *Ten Great Public Health Achievements in the 20th Century* [Online]. Available at www.cdc.gov/about/history/tengpha. htm (Accessed 10 January 2017).

02] Fine, P., Eames, K. and Heymann, D. L. (2011) '"Herd immunity": a rough guide', *Clinical Infectious Diseases*, vol. 52, no. 7, pp. 911–916.

03] Reichert, T. A., Sugaya, N., Fedson, D. S., Glezen, W. P., Simonsen, L. and Tashiro, M. (2001) 'The Japanese experience with vaccinating schoolchildren against influenza', *New England Journal of Medicine*, vol. 344, no. 12, pp. 889–896.

04] Lombard, M., Pastoret, P. P. and Moulin, A. M. (2007) 'A brief history of vaccines and vaccination', *Revue Scientifique et Technique*, vol. 26, no. 1, pp. 29–48.

05] Nunes, J. K., Woods, C., Carter, T., Raphael, T., Morin, M. J., Diallo, D., Leboulleux, D., Jain, S., Loucq, C., Kaslow, D. C. and Birkett, A. J. (2014) 'Development of a transmission-blocking malaria vaccine: progress, challenges, and the path forward', *Vaccine*, vol. 32, no. 43, pp. 5531–5539.

06] Wolfe, R. M. and Sharp, L. K. (2002) 'Anti-vaccinationists past and present', *British Medical Journal (Clinical research ed.)*, vol. 325, no. 7361, pp. 430–432.

07] Busse, J. W., Morgan, L. and Campbell, J. B. (2005) 'Chiropractic antivaccination arguments', *Journal of Manipulative and Physiological Therapeutics*, vol. 28, no. 5, pp. 367–373.

08] Colley, F. and Haas, M. (n.d.) 'Attitudes on immunization: a survey of American chiropractors', *Journal of Manipulative and Physiological Therapeutics*, vol. 17, no. 9, pp. 584–590.

09] Evans, M. W., Breshears, J., Campbell, A., Husbands, C. and Rupert, R. (2007) 'Assessment and risk reduction of infectious pathogens on chiropractic treatment tables', *Chiropractic and Osteopathy*, vol. 15, no. 1, p. 8.

10] Hall, H. (2009) '"I Reject Your Reality" – Germ Theory Denial and Other curiosities', *Science-based Medicine*, 9 December [Blog]. Available at www.sciencebasedmedicine.org/i-reject-your-reality (Accessed 20 January 2016).

11] British Homeopathic Society BHS (n.d.) *FAQs* [Online]. Available at www.britishhomeopathic.org/faqs (Accessed 20 January 2016).

12] Schmidt, K., Ernst, E. and Andrews (2002) 'Aspects of MMR. Survey shows that some homoeopaths and chiropractors advise against MMR', *British Medical Journal*, vol. 325, no. 7364, p. 597.

13] Flaherty, D. K. (2011) 'The vaccine-autism connection: a public health crisis caused by unethical medical practices and fraudulent science', *Annals of Pharmacotherapy*, vol. 45, no. 10, pp. 1302–1304.

14] O' Driscoll, C. (2005) *Pet Vaccination: An Institutionalised Crime* [Online].

Available at www.canine-health-concern.org.uk/PetVaccination.html (Accessed 23 January 2016).

15] Smith Squire, A. (2010) 'Vaccines "are making our dogs sick as vets cash in"', *Daily Mail*, 6 March [Online]. Available at www.dailymail.co.uk/news/article-1255863/Vaccines-making-dogs-sick-vets-cash-in.html (Accessed 10 January 2017).

16] O' Driscoll, C. (n.d.) *Canine Vaccine Survey* [Online]. Available at www.canine-health-concern.org.uk/caninevaccinesurvey.html (Accessed 10 January 2017).

17] Edwards, D.S., Henley, W.E., Ely, E. R. and Wood, J.L.N. (2004) 'Vaccination and ill-health in dogs: a lack of temporal association and evidence of equivalence', *Vaccine*, vol. 22, nos. 25–26, pp. 3270–3273.

18] Moore, G. E., Guptill, L. F., Ward, M. P., Glickman, N. W., Faunt, K. K., Lewis, H. B. and Glickman, L. T. (2005) 'Adverse events diagnosed within three days of vaccine administration in dogs', *Journal of the American Veterinary Medical Association*, vol. 227, no. 7, pp. 1102–1108.

19] Miyaji, K., Suzuki, A., Shimakura, H., Takase, Y., Kiuchi, A., Fujimura, M., Kurita, G., Tsujimoto, H. and Sakaguchi, M. (2012) 'Large-scale survey of adverse reactions to canine non-rabies combined vaccines in Japan', *Veterinary Immunology and Immunopathology*, vol. 145, no. 1, pp. 447–452.

20] Duval, D. and Giger, U. (1996) 'Vaccine-associated immune-mediated hemolytic anemia in the dog', *Journal of Veterinary Internal Medicine*, vol. 10, no. 5, pp. 290–295.

21] Carr, A. P., Panciera, D. L. and Kidd, L. (2002) 'Prognostic factors for mortality and thromboembolism in canine immune-mediated hemolytic anemia: a retrospective study of 72 dogs', *Journal of Veterinary Internal Medicine*, vol. 16, no. 5, pp. 504–509.

22] Burgess, K., Moore, A., Rand, W. and Cotter, S. M. (2000) 'Treatment of immune-mediated hemolytic anemia in dogs with cyclophosphamide', *Journal of Veterinary Internal Medicine*. vol. 14, no. 4, pp. 456–462.

23] Swann, J. W. and Skelly, B. J. (2015) 'Systematic review of prognostic factors for mortality in dogs with immune-mediated hemolytic anemia', *Journal of Veterinary Internal Medicine*, vol. 29, no. 1, pp. 7–13.

24] Day, M. J., Horzinek, M. C., Schultz, R. D. and Squires, R. A. (2016) 'WSAVA Guidelines for the vaccination of dogs and cats', *Journal of Small Animal Practice*, vol. 57, no. 1, pp. E1–E45.

25] Patel, M., Carritt, K., Lane, J., Jayappa, H., Stahl, M. and Bourgeois, M. (2015) 'Comparative efficacy of feline leukemia virus (FeLV) inactivated whole-virus vaccine and canarypox virus-vectored vaccine during virulent FeLV challenge and immunosuppression', *Clinical and Vaccine Immunology*, vol. 22, no. 7, pp. 798–805.

26] Sánchez-Vizcaíno, F., Jones, P. H., Menacere, T., Heayns, B., Wardeh, M., Newman, J., Radford, A. D., Dawson, S., Gaskell, R., Noble, P. J. M., Everitt, S., Day, M. J. and McConnell, K. (2015) 'Small animal disease surveillance', *Veterinary Record*, vol. 177, no. 23, pp. 591–594.

27] Hosie, M. J., Robertson, C. and Jarrett, O. (1989) 'Prevalence of feline leukaemia virus and antibodies to feline immunodeficiency virus in cats in the United Kingdom', *Veterinary Record*, vol. 125, no. 11, pp. 293–297.

28] Darkaoui, S., Fassi Fihri, O., Schereffer, J. L., Aboulfidaa, N., Wasniewski, M., Zouine, K., Bouslikhane, M., Yahia, K. I. S. and Cliquet, F. (2016) 'Immunogenicity and efficacy of Rabivac vaccine for animal rabies control in Morocco', *Clinical and Experimental Vaccine Research*, vol. 5, no. 1, pp. 60–69.

29] Spibey, N., Greenwood, N. M., Sutton, D., Chalmers, W. S. K. and Tarpey, I. (2008) 'Canine parvovirus type 2 vaccine protects against virulent challenge with type 2c virus', *Veterinary Microbiology*, vol. 128, nos. 1–2, pp. 48–55.

30] Abdelmagid, O. Y., Larson, L., Payne, L., Tubbs, A., Wasmoen, T. and Schultz, R. (2004) 'Evaluation of the efficacy and duration of immunity of a canine combination vaccine against virulent parvovirus, infectious canine hepatitis virus, and distemper virus experimental challenges', *Veterinary Therapeutics*, vol. 5, no. 3, pp. 173–186.

31] Hogenesch, H., Azcona-Olivera, J., Scott-Moncrieff, C., Snyder, P. W. and Glickman, L. T. (1999) 'Vaccine-induced autoimmunity in the dog', *Advances in Veterinary Medicine*, vol. 41, pp. 733–747.

32] Patel, M., Carritt, K., Lane, J., Jayappa, H., Stahl, M. and Bourgeois, M. (2015) 'Comparative efficacy of feline leukemia virus (FeLV) inactivated whole-virus vaccine and canarypox virus-vectored vaccine during virulent FeLV challenge and immunosuppression', *Clinical and Vaccine Immunology*, vol. 22, no. 7, pp. 798–805.

33] See: www.dogsnaturallymagazine.com/why-vets-are-getting-away-with-murder

§

## Chapter Ten – Homeopathy

01] Saxton, J. (2006) *Miasms as Practical Tools: A Homeopathic Approach to Chronic Disease*, Beaconsfield, Beaconsfield Publishers Ltd., pp. 8–9.

02] Campbell, A. (2013) *Homeopathy in Perspective: A Critical Appraisal*, Milton Keynes, Lightning Source UK Ltd., pp. 36–38.

03] Saxton, J. (2006) *Miasms as Practical Tools: A Homeopathic Approach to Chronic Disease*, p. 42.

04] Saxton, J. (2006) *Miasms as Practical Tools: A Homeopathic Approach to Chronic Disease*, p. 29.

05] Campbell, A. (2013) *Homeopathy in Perspective: A Critical Appraisal*, pp. 2–4.

06] Saxton, J. and Gregory, P. (2005) *Textbook of Veterinary Homeopathy*, Beaconsfield, Beaconsfield Publishers Ltd., p. 49.

07] Cherry, F. C. (1829) 'Case treated by vigorous depletion unsuccessful', *Farrier and Naturalist*, vol. 2, pp. 10–11.

08] Humphreys, F. (1860) *Manual of Veterinary Specific Homeopathy*, 3rd edn, New Delhi, Isha books (this edition 2013), p. 119.

09] Humphreys, F. (1860) *Manual of Veterinary Specific Homeopathy*, p. iii.

10] Mayhew, E. (1888) *The Illustrated Horse Doctor*, 16th edn, London, Wm. H. Allen & Co., p. 133.

11] Haehl, R. (1971 [1922]) *Samuel Hahnemann: His Life and Work*, Volume I (trans. M.L. Wheeler and F.J. Wheeler), New Delhi, B. Jain Publishers (P) Ltd., 11th impression (2013), pp. 10–11.

12] Haehl, R. (1971 [1922]) *Samuel Hahnemann: His Life and Work*, Volume I, pp. 35–36.

13] Haehl, R. (1971 [1922]) *Samuel Hahnemann: His Life and Work*, Volume I, p. 41.

14] Haehl, R. (1971 [1922]) *Samuel Hahnemann: His Life and Work*, Volume I, pp. 37–38.

15] Haehl, R. (1971 [1922]) *Samuel Hahnemann: His Life and Work*, Volume I, p. 66.

16] Campbell, A. (2013) *Homeopathy in Perspective: A Critical Appraisal*, pp. 19–22.

17] Haehl, R. (1971 [1922]) *Samuel Hahnemann: His Life and Work*, Volume I, pp. 317–320.

18] Hahnemann, S. (1983 [1921]) *Organon of Medicine*, 6th edn (trans. J. Kunzli, A. Naude and P. Pendleton), London, Orion, p. 18.

19] Haehl, R. (1971 [1922]) *Samuel Hahnemann: His Life and Work*, Volume I, pp. 322–323.

20] Hahnemann, S. (1983 [1921]) *Organon of Medicine*, p. 191, footnote c.

21] Hahnemann, S. (1983 [1921]) *Organon of Medicine*, p. 172.

22] Hahnemann, S. (1983 [1921]) *Organon of Medicine*, p. 191.

23] Haehl, R. (1971 [1922]) *Samuel Hahnemann: His Life and Work*, Volume I, p. 324.

24] Haehl, R. (1971 [1922]) *Samuel Hahnemann: His Life and Work*, Volume I, p. 38.

25] Park, R. L. (2000) *Voodoo Science: The Road From Foolishness to Fraud*, Oxford, New York, Oxford University Press, p. 52–58.

26] Haehl, R. (1971 [1922]) *Samuel Hahnemann: His Life and Work*, Volume I, p. 322.

27] Hahnemann, S. (1983 [1921]) *Organon of Medicine*, p. 189–190.

28] Saxton, J. and Gregory, P. (2005) *Textbook of Veterinary Homeopathy*, p. 31.

29] Chikramane, P. S., Suresh, A. K, Bellare, J. R. and Kane, S. G. (2010) 'Extreme homeopathic dilutions retain starting materials: A nanoparticulate perspective', *Homeopathy*, vol. 99, pp. 231–242.

30] Soil Association (2016) *Organic Standards Farming and Growing*, revision 17.4 August, [Online]. Available at https://www.soilassociation.org/media/1220/farming-and-growing-v17-4-august-2016.pdf (Accessed 15 April 2017).

31] Veterinary Medicines Directorate VMD (2016) *Guidance on applying to register, renew, or vary a Veterinary Homeopathic Remedy* [Online]. Available at https://www.gov.uk/guidance/apply-to-register-a-veterinary-homeopathic-remedy (Accessed 13 November 2016).

32] Colquhoun, D. (2012) *Another crackpot idea from homeopaths* [Online] Available at http://www.dcscience.net/improbable.html#water1 (Accessed 20 June 2016).

33] Wilson, R. W. (2005) *Homeopathic Pharmacy Notes on 'Dynamization'*, [Online].

Available at www.naturalworldhealing.com/notes-on-dynamization.htm (Accessed 20 June 2016).

34] Munns, C. (2014) *Revised theory of the quantum physics of potentisation of homeopathic medicine* [Online] Available at vixra.org/pdf/1312.0024v2.pdf (Accessed 20 June 2016).

35] Nordwall, S. (1981) *The potentiation problem: Some viewpoints from an anthroposophical perspective* [Online] Available at www.thebee.se/SCIENCE/Potprobl.htm (Accessed 20 June 2016).

36] Dayenas, E., Beauvais, F., Amara, J., Oberbaum, M., Robinzon, B., Miadonna, A., Tedeschit, A., Pomeranz, B., Fortner, P., Belon, P., Sainte-Laudy, J., Poitevin, B. and Benveniste, J. (1988) 'Human basophil degranulation triggered by very dilute antiserum against IgE', *Nature*, vol. 333, no. 30, pp. 816–818.

37] Maddox, J., Randi, J. and Stewart, W. W. (1988) 'High-dilution experiments a delusion', *Nature*, vol. 334, pp. 287–291.

38] Benveniste, J., Jurgens, P., Hsueh, W. and Aissa, J. (1997) 'Transatlantic Transfer of Digitized Antigen Signal by Telephone Link', *Journal of Allergy and Clinical Immunology*, vol. 99, no. 2, p. 75, (abstract 705).

39] Rao, M. L., Roy, R., Bell, I. R. and Hoover, R. (2007) 'The defining role of structure (including epitaxy) in the plausibility of homeopathy', *Homeopathy*, vol. 96, no. 3, pp. 175–182.

40] Kerr, M., Magrath, J., Wilson, P. and Hebbern, C. (2008) 'Comment on "The defining role of structure (including epitaxy) in the plausibility of homeopathy"', *Homeopathy*, vol. 97, no. 1, pp. 44–45.

41] Haehl, R. (1971 [1922]) *Samuel Hahnemann: His Life and Work*, Volume I, p. 322.

42] House of Lords Science and Technology Select Committee (2007) *6th Report of Session 2006–07 – Allergy. Volume II: Evidence* [Online], London, The Stationery Office Limited, p. 216, question 538. Available at www.publications.parliament.uk/pa/ld200607/ldselect/ldsctech/166/166ii.pdf (Accessed 18 November 2016).

43] Brien, S., Lewith, G. and Bryant, T. (2003) 'Ultramolecular homeopathy has no observable clinical effects. A randomized, double-blind, placebo-controlled proving trial of Belladonna 30C', *British Journal of Clinical Pharmacology*, vol. 56, no. 5, pp. 562–568.

44] Dantas, F. and Fisher, P. (2007) 'A systematic review of homeopathic pathogenetic trials ("provings") published in the United Kingdom from 1945 to 1995', *Homeopathy*, vol. 96, no. 1, pp. 4–16.

45] Goodyear, K., Lewith, G. and Low, J. L. (1998) 'Randomized double-blind placebo-controlled trial of homoeopathic "proving" for Belladonna C30', *Journal of the Royal Society of Medicine*, vol. 91, no. 11, pp. 579–582.

46] Vickers, A. J., Van Haselen, R. and Heger, M. (2001) 'Can homeopathically prepared mercury cause symptoms in healthy volunteers? A randomized, double-blind placebo-controlled trial', *Journal of Alternative and Complementary Medicine*, vol. 7, no. 2, pp. 141–148.

47] Walach, H. (1993) 'Does a highly diluted homeopathic drug act as a placebo in healthy volunteers? Experimental study of Belladonna 30C in a double blind crossover design – a pilot study', *Journal of Psychosomatic Research*, vol 37, no. 8, pp. 851–860.

48] Walach, H., Koster, H., Hennig, T. and Haag, G. (2001) 'The effects of homeopathic belladonna 30CH in healthy volunteers – a randomized, double-blind experiment', *Journal of Psychosomatic Research*, vol. 50, no. 3, pp. 155–160.

49] Walach, H., J Sherr, J., Schneider, R., Shabi, R., Bond, A. and Rieberer, G. (2004) 'Homeopathic proving symptoms: result of a local, non-local, or placebo process? A blinded, placebo-controlled pilot study', *Homeopathy*, vol. 93, pp. 179–185.

50] Walach, H. (2000) 'Magic of signs: a non-local interpretation of homeopathy', *British Homeopathic Journal*, vol. 89, pp.127–140. (Also published (1999) in *Journal of Scientific Exploration*, vol. 13, no. 2, pp. 291–315.)

51] Fraser, P. (2010) *Using Provings in Homeopathy*, London, Winter Press, pp. 14–16.

52] Scholten, J. (n.d.) *Dream proving* [Online]. Available at www.qjure.com/ remedy/dream-proving-0 (Accessed 14 November 2016).

53] Vithoulkas, G. (2008) 'British media attacks on homeopathy; Are they justified?', *Homeopathy*, vol. 97, no. 2, pp. 103–106.

54] Saxton, J. and Gregory, P. (2005) *Textbook of Veterinary Homeopathy*, p. 2.

55] HomeopathicVet.org (2014) *Veterinary Papers Peer Reviewed: Animal/Lab Studies by Name of Lead Author* [Online] Available at www.homeopathicvet.org/ Veterinary_Research_into_Homeopathy/Veterinary_Papers_Peer_Reviewed_ files/Animal%20Studies%20by%20Name%20of%20Lead%20Author.pdf (Accessed 23 December 2015).

56] Rational Veterinary Medicine (2011) *The best they can do* [Online] Available at www.rationalvetmed.org/the%20best%20they%20can%20do.html (Accessed 21 June 2016).

57] Hill, P. B., Hoare, J., Lau-Gillard, P., Rybnicek, J. and Mathie, R. T. (2009) 'Pilot study of the effect of individualised homeopathy on the pruritus associated with atopic dermatitis in dogs', *Veterinary Record*, vol. 164, pp. 364–370.

58] Egan, J. (1995) 'Evaluation of a homoeopathic treatment for subclinical mastitis', *Veterinary Record*, vol.137, p. 48.

59] Hektoen, L., Larsen, S., Ødegaard, S. A. and Løken, T. (2004) 'Comparison of homeopathy, placebo and antibiotic treatment of clinical mastitis in dairy cows – methodological issues and results from a randomized-clinical trial', *Journal of Veterinary Medicine*, series A, vol. 51, pp. 439–446.

60] Holmes, M. A., Cockcroft, P. D., Booth, C. E. and Heath, M. F. (2005) 'Controlled clinical trial of the effect of a homoeopathic nosode on the somatic cell counts in the milk of clinically normal dairy cows', *Veterinary Record*, vol. 156, pp. 565–567.

61] Scott, D. W., Miller, W. H., Senter, D. A., Cook, C. P, Kirker, J. E. and Cobb, S. M. (2002) 'Treatment of canine atopic dermatitis with a commercial homeopathic remedy: a single-blinded, placebo-controlled study', *Canadian Veterinary Journal*, vol. 43, no. 8, pp. 601–603.

62] de Verdier, K., Öhagen, P. and Alenius, S. (2003) 'No effect of a homeopathic preparation on neonatal calf diarrhoea in a randomised double-blind, placebo-controlled clinical trial', *Acta Veterinaria Scandinavica*, vol. 44, pp. 97–101.

63] Taylor, S. M., Mallon, T. R. and Green, W. P. (1989) 'Efficacy of a homoeo-pathic prophylaxis against experimental infection of calves by the bovine lung-worm *Dictyocaulus viviparus*', *Veterinary Record*, vol. 124, no. 1, pp. 15–17.

64] Day, C. E. (1984) 'Prevention of stillbirth in pigs using homoeopathy', *Veterinary Record*, vol. 114, p. 216.

65] Kleijnen, J., Knipschild, P. and ter Riet, G. (1991) 'Clinical trials of homoeopa-thy', *British Medical Journal*, vol. 9, no. 302, pp. 316–323.

66] Boissel, J. P., Cucherat, M., Haugh, M. and Gauthier, E. (1996) 'Critical litera-ture review on the effectiveness of homoeopathy: overview of data from homoeo-pathic medicine trials', In: *Homoeopathy Medicine Research Group: report to the European Commission Directorate General XII: science, research and development.* Brussels, Belgium pp. 195–210.

67] Linde, K. and Melchart, D. (1998) 'Randomized controlled trials of indi-vidualized homeopathy: a state-of-the-art review', *Journal of Alternative and Complementary Medicine*, vol. 4, no.4, pp. 371–388.

68] Cucherat, M., Haugh, M. C., Gooch, M. and Boissel, J. P. (2000) 'Evidence of clinical efficacy of homeopathy. A meta-analysis of clinical trials. HMRAG. Homeopathic Medicines Research Advisory Group', *European Journal of Clinical Pharmacology*, vol. 56, no. 1, pp. 27–33.

69] Shang, A., Huwiler-Müntener, K., Nartey, L., Jüni, P., Dörig, S., Sterne, J. A. C., Pewsner, D. and Egger, M. (2005) 'Are the clinical effects of homoeopathy placebo effects? Comparative study of placebo-controlled trials of homoeopathy and allopathy', *Lancet*, vol. 366, pp. 726–732.

70] Goldacre, B. (2007) 'Benefits and risks of homoeopathy (comment)', *Lancet*, vol. 370, pp. 1672–1673.

71] Olsen, O., Middleton, P., Ezzo, J., Gøtzsche, P. C., Hadhazy, V., Herxheimer, A., Kleijnen, J. and McIntosh, H. (2001) 'Quality of Cochrane reviews: assess-ment of sample from 1998', *British Medical Journal*, vol. 323, no. 7317, pp. 829–832.

72] Ernst, E. (2010) 'Homeopathy: what does the "best" evidence tell us? A Systematic Review', *Medical Journal of Australia*, vol. 192, no. 8, pp. 458–460.

73] Mathie, R. T., Frye, J. and Fisher, P. (2012) Homeopathic Oscillococcinum® for preventing and treating influenza and influenza-like illness, *Cochrane Database of Systematic Reviews 2012*, Issue 12, Art. No.: CD001957 [Online] DOI: 10.1002/14651858.CD001957.pub5 (Accessed 17 November 2016).

74] Mathie, R. T. and Clausen, J. (2014) 'Veterinary homeopathy: systematic review of medical conditions studied by randomised placebo-controlled trials', *Veterinary Record*, vol. 175, no. 15, pp. 373–381.

75] Hektoen, L., Larsen, S., Ødegaard, S.A. and Løken, T. (2004) 'Comparison of homeopathy, placebo and antibiotic treatment of clinical mastitis in dairy cows – methodological issues and results from a randomized-clinical trial', *Journal of Veterinary Medicine*, series A, vol. 51, pp. 439–446.

76] Camerlink, I., Ellinger, L., Bakker, E. J. and Lantinga, E. A. (2010) 'Homeopathy as replacement to antibiotics in the case of *Escherichia coli* diarrhoea in neonatal piglets', *Homeopathy*, vol. 99, no. 1, pp. 57–62.

77] Whitehead, M. (2015) *A critique of Camerlink et al (2010) Homeopathy 99:57–62* [Online]. Available at www.vetsurgeon.org/microsites/private/rational-medicine/p/homeopathy-critique.aspx (Accessed 21 June 2016).

78] HomeopathicVet.org (2014) *Systematic review counters argument of 'no reliable evidence' in veterinary homeopathy* [Online] Available at www.homeopathicvet. org/Veterinary_Research_into_Homeopathy/Welcome.html (Accessed 21 June 2016).

79] Mathie, R. T. and Clausen, J. (2015) 'Veterinary homeopathy: Systematic review of medical conditions studied by randomised trials controlled by other than placebo', *BioMedCentral Veterinary Research*, vol. 11, no. 236.

80] House of Commons Science and Technology Committee (2010) *Fourth Report of Session 2009–10 – Evidence Check 2: Homeopathy* [Online]. London, The Stationery Office Limited, pp. 28–29. Available at www.publications.parliament.uk/pa/cm200910/cmselect/cmsctech/45/45.pdf (Accessed 21 June 2016).

81] National Health and Medical Research Council NHMRC (2015) *Statement on Homeopathy and NHMRC Information Paper – Evidence on the effectiveness of homeopathy for treating health conditions* [Online] Available at https://www. nhmrc.gov.au/guidelines-publications/cam02 (Accessed 21 June 2016).

82] Robbins, M. (2010) 'Homeopathic association misrepresented evidence to MPs', *Guardian*, 5 February [Online] Available at https://www.theguardian. com/science/blog/2010/feb/04/homeopathic-association-evidence-commons-committee (Accessed 21 June 2016).

83] Schmidt, K. and Ernst, E. (2003) 'MMR vaccination advice over the internet', *Vaccine*, vol. 21, pp. 1044–1047.

84] Newcombe, J. R., East, J., McCartan, C. G., Staniek, G. and Jolley, S. A. (2003) 'Time for statement on unproven medicines', *Veterinary Times*, vol. 33, no. 9, p. 2.

85] Farr, S. (2003) 'Homoeopathic vaccine led to puppy deaths', *Veterinary Times*, vol. 33, no. 13, p. 8.

86] Bach, E. (1933) *The Twelve Healers and Other Remedies*, 2nd edn, Ashingdon, The CW Daniel Company Ltd., p. 3.

87] Resende, M. M., Costa, F. E., Gardona, R. G., Araújo, R. G., Mundim, F. G. and Costa, M. J. (2014) 'Preventive use of Bach flower Rescue Remedy in the control of risk factors for cardiovascular disease in rats', *Complementary Therapies in Medicine*, vol. 4, pp. 719–723.

88] Bach, E. (1933) *The Twelve Healers and Other Remedies*, p. 11.

89] Bach, E. (1933) *The Twelve Healers and Other Remedies*, p. 16.

90] Discover Homeopathy (2016) *Victims: Death by homeopathy* [Online]. Available at http://discoverhomeopathy.co.uk/victims-2 (Accessed 21 June 2016).

91] What's the Harm? (2016) *What's the harm in homeopathy?* [Online]. Available at http://whatstheharm.net/homeopathy.html (Accessed 21 June 2016).

92] Baker, S. J. and Baker, C. R. (2003) 'Rose-tinted view no longer tenable' (letter), *Veterinary Times*, vol. 33, no. 25, p. 3–4.

93] Vithoulkas, G. (1980) *The Science of Homeopathy*, New Delhi, B. Jain Publishers Ltd. (this edition 1998), p. 241–242.

94] Academy of Veterinary Homeopathy AVH (2014) *What is Homeopathy?* [Online]. Available at http://theavh.org/what-is-homeopathy/ (Accessed 27 June 2016).

95] *Phillipa* [sic] *Rodale – Homeopathy with Animals* (2013) YouTube video, added by Awakening TV [Online]. Available at https://www.youtube.com/watch?v=Ly7XWQt-9S8 (Accessed 23 June 2016).

96] Frampton, W. (2015) 'Vet found guilty of cruelty after dog with broken back left "in agony"', *Bournemouth Echo*, 4 December [Online]. Available at www.bournemouthecho.co.uk/news/14125523.Vet_found_guilty_of_cruelty_after_dog_with_broken_back_left__in_agony_ (Accessed 21 June 2016).

97] British Association of Homeopathic Veterinary Surgeons BAHVS (2015) *Statement Regarding Vet Prosecuted by RSPCA* [Online]. Available at www.bahvs.com/statement-regarding-vet-prosecuted-by-rspca (Accessed 21 June 2016).

98] Jordan, P. (2015) 'The Use of Homeopathic Medicines in Cleft Palate: A Case Report', *Journal of The Academy Of Veterinary Homeopathy*, Summer, pp. 8–9.

99] Coulter, H. L. (1980) *Homoeopathic Science and Modern Medicine*, Berkley, North Atlantic Books, pp. 8–9 and p. 94.

100] Nightingale Collaboration (2015) *On a downward spiral* [Online] Available at www.nightingale-collaboration.org/news/180-on-a-downward-spiral.html (Accessed 23 June 2016).

101] Anekwe, L. (2010) 'Ten PCTs pull NHS funding for homeopathy', *Pulse Today*, 19 August [Online]. Available at www.pulsetoday.co.uk/ten-pcts-pull-nhs-funding-for-homeopathy/11038927.fullarticle (Accessed 23 June 2016).

102] Bessant, C. et al. (2014) 'Vaccinations and boarding', *Veterinary Times*, vol. 44, no. 36, p. 18.

103] British Veterinary Association BVA (2014) *Policy – Veterinary medicines: Homeopathic medicines* [Online]. Available at www.bva.co.uk/News-campaigns-and-policy/Policy/Medicines/Veterinary-medicines/#homeopathic (Accessed 23 June 2016).

104] Gardiner, B. (2012) *Ineffective therapies* [Online]. Available at www.ava.com.au/12057 (Accessed 23 June 2016).

105] Horzinek, M. C. and Haagen, A. V. (2006) 'European veterinary specialists denounce alternative medicine', *Veterinary Sciences Tomorrow*, [Online] Available at vetsite.org/files/pdf/000059.pdf (Accesed 23 June 2016).

106] Guthrie, A. (2013) 'Vets say homeopathy isn't even good enough for the dog', *Press Dispensary*, 30 July [Online] Available at https://pressdispensary.co.uk/releases/c993700/Vets-say-homeopathy-isnt-even-good-enough-for-the-dog.html (Accessed 24 June 2016).

107] See: https://www.vetsurgeon.org/microsites/private/rational-medicine

108] Knapton, S. (2016) 'Homeopathy can kill pets and should be banned, say vets', *Telegraph*, 24 June [Online]. Available at www.telegraph.co.uk/

science/2016/06/24/homeopathy-can-kill-pets-and-should-be-banned-say-vets (Accessed 20 November 2016).

109] Viner, B. (2016) 'Homeopathy and Cancer', *Veterinary Record*, vol. 179, no. 3, p. 79.

110] Skeptvet (2013) 'Discussion of Homeopathy Continues in the AVMA', *The SkeptVet*, 3 April [Blog]. Available at http://skeptvet.com/Blog/2013/04/discussion-of-homeopathy-continues-in-the-avma (Accessed 24 June 2016).

111] Knapton, S. and Orange, R. (2015) 'EU orders Britain's organic farmers to treat sick animals with homeopathy', *Telegraph*, 24 April, [Online] Available at www.telegraph.co.uk/news/earth/agriculture/farming/11562234/EU-orders-Britains-organic-farmers-to-treat-sick-animals-with-homeopathy.html (Accessed 24 June 2016).

112] King, M. A. (2015) 'Horrified over EU directive on homeopathy', *Veterinary Times*, vol. 45, no. 20, p. 35.

113] Sehon, S. and Stanley, D. (2010) 'Evidence and simplicity: why we should reject homeopathy', *Journal of Evaluation in Clinical Practice*, vol. 16, no. 2, pp. 276–281.

114] Sober, E. (1992) 'Simplicity', in Dancy, J. and Sosa, E. (eds) *A Companion to Epistemology*, Oxford, Blackwell Publishers Ltd., pp. 477–478.

§

## Chapter Eleven – Manipulation Treatments

01] Mayes, B. (2015) 'Vet futures: Changes affecting the equine sector', *Veterinary Record*, vol. 176, pp. 457460.

02] House of Lords Science and Technology Select Committee (2000) *6th Report of Session 1999–2000 – Complementary and Alternative Medicine* [Online], Chapter 2: Disciplines Examined. Available at www.publications.parliament.uk/pa/ld199900/ldselect/ldsctech/123/12301.htm (Accessed 10 September 2016).

03] Great Britain. *Chiropractors Act 1994: Elizabeth II. Chapter 17* (1994) London, Her Majesty's Stationery Office, [Online]. Available at www.legislation.gov.uk/ukpga/1994/17/contents (Accessed 16 October 2016).

04] World Federation of Chiropractic (2012) *The Current Status of the Chiropractic Profession: Report to the World Health Organization* [Online]. Available at https://www.wfc.org/website/images/wfc/WHO_Submission-Final_Jan2013.pdf (Accessed 16 October 2016).

05] Ernst, E. (2008) 'Chiropractic: a critical evaluation', *Journal of Pain and Symptom Management*, vol. 35, no. 5, pp. 544–562.

06] Smith, R. L. (1969) *At You Own Risk: The Case Against Chiropractic*, New York, Simon and Schuster, p. 113.

07] Palmer, B. J. (1921) *The Chiropractic Adjuster*, Davenport, Palmer School of Chiropractic, pp 847–900.

08] Palmer, B. J. (1921) *The Chiropractic Adjuster*, p. 129.

09] Keating, J. C., Cleveland, C. S. and Menke, M. (2004) *Chiropractic History:*

a *Primer* [Online]. Available at www.historyofchiropractic.org/app/download/8299364/ChiroHistoryPrimer.pdf (Accessed 16 October 2016), p 26.

10] Palmer, B. J. (1921) *The Chiropractic Adjuster*, p. 44.

11] Palmer, B. J. (1906) *The Science of Chiropractic: Its Principles and Adjustments*, Davenport, Palmer School of Chiropractic, p. 24.

12] Smith, R. L. (1969) *At You Own Risk: The Case Against Chiropractic*, p. 8.

13] Palmer, B. J. (1906) *The Science of chiropractic: Its Principles and Adjustments*, p. 28.

14] Palmer, D. D. (1911) Letter to Johnson, P.W. [Online] Available at www.chiro.org/Plus/History/Persons/PalmerDD/PalmerDD%27s_Religion-of-Chiro.pdf (Accessed 15 April 2017).

15] Palmer, B. J. (1906) *The Science of Chiropractic: Its Principles and Adjustments*, p. 3.

16] Barge, F. H. (1996) in Shifflett, M. B. (2011) 'Rats in a Dump' *purechiro*, 30 September [Blog]. Available at http://purechiro.weebly.com/big-ideas-blog/rats-in-a-dump (Accessed 15 April 2017).

17] Peever, C. (2014) 'Rats in a Dump', *DrPeever.com*, 3 September [Blog]. Available at www.drpeever.com/chiropractic/rats-in-a-dump (Accessed 16 October 2016).

18] Lamar, T. R. (2013) 'Rats in a Dump', *Dr Lamar's SPINAL Column* January [Blog]. Available at https://spinalcolumnblog.com/2013/10/11/rats-in-a-dump (Accessed 16 October 2016).

19] Middleton, D. A. (2009) 'The Germ Theory: A Chiropractic Look at the Germ Theory' *Pathways to Family Wellness*, no. 23 [Online]. Available at http://pathwaystofamilywellness.org/Wellness-Lifestyle/a-chiropractic-look-at-the-germ-theory.html (Accessed 16 October 2016).

20] Wiese, G. (1996) 'Chiropractic's tension with the germ theory of disease', *Chiropractic History*, vol. 16, no. 1, pp. 72–87.

21] Smith, R. L. (1969) *At You Own Risk: The Case Against Chiropractic*, p. 18.

22] Keating, J. C. and Ramey, D. (2000) 'Further comments on veterinary chiropractic', *Canadian Veterinary Journal*, vol. 41, p. 518.

23] Keating, J. C., Bergmann, T. F., Jacobs, G. E., Finer, B. A. and Larson, K. (1990) 'Interexaminer reliability of eight evaluative dimensions of lumbar segmental abnormality', *Journal of Manipulative and Physiological Therapeutics*, vol. 13, no. 8, pp. 463–470.

24] French, S. D., Green, S., Forbes, A. (2000) 'Reliability of chiropractic methods commonly used to detect manipulable lesions in patients with chronic low-back pain', *Journal of Manipulative Physiological Therapeutics*, vol. 23, no 4, pp. 231–238.

25] Hestbaek, L. and Leboeuf-Yde, C. (2000) 'Are chiropractic tests for the lumbo-pelvic spine reliable and valid? A systematic critical review', *Journal of Manipulative Physiological Therapeutics*, vol. 23, no. 4, pp. 258–275.

26] Moore, S. A., Early, P. J. and Hettlich, B. F. (2016) 'Practice patterns in the management of acute intervertebral disc herniation in dogs', *Journal of Small Animal Practice*, vol. 57, no. 8, pp. 409–415.

27] www.chiropractic.org

28] www.acatoday.org

29] Wardwell, W. I. (1988), 'Chiropractors: Evolution to Acceptance', in Gevitz, N. (ed) *Other Healers – Unorthodox Medicine in America*, Baltimore, The Johns Hopkins University Press, p. 185.

30] Singh, S. and Ernst, E. (2008) *Trick or Treatment? Alternative Medicine on Trial*, London, Random house, p. 87.

31] Taylor, L. L and Romano, L. (1999) 'Veterinary chiropractic', *Canadian Veterinary Journal*, vol. 40, pp. 732–735.

32] Koren, T. (2003) *Does the Vertebral Subluxation Exist?* [Online] Available at www.chiro.org/LINKS/ABSTRACTS/Does_VS_Exist.shtml (Accessed 25 August 2016).

33] Sikorski, D. M. and Grod, J. P. (2003) 'The Unsubstantiated Web Site Claims of Chiropractic Colleges in Canada and the United States', *The Journal of Chiropractic Education*, vol. 17, no. 2, pp. 113–119.

34] Pollentier, A. and Langworthy, J. M. (2006) 'The scope of chiropractic practice: A survey of chiropractors in the UK', *Clinical Chiropractic*, vol. 10, pp. 147–155.

35] Stillings, D. (2011) 'Getting Involved Isn't the Solution: We Need a Paradigm Shift', *Dynamic Chiropractic*, vol. 29, no. 22 [Online] Available at www.dynamicchiropractic.com/mpacms/dc/article.php?id=55589 (Accessed 25 August 2016).

36] Societe Franco-Europeenne de Chiropraxie SOFEC (2015) *Clinical and Professional Chiropractic Education: a Position Statement* [Online] Available at http://vertebre.com/charte-pour-l-education-chiropratique-en-europe-8163 (Accessed 25 August 2016).

37] General Chiropractic Council GCC (2010) *Guidance on claims made for the chiropractic vertebral subluxation complex* [Online] Available at www.gcc-uk.org/UserFiles/Docs/Vertebralsublux2013revised.pdf (Accessed 25 August 2016).

38] Keating, J. C., Charlton, K. H., Grod, J. P., Perle, S. M., Sikorski, D., Winterstein, J. F., (2005) 'Subluxation: dogma or science?', *Chiropractic and Osteopathy*, vol. 13, no. 17.

39] Murphy, D. R., Schneider, M. J., Seaman, D. R., Perle, S. M., Nelson, C.F. (2008) 'How can chiropractic become a respected mainstream profession? The example of podiatry', *Chiropractic and Osteopathy*, vol. 16, no. 10.

40] Wardwell, W. I. (1988), 'Chiropractors: Evolution to Acceptance', in Gevitz, N. (ed.) *Other Healers – Unorthodox Medicine in America*, Baltimore, The Johns Hopkins University Press, pp. 189–190.

41] Singh, S. (2008) 'Beware the Spinal Trap', *Guardian*, 19 April [Online]. Available at https://www.theguardian.com/commentisfree/2008/apr/19/controversiesinscience-health (Accessed 23 June 2016).

42] Boseley, S. (2010) 'Simon Singh libel case dropped', *Guardian*, 15 April [Online]. Available at https://www.theguardian.com/science/2010/apr/15/simon-singh-libel-case-dropped (Accessed 16 October 2016).

43] Robbins, M. (2010) 'Furious backlash from Simon Singh libel case puts chiropractors on ropes', *Guardian*, 1 March [Online]. Available at https://www.

theguardian.com/science/2010/mar/01/simon-singh-libel-case-chiropractors (Accessed 16 October 2016).

44] Royal College of Veterinary Surgeons (RCVS) (2016) *Code of Professional Conduct for Veterinary Surgeons – Support Guidance: Treatment of animals by unqualified persons* [Online]. Available at www.rcvs.org.uk/advice-and-guidance/code-of-professional-conduct-for-veterinary-surgeons/supporting-guidance/treatment-of-animals-by-unqualified-persons (Accessed 16 October 2016).

45] Volhard, W. and Brown, K. L. (2000) *Holistic Guide for a Healthy Dog*, New Jersey, Wiley Publishing inc..

46] Glaister, D. (2016) 'I've been a homeopathic vet for 40 years, so how can I be seen as a fraud', *Guardian*, 17 July [Online]. Available at https://www.theguardian.com/science/2016/jul/16/vet-homeopathy-medicine-royal-college (Accessed 18 July 2016).

47] Homola, S. (2014) 'Neck manipulation, stroke and the precautionary principle', *Focus on Alternative and Complementary Therapies*, vol. 19, no. 4, pp. 208–211.

48] Biller, J., Sacco, R. L., Albuquerque, F. C. et al (2014) 'Cervical Arterial Dissections and Association with Cervical Manipulative Therapy', *AHA/ASA Scientific Statement*.

49] Epstein, N. E. and Forte, C. L. (2013) 'Medicolegal corner: Quadriplegia following chiropractic manipulation', *Surgical Neurology International*, vol. 4, no. 5.

50] Ernst, E. (2007) 'Adverse effects of spinal manipulation: a systematic review', *Journal of the Royal Society of Medicine*, vol. 100, no. 7, pp. 330–338.

51] Assendelft, W. J. J., Bouter, L. M. and Knipschild, P. G. (1996) 'Complications of spinal manipulation: A comprehensive review of the literature', *Journal of Family Practice*, vol. 42, pp. 475–480.

52] Stewart, B. (2002) 'Foreword', in Benedetti, P. and MacPhail, W. Spin Doctors: *The Chiropractic Industry Under Examination*, Toronto, Dundurn, p. 12.

53] Kjellin, R. E. and Kjellin, O. (2012) 'An Appraisal of Courses in Veterinary Chiropractic', *Science Based Medicine*, 16 March [Blog]. Available at https://www.sciencebasedmedicine.org/an-appraisal-of-courses-in-veterinary-chiropractic (Accessed 26 September 2016).

54] Cao, D. Y. and Pickar, J. G. (2014) 'Effect of spinal manipulation on the development of history-dependent responsiveness of lumbar paraspinal muscle spindles in the cat', *Journal of the Canadian Chiropractic Association*, vol. 58, no. 2, pp. 149–159.

55] Ianuzzi, A., Pickar, J. G. and Khalsa, P. S. (2010) 'Validation of the Cat as a Model for the Human Lumbar Spine During Simulated High-Velocity, Low-Amplitude Spinal Manipulation', *Journal of Biomechanical Engineering*, vol. 132, no. 7.

56] Keller, T. S., Colloca, C. J., Moore, R. J., Gunzburg, R., Harrison, D. E., Harrison, D. D., (2006) 'Three-dimensional vertebral motions produced by mechanical force spinal manipulation', *Journal of Manipulative Physiological Therapeutics*, vol. 29, no. 6, pp. 425–436.

57] Pickar, J. G. and McLain, R. F. (1995) 'Responses of mechanosensitive afferents to manipulation of the lumbar facet in the cat', *Spine*, vol. 20, no. 22, pp. 2379–2385.

58] Pickar, J. G. and Wheeler, J. D. (2001) 'Response of muscle proprioceptors to spinal manipulative-like loads in the anesthetized cat', *Journal of Manipulative Physiological Therapeutics*, vol. 24, no. 1, pp. 2–11.

59] Reed, W. R., Pickar, J. G. (1976) 'Paraspinal Muscle Spindle Response to Intervertebral Fixation and Segmental Thrust Level During Spinal Manipulation in an Animal Model', *Spine*, vol. 40, no. 13.

60] Reed, W. R., Cao, D. Y., Ge, W. and Pickar, J. G. (2013) 'Using vertebral movement and intact paraspinal muscles to determine the distribution of intrafusal fiber innervation of muscle spindle afferents in the anesthetized cat', *Experimental Brain Research*, vol. 225, no. 2, pp. 205–215.

61] Reed, W. R., Liebschner, M. A., Sozio, R. S., Pickar, J. G. and Gudavalli, M. R. (2015) 'Neural Response During a Mechanically Assisted Spinal Manipulation in an Animal Model: A Pilot Study', *Journal of Novel Physiotherapy and Physical Rehabilitation*, vol. 2, no. 2, pp. 20–27.

62] General Chiropractic Council GCC (2010) *Guidance on claims made for the chiropractic vertebral subluxation complex* [Online] Available at www.gcc-uk.org/UserFiles/Docs/Vertebralsublux2013revised.pdf (Accessed 25 August 2016).

63] Mirtz, T. A., Morgan, L., Wyatt, L. H. and Greene, L. (2009) 'An epidemiological examination of the subluxation construct using Hill's criteria of causation', *Chiropractic and Osteopathy*, vol. 17, no. 13.

64] Russell, M. L., Injeyan, H. S., Verhoef, M. J. and Eliasziw, M. (2004) 'Beliefs and behaviours: understanding chiropractors and immunization', *Vaccine*, vol. 23, no. 3, pp. 372–379.

65] Pollentier, A. and Langworthy, J. M. (2006) 'The scope of chiropractic practice: A survey of chiropractors in the UK', *Clinical Chiropractic*, vol. 10, pp. 147–155.

66] Balon J, et al. (1998) 'A comparison of active and simulated chiropractic manipulation as adjunctive treatment for childhood asthma', *New England Journal of Medicine*, vol. 339, no. 15, pp. 1013–1020.

67] Kjellin, R. E., and Kjellin, O. (2010) 'Is animal chiropractic in accordance with best practice?', *Svensk Veterinartidning*, vol. 62, no. 6, pp. 19–24.

68] Keating, J. C. and Ramey, D. (2000) 'Further comments on veterinary chiropractic', *Canadian Veterinary Journal*, vol. 41, p. 518.

69] Findley, J. and Singer, E. (2016) 'Equine back disorders 2. Treatment options', *In Practice*, vol. 38, pp. 33–38.

70] Rome, P. L. and McKibbin, M. (2011) 'A Review of Chiropractic Veterinary Science: An Emerging Profession With Somatic and Somatovisceral Anecdotal Histories', *Chiropractic Journal of Australia*, vol. 41, pp. 127–139.

71] Rome, P. L. (2012) 'Animal chiropractic neutralises the claim of placebo effect of spinal manipulation: Historical perspectives', *Chiropractic Journal of Australia*, vol. 42, no. 1, pp. 15–20.

72] Aharon, D. C., Heukels, J., Buntsma, R. (2016) 'Orthomanual therapy as treatment for suspected thoracolumbar disc disease in dogs', *European Journal of Companion Animal Practice*, vol. 26, no. 1, p. 42.

73] Madigan, J. E. and Bell, S. A. (2001) 'Owner survey of headshaking in horses', *Journal of the American Veterinary Association*, vol. 219, no. 3, pp. 334–337.

74] Thude, T. R. (2015) 'Chiropractic abnormalities of the lumbar spine significantly associated with urinary incontinence and retention in dogs', *Journal of Small Animal Practice*, vol. 56, no. 12, pp 693–697.

75] Beal, T. (2013) 'Yoga – with dogs', *BBC News*. 20 September [Online]. Available at www.bbc.co.uk/news/magazine-24129764 (Accessed 14 August 2016).

76] www.therealdogyoga.co.uk

77] Tellington-Jones, L. (1993) *The Tellington TTouch*, New York, Penguin Books.

78] Tellington-Jones, L. (2001) *Getting in Touch with Your Dog*, Buckingham, Kenilworth Press Ltd.

79] Corti, L. (2014) 'Massage therapy for dogs and cats', *Topics in Companion Animal Medicine*, vol. 29, no. 2, pp. 54–57.

80] Haussler, K. K. (2010) 'The role of manual therapies in equine pain management', *Veterinary Clinics of North America: Equine Practice*, vol. 26, pp. 579–601.

81] Saxton, J. G. G. (2000) 'Pure Energy Medicine – Radionics and Pranamonics', *Radionic Journal*, vol. 46, no. 3, p. 11.

82] Ball, P. (2004) 'The memory of water', *Nature* [Online] Available at www.nature.com/news/2004/041004/full/news041004-19.html (Accessed 25 August 2016).

83] Eagle, R. (1980) *A Guide to Alternative Medicine*, London, British Broadcasting Corporation, pp. 27–28.

84] Eagle, R. (1980) *A Guide to Alternative Medicine*, p. 29.

85] Elliott, M. (2001) 'What is Radionics?', *Horsemanship Magazine*, October–November [Online]. Available at www.horsemanshipmagazine.co.uk/magazines/2001/oct-nov-01/664-radionics-8 (Accessed 25 August 2016).

86] Saxton, J. G. G. (2000) 'Pure Energy Medicine—Radionics and Pranamonics', *Radionic Journal*, vol. 46, no. 3, p. 16.

87] Smith, R. L. (1969) *At you own risk: The Case against Chiropractic*, pp. 53–54.

88] Lee-Treweek, G., (2005) 'Knowledge, names, fraud and trust', in Lee-Treweek G., Heller T., MacQueen, H., Stone, J. and Spurr, S. (eds) *Complementary and Alternative Medicine: Structures and Safeguards*, Abingdon, Routledge, Taylor and Francis/Milton Keynes, The Open University, pp. 20–21.

89] Stone, J. and Katz, J. (2005) 'Understanding Health and Healing', in Heller, T., Lee-Treweek, G., Katz, J., Stone, J. and Spurr, S. (eds) *Perspectives on Complementary and Alternative Medicine*, Abingdon, Routledge, Taylor and Francis/Milton Keynes, The Open University, p. 163.

90] Lloyd, S., and Martin, S. A. (2006) 'Controlled trial on the effects of radionic healing and anthelmintics on faecal egg counts in horses', *Veterinary Record*, vol. 158, pp. 734–737.

91] Birke, L. (1987) 'An open mind in the veterinary surgery', *New Scientist*, vol. 115, pp. 34–36.

92] Lee, M. S. (2008) 'Is reiki beneficial for pain management?', *Focus on Alternative and Complementary Therapies*, vol. 13, no. 2, pp. 78–81.

93] Joyce, J. and Herbison, G.P. (2015) 'Reiki for depression and anxiety', *Cochrane*

*Database of Systematic Reviews 2015*, Issue 4, Art. no.: CD006833 [Online] DOI: 10.1002/14651858.CD006833.pub2 (Accessed 16 October 2016).

94] McCarney, R., Fisher, P., Spink, F., Flint, G. and van Haselen, R. (2002) 'Can homeopaths detect homeopathic medicines by dowsing? A randomised, double-blind, placebo-controlled trial', *Journal of the Royal Society of Medicine*, vol. 95, pp. 189–191.

95] Elliott, M. (2001) 'Cushing's disease: a new approach to therapy in equine and canine patients', *British Homeopathic Journal*, vol. 90, no. 1, pp. 33–36.

96] Rosa, L., Rosa, E., Larry Sarner, L. and Barrett, S. (1998) 'A Close Look at Therapeutic Touch', *Journal of the American Medical Association*, vol. 279, no. 13, pp. 1005–1010.

97] Saxton, J. G. G. (2000) 'Pure Energy Medicine—Radionics and Pranamonics', p. 14.

98] Stone, J. and Katz, J. (2005b), 'Can complementary and alternative medicine be classified?', in Heller, T., Lee-Treweek, G., Katz, J., Stone, J. and Spurr, S. (eds) *Perspectives on Complementary and Alternative Medicine*, Abingdon, Routledge, Taylor and Francis/Milton Keynes, The Open University, p. 48.

99] Rome, P. L. and McKibbin, M. (2011) 'A Review of Chiropractic Veterinary Science: An Emerging Profession With Somatic and Somatovisceral Anecdotal Histories', *Chiropractic Journal of Australia*, vol. 41, pp. 127–139.

§

## Chapter Twelve – Diagnostics

01] School of Homeopathy (2017) *Teachers* [Online], Available at www.homeopathyschool.com/the-school/faculty/teachers (Accessed 22 January 2017).

02] Hogeboom, C. J., Sherman, K. J. and Cherkin, D. C. (2001) 'Variation in diagnosis and treatment of chronic low back pain by traditional Chinese medicine acupuncturists', *Complementary Therapies in Medicine*, vol. 9, no. 3, pp. 154–166.

03] Zhang, G. G., Lee, W., Bausell, B., Lao, L., Handwerger, B. and Berman, B. (2005) 'Variability in the traditional Chinese medicine (TCM) diagnoses and herbal prescriptions provided by three TCM practitioners for 40 patients with rheumatoid arthritis', *Journal of Alternative and Complementary Medicine*, vol. 11, no. 3, pp. 415–421.

04] Simon, A., Worthen, D. M. and Mitas, J. A. (1979) 'An evaluation of iridology', *Journal of the American Medical Association*, vol. 242, no. 13, pp. 1385–1389.

05] Ernst, E. (2000) 'Iridology: not useful and potentially harmful', *Archives of Ophthalmology*, vol. 118, no. 1, pp. 120–121.

06] Schwartz, S. A., Utts, J., Spottiswoode, S. J. P., Shade, C. W., Tully, L., Morris, W. F. and Nachman, G. (2014) 'A double-blind, randomized study to assess the validity of applied kinesiology (AK) as a diagnostic tool and as a nonlocal proximity effect', *Explore*, vol. 10, no. 2, pp. 99–108.

07] Hall, H. (2011) 'Electrodermal Testing Part I: Fooling Patients with a Computerized Magic Eight Ball', *Science-Based Medicine*, 5 July [Blog]. Available at https://sciencebasedmedicine.org/13926 (Accessed 22 January 2017).

08] Barrett, S. (2016) *Regulatory Actions Related to EAV Devices* [Online]. Available at http://www.quackwatch.org/02ConsumerProtection/eav.html (Accessed 22 January 2017).

09] Meacock, R. S. (2006) *Energy Balancing with the e-Lybra 8 System* [Online]. Available at www.positivehealth.com/article/animals/energy-balancing-with-the-e-lybra-8-system (Accessed 22 January 2017).

10] Lewith, G. T., Kenyon, J. N., Broomfield, J., Prescott, P., Goddard, J. and Holgate, S.T. (2001) 'Is electrodermal testing as effective as skin prick tests for diagnosing allergies? A double blind, randomised block design study', *British Medical Journal*, vol. 322, no. 7279, pp. 131–134.

11] Semizzi, M., Senna, G., Crivellaro, M, Rapacioli, G., Passalacqua, G., Canonica, W. G. and Bellavite, P. (2002) 'A double blind placebo controlled study on the diagnostic accuracy of an electrodermal test in allergic subjects', *Clinical and Experimental Allergy*, vol. 32, pp. 928–932.

12] *Inside Out – South* (2003) BBC 1, 17 February [Online]. Available at www.bbc.co.uk/insideout/south/series2/food_sensitivity_allergy_vega_tests.shtml (Accessed 22 January 2017).

13] Barrett, S. (2016) *Quack 'Electrodiagnostic' Devices* [Online]. Available at www.quackwatch.com/01QuackeryRelatedTopics/electro.html (Accessed 22 January 2017).

§

## Chapter Thirteen – The Rest

01] Politifact (2016) *Donald Trump's File* [Online]. Available at www.politifact.com/personalities/donald-trump (Accessed 7 January 2017).

02] Deacon, M. (2016) 'In a world of post-truth politics, Andrea Leadsom will make the perfect PM', *Telegraph*, 9 July [Online]. Available at www.telegraph.co.uk/news/2016/07/09/in-a-world-of-post-truth-politics-andrea-leadsom-will-make-the-p (Accessed 23 January 2017).

03] Rabischong, P. and Terral, C. (2014) 'Scientific Basis of Auriculotherapy: State of the Art', *Medical Acupuncture*, vol. 26, no. 2, pp. 84–96.

04] Di, Y. M., May, B. H., Zhang, A. L., Zhou, I. W., Worsnop, C. and Xue, C. C. L. (2014) 'A meta-analysis of ear-acupuncture, ear-acupressure and auriculo-therapy for cigarette smoking cessation', *Drug and Alcohol Dependence*, vol. 142, pp. 14–23.

05] White, A. R., Rampes, H., Liu, J. P., Stead, L. F. and Campbell, J. (2014) 'Acupuncture and related interventions for smoking cessation', *Cochrane Database of Systematic Reviews 2011*, Issue 1, Art. No.: CD000009 [Online] DOI: 10.1002/14651858.CD000009.pub3 (Accessed 28 January 2017).

06] Asher, G. N., Jonas, D. E., Coeytaux, R. R., Reilly, A. C., Loh, Y. L.,

Motsinger-Reif, A. A. and Winham, S. J. (2010) 'Auriculotherapy for Pain Management: A Systematic Review and Meta-Analysis of Randomized Controlled Trials', *The Journal of Alternative and Complementary Medicine*, vol. 16, no. 10, pp. 1097–1108.

07] Zhao, H.-J., Tan, J.-Y., Wang, T. and Jin, L. (2015) 'Auricular therapy for chronic pain management in adults: A synthesis of evidence', *Complementary Therapies in Clinical Practice*, vol. 21, no. 2, pp. 68–78.

08] Still, J. (1995) 'Auriculodiagnosis of acute diarrhoea in the dog – an experimental study', *Journal of Auricular Medicine*, vol. 2, pp. 10–11.

09] Still, J. (1990) 'A clinical study of auriculotherapy in canine thoracolumbar disc disease', *Journal of the South African Veterinary Association*, vol. 61, no. 3, pp. 102–105.

10] Baggoley, C. (2015) *Review of the Australian government rebate on natural therapies for private health insurance* [Online], Australian Government Department of Health. Available at www.health.gov.au/internet/main/publishing.nsf/Content/0E9129B3574FCA53CA257BF0001ACD11/$File/Natural%20Therapies%20Overview%20Report%20Final%20with%20copyright%2011%20March.pdf (Accessed 7 January 2017).

11] Wells, D. L. (2006) 'Aromatherapy for travel-induced excitement in dogs', *Journal of the American Veterinary Medical Association*, vol. 229, no. 6, pp. 964–967.

12] Allport, R. (1987) *Heal Your Dog the Natural Way*, London, Mitchell Beazley, p. 10.

13] Krieger, F. (2004) 'Herbal hydrocarbons: the "natural alternative" to veterinary medicine?', *Veterinary Times*, vol. 34, no. 39, p. 12.

14] Posadzki, P., Alotaibi, A. and Ernst, E. (2012) 'Adverse effects of aromatherapy: a systematic review of case reports and case series', *The International Journal of Risk and Safety in Medicine*, vol. 24, no. 3, pp. 147–161.

15] Huang, Z., Ma, J., Chen, J., Shen, B., Pei, F. and Kraus, V. B. (2015) 'The effectiveness of low-level laser therapy for nonspecific chronic low back pain: a systematic review and meta-analysis', *Arthritis Research & Therapy*, vol. 17, no. 1, p. 360.

16] Chow, R. T., Johnson, M. I., Lopes-Martins, R. A. and Bjordal, J. M. (2009) 'Efficacy of low-level laser therapy in the management of neck pain: a systematic review and meta-analysis of randomised placebo or active-treatment controlled trials', *Lancet*, vol. 374, no. 9705, pp. 1897–1908.

17] Huang, Z., Chen, J., Ma, J., Shen, B., Pei, F. and Kraus, V. B. (2015) 'Effectiveness of low-level laser therapy in patients with knee osteoarthritis: a systematic review and meta-analysis', *Osteoarthritis and Cartilage*, vol. 23, no. 9, pp. 1437–1444.

18] Draper, W. E., Schubert, T. A., Clemmons, R. M. and Miles, S. A. (2012) 'Low-level laser therapy reduces time to ambulation in dogs after hemilaminectomy: a preliminary study', *Journal of Small Animal Practice*, vol. 53, no. 8, pp. 465–469.

19] French, C. C. and Williams, L. (1999) 'Crystal clear: Paranormal powers, placebo, or priming?', paper presented at *Sixth European Congress of Psychology*, Rome, 4–9 July 1999.

20] Allport, R. (1987) *Heal Your Dog the Natural Way*, pp. 32–34.

21] Sense about Science (2016) *Debunking Detox* [Online]. Available at http://archive.senseaboutscience.org/pages/debunking-detox.html (Accessed 7 January 2017).

22] Shapiro, R. (2008) '*Suckers: How Alternative Medicine Makes Fools of Us All*', London, Harvill Secker, p. 211.

23] Ameling, A. (2000) 'Prayer: an ancient healing practice becomes new again', *Holistic Nursing Practice*, vol. 14, no. 3, pp. 40–48.

24] Olver, I. N. and Dutney, A. (2012) 'A randomized, blinded study of the impact of intercessory prayer on spiritual well-being in patients with cancer', *Alternative Therapies in Health and Medicine,* vol. 18, no. 5, pp. 18–27.

25] Harris, W. S., Gowda, M., Kolb, J. W., Strychacz, C. P., Vacek, J. L., Jones, P. G., Forker, A., O'Keefe, J. H. and McCallister, B. D. (1999) 'A randomized, controlled trial of the effects of remote, intercessory prayer on outcomes in patients admitted to the coronary care unit', *Archives of Internal Medicine*, vol. 159, no. 19, pp. 2273–2278.

26] Roberts, L., Ahmed, I. and Hall, S. (2007) 'Intercessory prayer for the alleviation of ill health', *Cochrane Database of Systematic Reviews 2007*, Issue 1, Art. No.: CD000368 [Online] DOI: 10.1002/14651858.CD000368.pub2 (Accessed 28 January 2017).

27] Jørgensen, K. J., Hróbjartsson, A. and Gøtzsche, P. C. (2009) 'Divine intervention? A Cochrane review on intercessory prayer gone beyond science and reason', *Journal of Negative Results in Biomedicine*, vol. 8, no. 1, p. 7.

28] Gentle Care Pet Products (2016) *Distant Pet Homeopathic Transmission Therapy* [Online]. Available at www.gentlecarepet.com/distance_pet_healing (Accessed 7 January 2017).

29] Braithwaite, E. (2016) *Distant healing for a dog* [Online]. Available at http://thehealingvet.com/vet-stories/distant-healing-dog (Accessed 7 January 2 017).

30] Grey, S. (2016) *Susan Grey's Distance Animal Healing* [Online]. Available at www.distancehealer.net/animal-healing.htm (Accessed 7 January 2017).

31] Astin, J. A., Harkness, E. and Ernst, E. (2000) 'The efficacy of "distant healing": a systematic review of randomized trials', *Annals of Internal Medicine,* vol. 132, no. 11, pp. 903–910.

32] Ernst, E. (2003) 'Distant healing – an "update" of a systematic review', *Wiener Klinische Wochenschrift*, vol. 115, nos. 7–8, pp. 241–245.

33] Rogachefsky, R. A., Altman, R. D., Markov, M. S. and Cheung, H. S. (2004) 'Use of a permanent magnetic field to inhibit the development of canine osteoarthritis', *Bioelectromagnetics*, vol. 25, no. 4, pp. 260–270.

34] Bigham-Sadegh, A., Ghasemi, S., Karimi, I., Mirshokraei, P., Nazari, H. and Oryan, A. (2015) 'Tendon Healing with Allogenic Fibroblast and Static Magnetic Field in Rabbit Model', *Iranian Journal of Veterinary Surgery*, vol. 10, no. 2, pp. 11–19.

35] Hoque, M., Maiti, S. K., Aithal, H. P., Singh, G. R., Kumar, N., Singh, P. and Charan, K. (2003) 'Effects of static magnetic field in fracture healing in goats: An experimental study', *Indian Journal of Animal Science*, vol. 73, no. 3, pp. 275–277.

36] Edner, A., Lindberg, L.-G., Broström, H. and Bergh, A. (2015) 'Does a magnetic blanket induce changes in muscular blood flow, skin temperature and muscular tension in horses?', *Equine Veterinary Journal*, vol. 47, pp. 302–307.

37] Shafford, H. L., Hellyer, P. W., Crump, K. T., Wagner, A. E., Mama, K. R. and Gaynor, J. S. (2002) 'Use of a pulsed electromagnetic field for treatment of post-operative pain in dogs: a pilot study'. *Veterinary Anaesthesia and Analgesia*, vol. 29, pp. 43–48.

38] Pittler, M. H., Brown, E. M. and Ernst, E. (2007) 'Static magnets for reducing pain: systematic review and meta-analysis of randomized trials', *Canadian Medical Association Journal*, vol. 177, no. 7, pp. 736–742.

39] Nogales, C. G., Ferrari, P. H., Kantorovich, E. O. and Lage-Marques, J. L. (2008) 'Ozone therapy in medicine and dentistry', *Journal of Contemporary Dental Practice*, vol. 9, no. 4, pp. 75–84.

40] Mohamed, A., Goodin, K., Pope, R., Hubbard, M. and Levine, M. (2016) 'Association between asthma hospital visits and ozone concentration in Maricopa County, Arizona (2007–2012)', *Journal of Environmental Health*, vol. 78, no. 9, pp. 8–13.

41] Food and Drug Administration USA (2015) Code of Federal Regulations – Maximum acceptable level of ozone. PART 801 – LABELING, Subpart H – Special Requirements for Specific Devices, Sec. 801.415

42] Azarpazhooh, A. and Limeback, H. (2008) 'The application of ozone in dentistry: A systematic review of literature', *Journal of Dentistry*, vol. 36, no. 2, pp. 104–116.

43] Sweet, F., Kao, M. S., Lee, S. C., Hagar, W. L. and Sweet, W. E. (1980) 'Ozone selectively inhibits growth of human cancer cells', *Science*, vol. 209, no. 4459, pp. 931–933.

44] Ozkan, H., Ekinci, S., Uysal, B., Akyildiz, F., Turkkan, S., Ersen, O., Koca, K. and Seven, M. M. (2015) 'Evaluation and comparison of the effect of hypothermia and ozone on ischemia-reperfusion injury of skeletal muscle in rats', *Journal of Surgical Research*, vol. 196, no. 2, pp. 313–319.

45] Kocaman, H., Erginel, B., Onder, S. Y., Soysal, F. G., Keskin, E., Celik, A. and Salman, T. (2016) 'The role of ozone therapy in hepatic fibrosis due to biliary tract obstruction', *European Journal of Pediatric Surgery*, vol. 26, no. 1, pp. 133–137.

46] Ozbay, I., Ital, I., Kucur, C., Akcılar, R., Deger, A., Aktas, S. and Oghan, F. (2016) 'Effects of ozone therapy on facial nerve regeneration', *Brazilian Journal of Otorhinolaryngology*, doi: 10.1016/j.bjorl.2016.02.009. [Epub ahead of print].

47] Magalhaes, F. N. D. O., Dotta, L., Sasse, A., Teixera, M. J. and Fonoff, E. T. (2016) 'Ozone therapy as a treatment for low back pain secondary to herniated disc: a systematic review and meta-analysis of randomized controlled trials', *Pain Physician*, vol. 15, no. 2, pp. E115–129.

48] Brazzelli, M., McKenzie, L., Fielding, S., Fraser, C., Clarkson, J., Kilonzo, M.

and Waugh, N. (2006) 'Systematic review of the effectiveness and cost-effectiveness of HealOzone for the treatment of occlusal pit/fissure caries and root caries', *Health Technology Assessment*, vol. 10, no. 16, pp. iii–iv, ix–80.

49] Liu, J., Zhang, P., Tian, J., Li, L., Li, J., Tian, J. H. and Yang, K. (2015) 'Ozone therapy for treating foot ulcers in people with diabetes', *Cochrane Database of Systematic Reviews 2015*, Issue 10, Art. No.: CD008474 [Online] DOI: 10.1002/14651858.CD008474.pub2 (Accessed 28 January 2017).

50] Azarpazhooh, A. and Limeback, H. (2008) 'The application of ozone in dentistry: A systematic review of literature', *Journal of Dentistry*.

51] Martínez-Sánchez, G., Delgado-Roche, L., Díaz-Batista, A., Pérez-Davison, G. and Re, L. (2012) 'Effects of ozone therapy on haemostatic and oxidative stress index in coronary artery disease', *European Journal of Pharmacology*, vol. 691, nos. 1–3, pp. 156–162.

52] Clavo, B., Ceballos, D., Gutierrez, D., Rovira, G., Suarez, G., Lopez, L., Pinar, B., Cabezon, A., Morales, V., Oliva, E., Fiuza, D. and Santana-Rodriguez, N. (2013) 'Long-term control of refractory hemorrhagic radiation proctitis with ozone therapy', *Journal of Pain and Symptom Management*, vol. 46, no. 1, pp. 106–112.

53] Roman, M. (2013) *Ozone Therapy in the Veterinary Practice* [Online]. Available at: http://ivcjournal.com/ozone-therapy-in-the-veterinary-practice (Accessed 7 January 2017).

54] Đurii, D., Valpoti, H., Žura Žaja, I. and Samardžija, M. (2016) 'Comparison of intrauterine antibiotics versus ozone medical use in sheep with retained placenta and following obstetric assistance', *Reproduction in Domestic Animals*, vol. 51, no. 4, pp. 538–540.

55] Teixeira, L. R., Luna, S. P. L., Taffarel, M. O., Lima, A. F. M., Sousa, N. R., Joaquim, J. G. F. and Freitas, P. M. C. (2013) 'Comparison of intrarectal ozone, ozone administered in acupoints and meloxicam for postoperative analgesia in bitches undergoing ovariohysterectomy', *Veterinary Journal*, vol. 197, no. 3, pp. 794–799.

56] Han, H.-J., Kim, J.-Y., Jang, H.-Y., Lee, B., Yoon, J.-H., Jang, S.-K., Choi, S. H. and Jeong, S.-W. (2007) 'Fluoroscopic-guided intradiscal oxygen-ozone injection therapy for thoracolumbar intervertebral disc herniations in dogs', *In Vivo*, vol. 21, no. 4, pp. 609–613.

57] Al Bedah, A. M. N., Khalil, M. K. M., Elolemy, A. T., Alrasheid, M. H. S., Al Mudaiheem, A. and Elolemy, T. M. B. (2013) 'Ozone therapy in postgraduate theses in Egypt: systematic review', *The Journal of the Egyptian Public Health Association*, vol. 88, no. 2, pp. 57–66.

58] Marchetti, D. and La Monaca, G. (2000) 'An unexpected death during oxygen-ozone therapy', *The American Journal of Forensic Medicine and Pathology*, vol. 21, no. 2, pp. 144–147.

59] Hidalgo-Tallón, J., Menéndez-Cepero, S., Vilchez, J. S., Rodríguez-López, C. M. and Calandre, E. P. (2013) 'Ozone therapy as add-on treatment in fibromyalgia management by rectal insufflation: an open-label pilot study', *Journal of Alternative and Complementary Medicine*, vol. 19, no. 3, pp. 238–242.

60] American Academy of Otolaryngology – Head and Neck Surgery AAO-HNS (2015) *Earwax and Care* [Online]. Available at www.entnet.org/content/earwax-and-care (Accessed 24 January 2017).

61] Seely, D. R, Quigley, S.M. and Langman, A. W. (1996) 'Ear candles – efficacy and safety', *Laryngoscope*, vol. 106, no. 10, pp. 1226–1229.

62] Schuett, K. (2012) 'A Case of Severe Pyometra in a Dog', *Hpathy Ezine*, June, [Online]. Available at http://hpathy.com/veterinary-homeopathy/a-case-of-severe-pyometra-in-a-dog/ (Accessed 24 January 2017).

63] Natural Paws Holistic Pet Care (2013) *Useful Information: Pyometra (uterus infection)* [Online]. Available at www.naturalpaws.com.au/pyometra-uterus-infection-usefulinfo-78-false.html (Accessed 24 January 2017).

§

## Conclusion

01] Oxford Dictionaries (2016) *Word of the Year 2016 is …* [Online]. Available at https://en.oxforddictionaries.com/word-of-the-year/word-of-the-year-2016 (Accessed 10 December 2016).

02] Meyjes, T. (2016) 'Vote Leave's £350 million NHS slogan bus is back and circling London', *Metro*, 16 July [Online]. Available at http://metro.co.uk/2016/07/16/vote-leaves-350million-nhs-slogan-bus-is-back-and-circling-london-6011056 (Accessed 10 December 2016).

03] Deacon, M. (2016) 'Michael Gove's guide to Britain's greatest enemy … the experts', *Telegraph*, 10 June [Online]. Available at www.telegraph.co.uk/news/2016/06/10/michael-goves-guide-to-britains-greatest-enemy-the-experts (Accessed 10 December 2016).

04] *Sherlock: 'The Reichenbach Fall'* (2012) BBC One, 15 January.

05] Imrie, R. H. and Ramey, D. W. (2000) 'The evidence for evidence based medicine', *Complementary Therapies in Medicine*, vol. 8, pp. 123–126.

06] Novella, S. (2015) 'It's time for science-based medicine', *Skeptical Inquirer*, vol. 39, no. 3.

07] Deacon, M. (2016) 'Michael Gove's guide to Britain's greatest enemy … the experts', *Telegraph*, 10 June [Online].

08] Orac (2015) 'The Food Babe: "There is just no acceptable level of any chemical to ingest, ever"', *Respectful Insolence*, 12 February [Blog]. Available at http://scienceblogs.com/insolence/2015/02/12/the-food-babe-there-is-just-no-acceptable-level-of-any-chemical-to-ingest-ever (Accessed 19 December 2016).

09] Wikipedia (2016) *Quinoa* [Online], 13 December 2016. Available at https://en.wikipedia.org/wiki/Quinoa (Accessed 19 December 2016).

10] Lewin, J. (n.d.) *BBC Good Food: Health benefits of … quinoa* [Online]. Available at http://www.bbcgoodfood.com/howto/guide/health-benefits-quinoa (Accessed 19 December 2016).

11] Gunnars, K, (2016) '11 Proven Health Benefits of Quinoa', *Authority Nutrition*,

[Blog]. Available at https://authoritynutrition.com/11-proven-benefits-of-quinoa (Accessed 19 December 2016).

12] Blythman, J. (2013) 'Can vegans stomach the unpalatable truth about quinoa?', *Guardian*, 16 January [Online]. Available at https://www.theguardian.com/commentisfree/2013/jan/16/vegans-stomach-unpalatable-truth-quinoa (Accessed 19 December 2016). [Authors' note: it's pronounced *keen-wa*, by the way, not *qui-no-a*].

13] Way, T. (2016) *Dihydrogen Monoxide Research Division* [Online]. Available at www.dhmo.org (Accessed 10 December 2016).

14] Bell, I. and Gold, P. (2016) *Homeopathy Research Evidence Base: References* [Online], The American Institute of Homeopathy. Available at homeopathyusa.org/uploads/Homeopathy_Research_Evidence_Base_7-7-16.pdf (Accessed 7 December 2016).

# Recommended Reading

Benson, O. and Stangroom, J. (2007) *Why Truth Matters*, London, Continuum.

Campbell, A. (2013) *Homeopathy in Perspective: A Critical Appraisal*, Milton Keynes, Lightning Source UK Ltd.

Diamond, J. (2001) *Snake Oil and other Preoccupations*, London, Vintage.

Gilovich, T. (1993) *How We Know What Isn't So*, New York, The Free Press.

Goldacre, B. (2009) *Bad Science*, London, Fourth Estate.

Gross, P. R. and Levitt, N. (1994) *Higher Superstition: The Academic Left and its Quarrels with Science*, Baltimore and London, The Johns Hopkins University Press.

Park, R. L. (2000) *Voodoo Science: The Road From Foolishness to Fraud*, Oxford, New York, Oxford University Press.

Ramey, D.W. and Rollin, B.E. (2004) *Complementary and Alternative Veterinary Medicine Considered*, Ames, Iowa State Press.

Shapiro, R. (2008) '*Suckers: How Alternative Medicine Makes Fools of Us All*, London, Harvill Secker.

Singh, S. and Ernst, E. (2008) *Trick or Treatment: Alternative Medicine on Trial*, London, Transworld Publishers.

Specter, M. (2010) *Denialism: How Irrational Thinking Harms the Planet and Threatens Our Lives*, London, Penguin.

# Appendix

## Opinions on Complementary and Alternative Veterinary Medicine

*A*N *interview with Dr Narda Robinson, by Alex Gough MA, VetMB, CertSAM, CertVC, PGCert MRCVS*
[This article was first published in the *Veterinary Times* on 5 December 2011 and is reproduced here with kind permission]

I first encountered Dr Robinson on an email list that examines the evidence for complementary and alternative veterinary medicine (CAVM). As the list was predominantly populated by sceptics, I found that Dr Robinson immediately stood out because of her CAVM background, and her advocacy of certain CAVM techniques. It soon became clear, though, that Dr Robinson had a very different approach to the observational and take-it-on-faith 'proofs' of CAVM. As an Assistant Professor at Colorado State University, a Director of the CSU Centre for Comparative and Integrative Pain Medicine, and boasting among her qualifications a Masters in Biomedical Sciences, Diplomate status through the American Board of Medical Acupuncture, and a Fellowship from the American Academy of Medical Acupuncture, her academic credentials are formidable. She leads research projects in acupuncture anatomy, herbal medicine and patient simulator development for acupuncture education, and writes a regular column on complementary medicine in the US publication, *Veterinary Practice News*.

However, her academic and evidence-based approach, and her views on CAVM, have often brought her into conflict with CAVM advocates, just as Edzard Ernst, the world's first Professor of Complementary Medicine, and a trained homeopath, has upset the human complementary and alternative

344

medicine (CAM) fraternity by questioning the evidence and rationale for many CAM techniques. Her call for Traditional Chinese Medicine (TCM) to be modernised has been branded as 'racist' and she has been accused of 'contempt prior to investigation', prejudice, and insulting fellow veterinarians. She has been the subject of numerous calls to have her fired from her column on CAVM in *Veterinary Practice News*, and to be replaced by someone more positive about the practices.

Dr Narda kindly agreed to answer some questions that, given the frequent discussions in the letters pages of *Veterinary Times*, I thought readers of this publication might find interesting.

§

**Alex Gough (AG):** Which CAVM modalities would you say have the best evidence to support their use, in terms of efficacy?

**Narda Robinson (NR):** Alex, thank you for the opportunity to discuss my views on the current state of CAVM. Regarding the best evidential support for a given modality as a whole, far and away it would be acupuncture. That said, however, certain botanical preparations have also been well characterised as to their mechanisms of action, safety profile (in humans, at least).

**AG:** Which CAVM modalities are proven to be or likely to be safe?

**NR:** It depends on whether we are talking about species-specific applications or general impressions. Again, acupuncture leads the way in having the most well understood mechanisms (in terms of neurophysiology, not mystical *Qi* or energy phenomena) and greatest margin of safety when performed by a medical professional with a solid educational background in anatomy. The mechanisms of massage are also becoming clearer, and when practised by a veterinary medical professional who has undergone properly supervised, hands-on training, is relatively safe. The evidence for massage, however, comes mainly from the human field. Certain herbs are safer than others, but again, we need more information on how these chemicals impact canine versus feline versus equine physiology, and what the downsides and interactions might be.

**AG:** What harm have you seen yourself from CAVM, direct or indirect, or had reported to you?

**NR:** I have received several reports of animals killed or injured by chiropractic. One horse was killed at a race track event, but I don't have specifics on that. Another received an upper spinal cord injury from recoiling

345

after an adjustment while the horse was in cross ties. I have had patients injured by excessive pressure by individuals (non-veterinarians) performing massage, such as one human physical therapist determined to put a Schnauzer's kidney 'back in place', leading to gastrointestinal and urinary bleeding. Another placed so much pressure on a Dalmatian's spine that the dog, who had pre-existing intervertebral disk disease, had trouble walking for a day or two. There are countless anecdotal reports and cases I've seen where herbs have caused negative reactions, evidenced either by altered liver values, bleeding times, or gastrointestinal function.

**AG:** You have been quoted as saying that the use of gold bead implants is not just quackery but malpractice. Could you expand on your reasons for saying this?

**NR:** I do ask whether gold bead implants are 'medicine or malpractice' in my article of the similar name found at https://curacore.org/gold-bead-implants-medicine-or-malpractice. Human medical literature on embedding acupuncture needles and metal fragments indicates that it is considered malpractice. The gold bead therapists claim that their beads either don't migrate (which is untrue) or don't interfere with diagnostic imaging (also untrue). Further, they promise high success rates for a number of conditions, but cannot point to any methodologically sound studies justifying that the benefits outweigh the risks. Why not just keep the procedure safe by employing needles that can be removed, as in normal acupuncture?

**AG:** How do you address critics of negative studies into homeopathy who say that homeopathy is not testable with conventional science, or double-blinded trials?

**NR:** Homeopathy doesn't seem to work in the way its proponents claim. I recognise that there may be effects from chemicals in small amounts, and their influence in the body may change depending on the dose. But veterinary homeopaths have re-invented even Hahnemann's homeopathy and applied it to animals without verifying safety or effectiveness. The 'provings' done on humans to characterise the influences of homeopathic remedies, to whatever sense they make in human medicine, have not been done in animals. Thus, recommending one remedy over another tends to stem either from untested extrapolation or de novo invention. My greatest concern with homeopathy is the delay of proper diagnosis and treatment. I have received complaints from veterinarians, even those trained in homeopathy. They cite instances where their homeopathic colleagues were withholding proper pain medicine, antibiotics, other appropriate medications, or surgery for weeks, as the animal's health status declines, waiting to stumble upon the 'correct' remedy. This is just plain wrong.

**AG:** Do you have an opinion on the use of raw food diets as a maintenance diet or a therapeutic?

**NR:** Sometimes raw food diets seem to help, but I don't think it's that they are raw, but instead that the food ingredients are of a higher quality than those found in some dog foods. Given the antibiotic resistance in our food supply because of chronically administered antibiotics, it's just not worth risking the animal's and human family members' health to introduce salmonella and E. coli-laden foods into the household on a regular basis.

**AG:** Do you feel that the evidence for acupuncture is unequivocally supportive that it has an effect, or do you still have room for doubt that it could be an elaborate placebo?

**NR:** Acupuncture is simply neuromodulation, as is placebo. While the brain pathways leading to effects related to placebos overlap with acupuncture, the peripheral and spinal nerve stimulation engendered by the somatic afferent stimulation of acupuncture is discrete, measurable, and purposeful. Both acupuncture and placebos can provide clinically meaningful benefits, but acupuncture impacts the neuromatrix in ways that provide a deeper and more long-lasting, as well as specific neuromodulatory, input.

**AG:** Can you give some examples of cases in which your opinions have led to you taking a lot of criticism personally, by either sceptics or proponents of CAVM? How do you handle such criticism?

**NR:** Currently, CAVM practitioners in the US are focused against me in their battling against the RACE (Registry of Approved Continuing Education) Committee's work. Our (the RACE committee's) task is to uphold the criteria and standards approved by the American Association of Veterinary State Boards, stipulating that continuing education should be scientifically based and evidentially supported. The holistic groups fighting this forward movement point to me and my role as a screener for the committee as the reason why some of their courses have not received RACE approval.

**AG:** Why do you feel that the discussion and criticism of CAVM arouses such vigorous and vitriolic defences?

**NR:** This is the problem with practising based on belief systems and appointing gurus that one follows without question. Medicine becomes a religion, and the teachers are regarded as 'wise sages', even though many times the information they are teaching has never been tested, cannot be supported, or could actually lead to dangerous outcomes.

**AG:** If there was one question in CAVM that you would like answered, what would it be?

**NR:** Where did critical thinking in our profession go?

# Glossary

**Anaerobic infection** – an infection with bacteria that require an oxygen-free environment to thrive. Such infections can be difficult to treat as they occur in areas with limited or no blood supply.

**Antineoplastons** – chemicals found in blood and urine that have been marketed for a number of years as a cure for cancer despite there being no proper evidence to support this claim and legal action being taken against those who promote it.

**Arrhythmia** – an irregular heartbeat, this is usually abnormal and can lead to heart failure and serious illness. One form, sinus arrhythmia, described as a 'regular irregularity', is normal, however.

**Ascites** – the accumulation of fluid in the abdomen, giving a pot-bellied appearance, ascites can be associated with a variety of serious diseases.

**Auscultation** – listening to the internal sounds of the body – occasionally gut, but more usually heart and lung. Typically a stethoscope would be used for this purpose.

**Biofield** – in radionics. A supposed energy field surrounding living things or occasionally non-living things. Sometimes electromagnetic, sometimes quantum, occasionally tachyon-based, also known as the Aura, sometimes 'subtle energy', sometimes 'morphogenic'. Allegedly capable of self-direction but only by those in the know. Radionics practitioners claim they can detect and manipulate this field over great distances to assess and correct imbalances at the flick of a switch or a wave of the hand.

**Blinding** – taking steps in a clinical trial to ensure patients are unaware whether they are receiving the substance under test or a blank placebo in case this unconsciously influences the results. In double- and triple-blinded trials the persons administering the remedies and those analysing the statistics afterwards are also kept 'blind'.

**British Association of Homeopathic Veterinary Surgeons (BAHVS)** – www.bahvs.com

**Cardiomyopathy** – disease affecting the heart muscle, it has a wide range of possible causes.

**Caregiver placebo effect** – the phenomenon where those close to an animal can become convinced there has been an improvement in that animal's medical condition even when objective measurements confirm there has been no such improvement or occasionally even a deterioration.

**Cholangiohepatitis** – inflammation of the liver and biliary tree. It is common in cats, often associated with pancreatitis and inflammatory bowel disease. It can be caused by infections ascending into the liver from the gut, or may be immune-mediated.

**Coliforms** – rod-shaped bacteria, universally found in faeces, the presence of which often indicates unsanitary conditions. *E. coli* is a typical coliform.

**Computed Tomography (CT)** – an advanced form of X-ray imaging giving cross-sectional views through the body.

**Crossover trial** – a study in which each subject receives a sequence of different treatments. In most crossover trials each subject receives all treatments being tested at different times (e.g. standard treatment and placebo). They can be either observational or controlled and are particularly useful in medicine.

**De Qi** – The sensations of needling, experienced by patients undergoing acupuncture, including pain and numbness. Sometimes regarded by acupuncturists as a sign they have 'hit the spot'.

**Double Blind Placebo Controlled Trial (DBPCT)** – a clinical trial where, in an attempt to eliminate unconscious bias, participants, investigators and analysts are prevented from knowing which groups have received the substance under test and which have received a blank placebo. Often referred to as the gold standard of clinical trials.

**Dry needling** – a Westernised form of acupuncture, rather poorly defined in the literature, but which employs needling based more on bio-scientific principles than those of Traditional Chinese Medicine.

**Dystocia** – difficulty giving birth.

**Endorphins** – naturally occurring painkillers produced by the body in response to stimulus. They are chemicals known as neuropeptides and are closely related to morphine and other opioids.

**Enteropathogenic bacteria** – harmful bacteria originating in the gut and which cause gastro-enteric diseases such as vomiting and diarrhoea.

**Gate control theory of pain** – where a non-painful stimulus blocks a more painful input, and prevents pain sensation from travelling to the central nervous system, thus 'closing the gate' to and suppressing pain.

**Heroic Medicine** – practised from the eighteenth to the early twentieth century, this form of medicine employed techniques including bleeding, purging, firing, blistering and the administration of toxic heavy metals in an attempt to treat illness.

**Homeostasis** – the regulation of the internal environment of the body by means of natural, physiological processes that ensure certain parameters (blood pressure, carbon dioxide levels, glucose levels and so on) are maintained within strict limits.

**Hyperthyroidism** – a condition, almost exclusively affecting elderly cats, resulting from an overactive thyroid gland that causes the sufferer to develop a rapid heart rate, lose weight, eat ravenously and become irascible. If untreated, although affected cats can live for some time, life is uncomfortable and many will die prematurely from heart failure.

**Imponderables** – homeopathic remedies prepared from immaterial base ingredients such as types of energy, natural phenomena and abstract concepts. Examples include the colour blue, eclipse, fire, shipwreck, dream, storm, African sun and anti-matter.

**In vitro** – literally 'in glass', an experiment or trial carried out in a laboratory container rather than directly on a living organism.

**In vivo** – literally 'in life', an experiment or trial carried out on a living organism or in a natural setting.

**Innate Intelligence** – in chiropractic a spirit-like force said to maintain health by travelling along nerves. Also: 'The Innate'.

**Laetrile** – a bogus cancer treatment made from the kernels of fruit stones containing cyanide and known to cause life-threatening toxicity that, despite being banned in the US for more than fifty years, nevertheless has thousands of advocates for its unrestricted use.

**Malassezia** – a type of yeast, previously known as Candida, which can cause disease of the skin and ear canals. Malassezia infections are characterised by a distinctive 'earthy' smell.

**Mast Cell Tumour (MCT)** – the cancerous growth of a type of white blood cell known as mast cells. There are different categories of MCT in animals, commonly dogs, but they are generally regarded as malignant.

**Mastitis** – inflammation (usually because of infection) of the mammary, or milk-producing, gland. A painful condition in any species, especially problematic in a dairy herd.

**Melanoma** – a form of cancer caused by the abnormal growth of pigment-producing cells (melanocytes).

**Meta-analysis** – a study that combines the data from multiple, smaller studies on a single subject. It is considered one of the strongest forms of evidence.

**Moxibustion** – the practice of burning fragrant herbs at acupuncture points.

**Murmur** – an abnormal sound heard during the heartbeat, it usually indicates a leak – either in a heart valve or occasionally through a hole in one of the walls separating the heart chambers. It can lead to heart failure. A harmless type of murmur is sometimes identified in young or athletic animals.

**Numinous** – pertaining to the spirit or the divine.

**Nutritional secondary hyperparathyroidism** – a disease of young, growing animals caused by low-calcium, high-phosphorus diets, such as all meat diets. Clinical signs include pain, depression and deformed, weak bones that are prone to fracturing.

**Oncology** – The study of cancer.

**Periodontal disease** – disease of the tissues around the tooth, including the gums and tooth socket.

**Placebo** – a substance or occasionally a medical intervention that itself is inert but is designed to mimic a real drug or intervention. Used in clinical trials to rule out unconscious bias as a result of the *placebo effect* where some patients will appear to show an improvement even after an ineffective treatment has been administered.

**Polyarthritis** – inflammation that affects multiple joints of the body at the same time. The cause is often a result of an abnormal immune system (e.g. rheumatoid arthritis) or occasionally because of infection.

**Psychic Surgery** – a form of alternative surgery, popular in South America, where the 'surgeon' introduces various pieces of animal organs by sleight of hand into a bogus surgical field and then passes them off as tumours or other masses, claiming to have removed them via an incision that heals instantly, leaving no trace. The practice is a simple conjuring trick and has been denounced by medical authorities as a hoax.

**Qi** – (also spelled *ch'i* in English, 氣 in traditional Chinese) a concept in Traditional Chinese Medicine representing an essence that pervades living things. Literally translated it means 'breath' or 'wind' and, in some forms, 'food'. Similar to the 'pneuma' of the ancient Greeks, *Qi* supposedly travels around the body in channels known as meridians and can be manipulated by various means, including using acupuncture needles.

**Regression to the mean** – in medicine, the phenomenon where if a condition goes untreated and symptoms reach the point of maximum intensity then in all likelihood at this point they are likely to regress; even on a purely statistical basis the likelihood of symptoms improving is far greater than that of them getting even worse. This can confound the perception of the effectiveness of treatment since, if intervention is delayed until the symptoms are at their most extreme then the chances are there would have been an improvement anyway, regardless of the merits of the treatment used.

**Royal College of Veterinary Surgeons (RCVS)** – the governing body for the veterinary profession in the UK (www.rcvs.org.uk).

**Second intention healing** – the means by which an open wound heals (involving gradual infilling with granulation tissue and later scar tissue), as opposed to first intention healing, the way a wound that has been surgically closed heals.

**Sepsis** – also known as septicaemia or blood poisoning. A condition where the body is overwhelmed by infection and bacteria are found in all areas of the body, including the bloodstream. Severe, life-threatening illness develops as a result of toxins released by the bacteria and often an inappropriate and damaging response from the body's immune system.

**Succussion** – in homeopathy, the vigorous banging of remedies on a leather pad during production that supposedly increases the strength of the final remedy.

**Surrogate outcome or endpoint** – 'In clinical trials, a surrogate endpoint is a measure of effect of a specific treatment that may correlate with a real clinical endpoint but does not necessarily have a guaranteed relationship' (en.wikipedia.org/wiki/Surrogate_endpoint).

**Systematic review** – a systematic, rigorous and explicit review of trials and other research addressing a specific subject with the intention of summarising relevant data to give a more comprehensive insight.

**Traumatic pericarditis** – in cows, this occurs after the accidental ingestion of a sharp foreign body such as a wire, which then penetrates through the wall of the stomach and into the adjacent tissues, eventually reaching the membrane surrounding the heart (pericardium) causing infection.

**Valvular insufficiency** – the sub-optimal performance of a heart valve resulting from damage that causes leaking. This will be heard as a murmur and can lead to heart failure.

**Vertebral Subluxation (VSL)** – in chiropractic, a supposed misalignment or abnormal movement of the bones of the spine, allegedly responsible for a number of health problems, not confined to the spine itself. The VSL has never been reliably demonstrated to exist and is regarded as pseudoscience by mainstream medicine.

**Veterinary Medicines Directorate (VMD)** – the UK government body responsible for assuring the safety, quality and efficacy of veterinary medicines (www.gov.uk/government/organisations/veterinary-medicines-directorate).

**Vital Force** – in homeopathy the spirit-like energy that it is claimed is contained within living things and homeopathic remedies themselves and which becomes disturbed ('untuned') in disease.

**Withholding (or withdrawal) times** – the period of time that must legally be allowed after the administration of a drug to an animal in order to allow it sufficient time to be eliminated from the system before its meat, milk or eggs can be consumed.

# Index